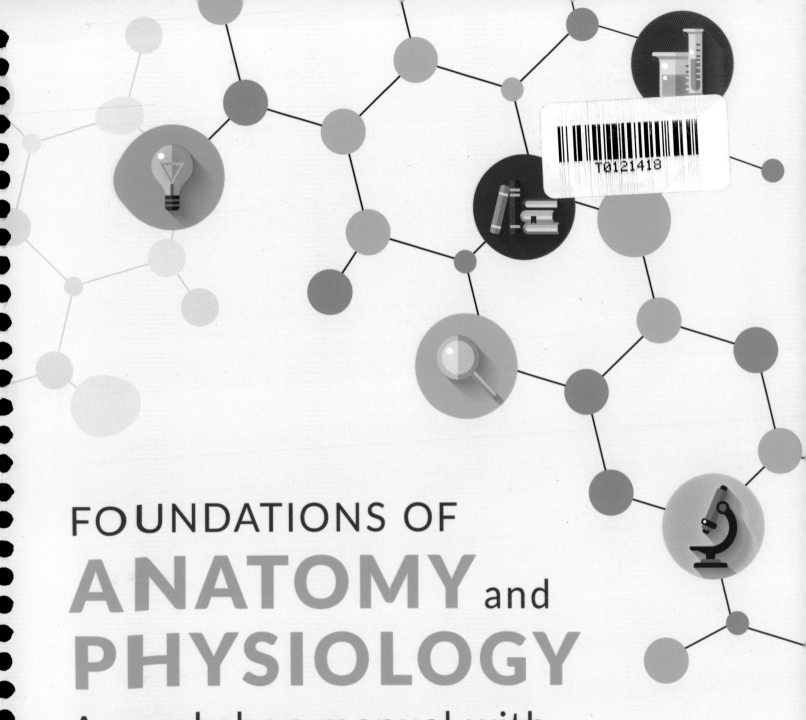

FOUNDATIONS OF
ANATOMY and
PHYSIOLOGY

A workshop manual with laboratory applications

Ellie Kirov
Alan Needham

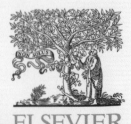

ELSEVIER

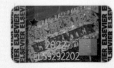

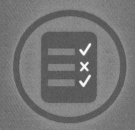

FOUNDATIONS OF
ANATOMY and
PHYSIOLOGY

FOUNDATIONS OF
ANATOMY and
PHYSIOLOGY

A workshop manual with laboratory applications

Ellie Kirov BSc (BiolSc) Hons, PhD
Unit Coordinator and Lecturer (Health Sciences)
School of Science
Edith Cowan University
Perth, Western Australia

Alan Needham BSc (Hons), PhD
Former Senior Lecturer and Course Coordinator
Edith Cowan University
Perth, Western Australia

ELSEVIER

ELSEVIER

Elsevier Australia. ACN 001 002 357
(a division of Reed International Books Australia Pty Ltd) Tower 1, 475 Victoria Avenue, Chatswood, NSW 2067

ISBN: 978-0-7295-4401-6

National Library of Australia Cataloguing-in-Publication Data

A catalogue record for this book is available from the National Library of Australia

Content Strategist: Natalie Hunt
Content Project Manager: Shubham Dixit
Edited by Margaret Trudgeon
Proofread by Melissa Faulkner
Permissions Editing and Photo Research: Arun Prasad Kandasamy
Cover design and Internal Design by Lisa Petroff
Index by Innodata
Typeset by GW Tech
Printed in China

Last digit is the print number: 9 8 7 6 5 4 3 2 1

Contents

Contents

Contents

Additional Activities (Available on Evolve)

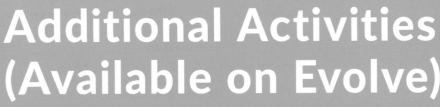

Preface

Foundations of Anatomy and Physiology: A Workshop Manual with Laboratory Applications is intended for students in introductory human anatomy and physiology courses. It is a unique resource in that it is not linked to a particular textbook, but is deliberately designed to be used alongside any of the major introductory anatomy and physiology texts currently available to students of nursing and the health sciences. This has given us the freedom to broaden the manual's content to the point where instructors and students have a wide range of activities to choose from, and the opportunity to adapt the use of the manual to their own course structure.

While all the organ systems of the body are covered in detail, many of the activities may also be found valuable as supplementary work in areas considered to be assumed knowledge but which students might struggle with. For example, Chapters 1 to 5 address Measurement and Scientific Mathematics, Basic Physics for Physiology, Basic Chemistry, Biological Chemistry, and Microscopy. These areas are not always included in introductory anatomy and physiology courses, so we have provided activities in those chapters to help students make more sense of the physiological principles and processes they will encounter later and to impart some practical laboratory skills. Each of the remaining 17 chapters comprehensively covers a major area of anatomy and physiology.

An important feature of this manual, in addition to the wide choice of activities available, is the range of activity types. We recognise that in many learning environments, laboratory facilities are limited or unavailable, so many activities have been designed to suit tutorial or private study settings. A total of 193 activities may be found in these pages, with another 81 available online, ranging from full laboratory experiences to textbook and library work. It has been our aim to make all activities both interesting and relevant to students' needs. Hands-on activities include examining models, performing dissections, using microscopes to study cells and tissues, conducting experiments, and investigating the body's chemical and physiological processes.

All health professionals live and work in an increasingly sophisticated scientific environment and need to feel both familiar and comfortable with the language and principles of the science they are applying. This can be challenging for students new to the discipline, so we have provided introductions to activities that explain key terms and concepts clearly and simply without sacrificing scientific rigour.

We hope that students will find this manual useful in a number of ways:

- as a stimulating companion to studies in anatomy and physiology,
- as a guide to essential knowledge in each subject area,
- as a means of learning techniques useful in a clinical setting, and
- as a handy revision aid when preparing for assessments. The lists of learning outcomes and key terms at the beginning of each chapter are designed to assist with this.

We sincerely hope you enjoy your studies in anatomy and physiology, and wish you every success with your course.

Ellie Kirov
Alan Needham
March 2023

Introduction to the Manual

Welcome to the first edition of *Foundations of Anatomy and Physiology: A Workshop Manual with Laboratory Applications*, an all-inclusive resource for health science and nursing students. This workshop manual is designed to provide students with the conceptual foundations of basic science, anatomy, and physiology, as well as the critical thinking skills they will need to apply theory to practice in real-life settings, irrespective of the facilities available. It caters to nursing, health science, and allied health students at varying levels of understanding and ability.

This manual was developed as a result of difficulties experienced in sourcing and accessing relevant learning activities for use across a number of learning applications (pre-, in-, post-class) and environments (online, classroom, standard laboratory) in the teaching of health science units. In this process, relevant instruction materials are often selected from a variety of sources and collated into study modules for their collective value, which is time-consuming, presents inconsistencies in language and content, and needs to be undertaken for individual units within a course. In addition, manuals accompanying textbooks are specific to the textbook and become redundant when another textbook is adopted, or where institutional facilities, instructor budgets, and study modes make some activities difficult to conduct.

Progression within a unit of study or through a course often relies on understanding key foundational concepts, which can then be scaffolded to introduce more complex concepts. By focusing on understanding foundational concepts, conceptual progression becomes easier for the instructor and student. This manual is a concept-based resource that facilitates this process. Learning activities are scaffolded to enable students to progress to more complex concepts once they have mastered the basics.

KEY FEATURES

Key features of the manual:
- May be used with any textbook or as a standalone – provides a flexible resource for teachers and students alike as it is concept-based.
- Adaptable to all learning environments, including a combination of classroom and laboratory-based activities, allowing for situations where standard laboratory facilities are not available.
- Scaffolded content – suitable for varying levels of student competency, learning requirements, available facilities, and within multiple units across courses.
- Concept-based activities – can be selected and adapted to align with different units across courses.
- Range of activities – supports understanding and builds knowledge, including theory, application, clinical scenarios, and experimentation.
- Activities can be aligned to learning requirements – can be selected to assist pre-class, in-class, post-class, and self-paced learning based on unit requirements and available resources.
- Easy to navigate – colourful icons identify content type in each activity as well as safety precautions.
- eBook access – included in all print purchases.

USING THE MANUAL

Activities within the manual are concept-based rather than being linked to chapters associated with a specific textbook, scaffolded to meet varied learning requirements, and designed to be tailored to suit a variety of teaching facilities.

Activities can be:
- selected to suit course structure, prescribed texts, or conceptual requirements.
- selected as required within and across chapters.
- assigned as pre-class, in-class, and post-class assignments.
- completed in-class with associated questions assigned as post-class follow-up.
- completed as demonstrations and/or filmed for online cohorts.
- used to form the basis for written or practical assessment.
- completed as a class with individual questions assigned to different groups and consolidated at the end of the session.

FEATURES OF THE MANUAL

Introductions

Each chapter commences with a main introduction to provide an overview and scope of the chapter content. The introduction also provides links to other chapters where relevant or to where linked content can be located. Each activity is also accompanied by a separate introduction outlining the conceptual relevance of the activity.

Learning Outcomes

Numbered learning outcomes at the beginning of each chapter provide an outline of the objectives achieved by the activities in the chapter. Activities are also accompanied by individual objectives which provide conceptual scope.

Key Terms

Key terms are provided at the beginning of each chapter and provide an overview of the concepts addressed by the activities within the chapter. Key terms are also provided in bold within activity introductions so that conceptual links can be made between the key terms and activity objectives.

Numbered Activities

Activities are numbered according to chapter and number for activities located within the manual, and chapter and letter for activities located on Evolve˙ (for example, Activity 6.2 and Activity 6D respectively).

Additional Activities

Additional activities have been provided to extend learning application, and are indicated within chapters by text boxes. These activities are numbered according to chapter and letter order to facilitate navigation (for example, Activity 6B). Additional activities can be accessed through Evolve˙.

Activity Icons

Each activity is accompanied by an icon which indicates the learning application and resources required. Some activities are accompanied by more than one icon to indicate that multiple concepts are covered within the activity.

 Indicates an activity that can be conducted at home or within a classroom environment, with few or no resources required. It is associated with activities requiring research, bookwork, and diagram interpretation.

 Indicates an activity that can be conducted within a classroom environment with some additional resources required, but does not require a standard laboratory environment. It is associated with activities indicating physical application of concepts.

 Indicates an activity that can be conducted within a classroom or traditional laboratory environment, but requires access to a microscope. It is associated with activities involving microscopy and requiring associated resources.

 Indicates an activity that should be conducted within a standard laboratory environment, with additional resources required. It signals activities that should not be conducted within a classroom setting or at home.

Associated with Apply the Concepts boxes. These boxed features provide questions and scenarios associated with applications of the activity or chapter concepts and usually require further research.

 Indicates potential warnings or risks associated with an activity. Please check the risk management and safety requirements of your institution prior to conducting these activities.

 Indicates an additional activity that is provided online and can be accessed through Evolve˙. Evolve˙ activities are also accompanied by the icons shown above.

Figures

Questions and activities are accompanied by full-colour figures to provide clarity, create a user-friendly manual, and enhance the learning experience

Answer Lines

Each question is accompanied by answer lines so that students can interact directly with the content in the manual. This also allows for activities to be used as pre-class, in-class and post-class activities or submitted as assessment items.

Additional Resources

A list of additional resources is located at the end of each chapter to provide access to further content for students to explore and interact with online. These can be used to supplement activities in the manual during class, form pre-class preparation or post-class follow-up, or to facilitate online learning.

Spiral Binding

The manual is provided as a spiral bound book for ease of use, allowing students to use it directly within the classroom or lab setting.

Page Perforations

Pages are perforated near the spiral binding so that they can be removed with ease. This allows for activities to be removed and submitted as assessed items or to be included as part of an external portfolio.

eBook on VitalSource

The manual is provided as an eBook on VitalSource to support varied modes of teaching and learning, and to allow for electronic submission. The eBook also supports technology-enabled learning, where personal devices or computer laboratory facilities form part of the learning environment, as well as in technology-enabled wet laboratories with inbuilt student tablets.

FOR INSTRUCTORS: RESOURCES ACCOMPANYING THE MANUAL

Answers to Activity Questions

Answers are provided for all activity questions on Evolve˙. Answers can be used by instructors to guide student responses and critical inquiry, as a marking guide where activities form assessment items, or released to students periodically as an adaptive learning tool.

Image Collection

All figures featured in the manual are available for download via Evolve˙. These can be used as learning tools or assessment items.

List of Suggested Materials and Set-Up Requirements for each Activity

Lists of suggested materials and set-up requirements for each activity (where required) are available for download via Evolve˙. These can be used to assist planning, budgeting, delivery, and set-up of activities for instructors and technicians.

About the Authors

Dr Ellie Kirov graduated from Edith Cowan University with Honours in Biological Science and a PhD in Biomedical Science. She is a Unit Coordinator and Lecturer in anatomy, physiology, chemistry and scientific method at Edith Cowan University. She has been deeply committed to engaging and inspiring future healthcare professionals majoring in nursing, biomedicine, and health science, through demonstration, critical thinking, and conceptual application for 25 years. She has authored and co-authored several publications in the fields of anatomy and physiology, pathophysiology, laboratory science, case studies and clinical care. Her key areas of interest include physiological mechanisms of action, pharmacology, and enhancing the learning experience through conceptual scaffolding, practical application, and integration to the clinical setting. Outside her academic pursuits, Ellie enjoys taking long nature walks, cooking with fresh market produce, and going in search of the perfect coffee.

Dr Alan Needham graduated from the University of New South Wales with first-class honours and a PhD in Comparative Physiology. In a 33-year teaching and research career at UNSW and ECU, he coordinated units in cell biology, human physiology, comparative physiology and nursing science. His special interests include cardiovascular and thermoregulatory physiology, and techniques for making science approachable and interesting to both undergraduates and members of the general community. These have included the design and delivery of bridging courses aimed at helping new students in clinical science courses succeed in their first year at university. Outside his academic pursuits, Alan gives community lectures, works for the conservation of endangered wildlife and directs musical theatre productions.

Reviewers

Evonne T Curran NursD
Honorary Senior Research Fellow – School of Health and
Life Sciences
Glasgow Caledonian University
Glasgow, United Kingdom

Ros Leahy RN, ME
Lecturer, Bachelor of Nursing Pacific
Whitieria Community Polytechnic
New Zealand

Stuart Shields BSc(HumBiol), GradDipEd(SecSci),
GradDipPsych, GradDipAdvPsych
Applecross Senior High School
Ardross, Western Australia, Australia

CHAPTER 1
Measurement and Scientific Mathematics

Any scientific discipline requires the making and recording of measurements, the manipulation of data and its conversion from one form to another, the use of formulae and equations, an understanding of tables and graphs, and the ability to work with very large and very small numbers. In the health sciences, skills such as being able to accurately estimate weight, volume, and time can be lifesaving. Health professionals need to be comfortable with the language of science and mathematics. It must come as naturally as any spoken language, and it must be completely free of ambiguity.

Scientific information is only reliable when the data collected have been accurately measured, recorded and presented. The use of incorrect units, the wrong formula or the wrong notation is confusing and potentially dangerous. It is for this reason that an international system of units and scientific notation has been developed. The language of mathematics is universal. A concentration of 6.38 mmol/L should make sense to anyone interested in blood glucose levels, and every haematologist in the world should be able to recognise that 3.20×10^9/mL is an unusually low red blood cell count.

LEARNING OUTCOMES

On completion of these activities, the student should be able to:

1. demonstrate familiarity with the SI system of units and with common non-SI units, and their multiplier and divisor prefixes.

2. convert measurements from one unit to another.

3. discuss sources of error in measurements and the ways of minimising them.

4. make accurate estimates of lengths, masses, volumes and time.

5. explain the correct use and limitations of laboratory equipment for measuring large and small quantities.

6. use scientific notation to represent large and small numbers.

7. explain the use of significant numbers to indicate levels of confidence in a measurement.

8. use and manipulate equations and formulae.

9. interpret data presented in graphical form and use graphs as a source of derived information.

KEY TERMS

Absolute value	Exponent	Quantitative measurement
Algebraic equation	Exponential notation	Random error
Accuracy	Formula	Rounding
Base unit	Graph	Scientific notation
Data	Independent variable	SI unit
Dependent variable	Length	Significant figure
Derived unit	Mass	Systematic error
Divisor prefixes	Metric unit	Time
Equation	Multiplier prefixes	Weight
Error	Precision	Volume
Estimate	Qualitative measurement	

ACTIVITY 1.1: MEASUREMENTS, UNITS AND CONVERTING QUANTITIES

People engaged in clinical and analytical work are often required to make measurements. Those measurements that rely on the subjective assessment or experience of the observer are **qualitative measurements**. **Quantitative measurements** are those made with a measuring instrument and have a precise value or number that provides the magnitude of a quantity as compared to a standard, for example, length, and is accompanied by a unit of measurement, for example, metres.

In science and health, the International System (Système Internationale), or SI System, is used; it is an extension of the metric system. The SI system makes use of seven **base units** from which **derived units**, involving the multiplication or division of base units by other units, can be derived (Table 1.1). Base units are fixed quantities that are defined independently of any other units, largely determined by their practicality. Some units commonly used in clinical practice are not **SI units** but **metric units** (Table 1.2). These include the litre (L) and the degree celsius (°C). The degree celsius actually has the same value as the SI unit of temperature, the kelvin, but the two units operate on different scales. Minutes and hours are also not SI units, although they are multiples of the second, which is an SI unit.

This activity explores measurements and units, and provides practice in unit conversions.

Part 1: Measurements and Units

Table 1.1 Base and derived units in the SI system

Quantity	Unit	Symbol
Base units		
length	metre	m
mass	kilogram	kg
time	second	s
electric current	ampere	A
temperature	kelvin	K

Part 1: Measurements and Units *Continued*

Table 1.1 Base and derived units in the SI system *Continued*

Quantity	Unit	Symbol
luminous intensity	candela	cd
amount of substance	mole	mol
Derived units		
area	square metre	m^2
volume	cubic metre	m^3
velocity	metre/second	m/s or ms^{-1}
acceleration	metre/second/second	m/s/s or ms^{-2}
force	newton	N
pressure	pascal	Pa
work and energy	joule	J

Table 1.2 Units commonly used in clinical practice

Quantity	Base unit	Symbol	System
length	metre	m	metric and SI
volume	litre	L	metric
mass	kilogram	kg	metric and SI
time	second	s	metric and SI
pressure	millimetres of mercury	mmHg	metric
temperature	degree celsius	°C	metric
number of particles	mole	mol	SI

1. Identify whether each of the following is an example of a qualitative or quantitative assessment:

   a. The boiling point of H_2O is greater than that of H_2

   _____

   b. The car travelled 12 ms^{-1}

   _____

   c. 12 cm is greater than 5 cm

   _____

   d. The bottle of H_2O is half-full

   _____

   e. Water boils at 100°C

   _____

2. Identify whether each of the following is an example of systematic or random error:

   a. Mixing up solutions with different concentrations

   _____

b. Mislabelling a test tube containing a special solution

_____

c. A measuring scale that measures 10 kg as 9.5 kg

_____

d. A computer fault causing loss of recorded data

_____

e. A disagreement between scientists on data

_____

3. Identify whether each of the following is an SI or metric unit:

a. metre _____

b. litre _____

c. gram _____

d. mole _____

e. °C _____

f. m^3_____

g. s_____

h. K _____

i. cm _____

j. kg _____

Part 2: Converting Quantities

Both base units and derived units are often inconveniently large or small to be used without modifying them. For example, the base unit of distance, the metre, is far too large to be applied to the diameter of a red blood cell, which is about 0.000008 m. It is more convenient to divide a metre into millionths and give the diameter of a red blood cell as 8 micrometres. Similarly, the metre is far too small to be applied to the distance from Sydney to London, which is about 17 000 000 m. It is more convenient to multiply the metre by a thousand or even a million, giving 17 000 kilometres or 17 megametres. This is achieved through multiplier prefixes and divisor prefixes (Table 1.3). Note the importance of using uppercase and lowercase letters correctly: Mm means megametre (not millimetre) and kJ means kilojoule (and not kelvin joule). Note: when communicating medical information, the abbreviation µg is now commonly replaced with the full name, microgram, to avoid possible confusion with milligram.

Table 1.3 Prefixes commonly used in clinical practice

Prefix	Symbol	Multiplication factor	Numeric multiplication factor
mega	M	million	1 000 000
kilo	k	thousand	1000
deca	da	ten	10
deci	d	one-tenth	1/10
centi	c	one-hundredth	1/100
milli	m	one-thousandth	1/1000
micro	μ^1	one-millionth	1/1 000 000
nano	n	one-thousand millionth	1/1 000 000 000

Note:

1. Micro should be spelt out in all instances to avoid being confused with milli. *Source: Australian Government TGA: www.tga.gov.au/ resources/resource/guidance/medicine-labels-guidance-tgo-91-and-tgo-92/1-using-orders*

1. Complete the following conversions, referring to Table 1.3 to assist:

a. 1 L= _____ mL

b. 1 mL = _____ µL

c. 20 L = _____ mL

d. 750 mL = _____ L

e. 2500 µL (microlitres) = _____ mL

2. Convert the following quantities and provide the correct symbols for each, referring to Table 1.3 to assist:

   a. 152 metres to millimetres

   _____

   b. 5 megametres to metres

   _____

   c. 18.4 centimetres to metres

   _____

   d. 1962.6 milligrams to grams

   _____

   e. 2.3 kilograms to grams

   _____

   f. 0.74 grams to micrograms

   _____

   g. 19.2 moles to millimoles

   _____

   h. 1766.7 micromoles to moles

   _____

   i. 38.9 seconds to milliseconds

   _____

   j. 68.4 seconds to microseconds

   _____

   k. 556 micrograms to grams

   _____

   l. 13.6 kilograms to megagrams

   _____

Apply the Concepts

1. Explain the importance of using SI units internationally.

   _____

   _____

   _____

2. Why is an understanding of unit conversion important?

   _____

   _____

   _____

3. A patient requires 1.5 g of an antibiotic, which is available in tablets each containing 250 mg.

   How many tablets are required?

   _____

   _____

4. A patient is ordered to take 0.5 mg of digoxin orally. The digoxin is available in tablets each containing 125 micrograms.

   How many tablets should be taken?

   _____

   _____

5. A patient needs an injection of 6 mg of morphine. The drug is available in ampoules containing 10 mg in 2 mL.

   What volume should be injected?

   _____

   _____

ACTIVITY 1.2: ESTIMATION, ACCURACY AND PRECISION

In the health sciences, the ability to **estimate** accurately is a valuable skill and can sometimes be lifesaving. Knowing the difference at a glance between 0.5 mL and 5.0 mL in an injection, being able to estimate heart or ventilation rates without a timing device, and estimating the **weight** of a patient for emergency medication, are all important skills. For any particular measurement there is an **absolute value**; however, it is never possible to achieve this value because there is always some source of uncertainty, or **error**.

There are two types of errors: **systematic errors**, which are due to some constant variation in the instrument, method used or operator and can usually be identified and controlled, and **random errors**, which are due to random variations of the instrument or operator and cannot be completely identified and controlled, but may be minimised by taking multiple measurements and averaging results. Errors affect accuracy and precision. **Accuracy** is the extent to which a measurement approaches the true value, while **precision** is the extent to which repeated measurements agree with each other. Absolute accuracy cannot be achieved because it is impossible to eliminate all sources of error, while high precision measurements can only be made if random errors are very small.

This activity provides practice in estimating the properties of objects and checking the accuracy of estimates.

Part 1: Estimation and Measurement of Length

The metric and SI base unit of **length** is the metre (m). For small but visible lengths, millimetres are more accurate, while for large distances, kilometres are more practical. Centimetres are an intermediate measurement between millimetres and metres, but are used when convenient.

1. Estimate the length of the lines below in mm by filling in the table below.

   a. _____

   b. _____

   c. _____

   d. _____

2. Once these have been estimated, measure each line with a ruler.

3. If the estimates were more than 10% inaccurate draw some more lines in the space below and practise estimating their lengths.

	Estimated length	Measured length
a.		
b.		
c.		
d.		

4. Estimate the following objects in centimetres and metres to the nearest 10 cm, then check by measuring each item with a ruler or tape measure and record your results in the table provided.

Object	Estimated		Measured	
	cm	m	cm	m
Length of laboratory bench				
Width of room				
Length of room				

5. If the estimates were more than 10% inaccurate, select different objects to measure for practice and record your results in the table provided.

Object	Estimated		Measured	
	cm	m	cm	m

6. Form a group of four and allocate a number (1–4) to each person in the group.

7. Estimate the height in centimetres of each group member, doing this independently of other group members.

Person 1 _____

Person 2 _____

Person 3 _____

Person 4 _____

8. Now measure the height of each person with a wall-mounted height gauge, recording your results in the table provided.

Individual	Measured height (cm)	Highest estimate	Lowest estimate	Difference
1				
2				
3				
4				

9. Compare your estimates with those of other group members and complete the table.

10. List the factors that affected accuracy and precision in the measurements taken.

Precision	Accuracy

Part 2: Estimation and Measurement of Volume

The metric unit of **volume** is the litre (L), whereas the SI base unit of volume is the cubic metre (m^3). Small volumes of liquids are usually measured by pipettes, which are available in various capacities. Some are graduated and can be used to measure different volumes, and some are calibrated to deliver a specific volume (Fig. 1.1). Larger volumes of liquids are usually measured in measuring cylinders (Fig. 1.2).

⚠ To conduct these activities it is important to ensure the following safety precautions:

- *Toxic or corrosive liquids should never be pipetted by mouth.*

- *A safety pipette fitted with a safety pump, or a measuring cylinder should be used.*

1. Observe the demonstration of the correct method of using a pipette.

2. Note that the volume of liquid is always read at the bottom of the meniscus (the curve in the liquid surface).

3. Note that not all pipettes are graduated right to the tip which means they do not have to be drained completely to deliver the stated volume.

4. Only pipettes labelled 'Blowout' should be blown out. Others are drained against the side of the receiving vessel.

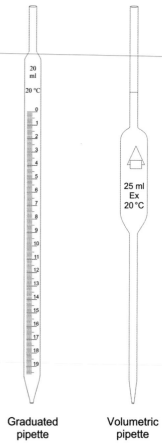

Graduated
pipette

Volumetric
pipette

Figure 1.1 Graduated and volumetric pipettes.
(Source: © Eni Generalić)

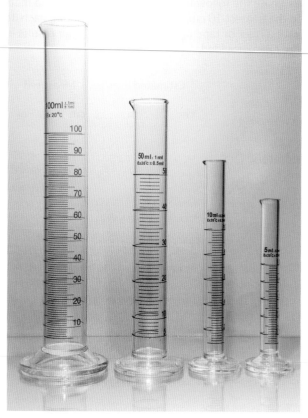

Figure 1.2 Measuring cylinders.

5. Examine the different pipettes available.

a. What different capacities of pipettes are in use in the laboratory?

_____

b. What volume is represented by the smallest graduations on a 1.0 mL pipette?

_____

c. What volume is represented by the smallest graduations on a 10 mL pipette?

_____

d. Identify the most appropriate pipette capacity to dispense a volume of:

    i. 8.3 mL _____

    ii. 0.1 mL _____

    iii. 4.8 mL _____

    iv. 5.0 mL _____

    v. 1.7 mL _____

e. Would it be suitable to use a 10 mL pipette to dispense 0.2 mL of a liquid into each of 10 test tubes? Explain.

_____

_____

6. Examine the different measuring cylinders available.

7. Note that the volume is read at the bottom of the meniscus. When reading volume, ensure that the measuring cylinder is standing on a flat surface and your eyes are level with the meniscus.

a. What different capacities of measuring cylinder are in use in the laboratory?

_____

b. What volume is represented by the smallest graduations on a 10 mL measuring cylinder?

_____

c. What volume is represented by the smallest graduations on a 100 mL measuring cylinder?

_____

d. Identify the most appropriate measuring cylinder capacity to dispense a volume of:

    i. 8 mL _____

    ii. 15 mL _____

    iii. 87 mL _____

    iv. 380 mL _____

8. Pipette the following volumes of tap water into a 25 mL measuring cylinder.

9. Note the capacity of each pipette used below:

    a. 1.0 mL _____

    b. 6.0 mL _____

    c. 5.5 mL _____

    d. 8.7 mL _____

    e. 3.3 mL _____

    f. 0.5 mL _____

    g. Calculate the total volume added: _____

    h. Read the final volume in the measuring cylinder:

    _____

    i. How precisely can this be read? _____

    j. Is it the same as the calculated total? _____

10. Pour what you estimate is 5 mL of water into a test tube.

    a. Measure the actual volume: _____ mL

11. Pour what you estimate is 30 mL of water into a cup.

    a. Measure the actual volume: _____ mL

12. Some beakers and flasks have graduations marked on them. To check the accuracy of these, fill a graduated beaker to one of the marks then check this volume by tipping it into a measuring cylinder.

    a. Volume according to graduated beaker:

    _____ mL

    b. Volume as read in measuring cylinder:

    _____ mL

13. Would it be suitable to use graduated beakers and flasks for accurate measuring? Explain.

_____

_____

_____

Part 3: Estimation and Measurement of Mass

The metric and SI base unit of **mass** is the kilogram (kg). The terms mass and weight are often used interchangeably; however, mass refers to the amount of matter in an object, whereas weight depends on the force of gravity acting upon a mass. Weight is most commonly used in relation to healthcare settings.

Rules for using balances:

- *Never weigh directly onto the balance pan; always use a suitable container. Anything spilt on the balance should be brushed or wiped off immediately.*

- *With a balance that is open to the air, record only two decimal places because air currents limit the accuracy of this type of balance.*

- *The tare facility saves having to subtract the mass of the container from the total mass. Simply place the container onto the balance pan, press the tare button and weigh.*

1. Observe the demonstration of the use of an electronic balance.

2. Place a small weigh tray on the balance pan and tare to zero.

3. Weigh 5.0 g sodium chloride into the weigh tray.

4. Look carefully at this amount of salt, then tip it back into the original container.

5. Check the tare of the weigh tray and remove it from the balance.

6. Place what you estimate to be 5.0 g of salt in it and replace it on the balance.

    a. Actual mass of salt = _____ g

7. Tip the salt back into the original container and check the tare of the weigh tray again.

8. Place what you estimate to be 1.0 g of salt in it and replace it on the balance.

    a. Actual mass of salt = _____ g

9. Repeat the procedure estimating 0.5 g.

    a. Actual mass of salt = _____ g

10. Repeat the procedure estimating 0.1 g.

    a. Actual mass of salt = _____ g

11. Use the scales provided to weigh yourself.

    a. Weight = _____ kg

12. Estimate the weights of three other students.

13. Record your estimates in the table provided, then measure the actual weights.

Student	Estimated weight	Actual weight
1		
2		
3		

14. If the estimates were more than 5 kg out, try some more for practice.

Part 4: Estimation and Measurement of Time

The metric and SI base unit of **time** is the second (s). For historical reasons, the normal prefixes are only employed for time intervals of less than 1 second. For time intervals greater than 60 seconds, the everyday measures of minutes, hours and days are employed. Normal clinical practice usually involves measuring time intervals to the nearest second. In addition, clinical practice often uses a 24-hour (international standard) clock for providing time measurements rather than the commonly used 12-hour (standard) clock (Fig. 1.3).

1. Use a digital stopwatch to estimate the following times, recording your results in the table provided, and repeating each estimate:

Time	Estimate 1	Estimate 2
0.5 s		
1 s		
5 s		
20 s		
60 s		

2. Examine the stopwatch and note that it can measure to an accuracy of 0.01 s (1 centisecond).

3. Start the watch and let it run for a few seconds then stop it.

    a. How many centiseconds does it show?

    _____

    b. How many milliseconds does this correspond to?

    _____

4. Working in pairs, locate the radial pulse of your partner by placing a finger on their wrist.

5. Using your other hand, start the stopwatch and without looking at it, stop it after your estimate of 60 seconds.

6. During this time, count the number of pulses in your partner's wrist and check the time elapsed.

    a. Time elapsed: _____ s

    b. Number of pulses: _____

7. Using these figures, calculate your partner's heart rate in beats per minute.

    a. Heart rate: _____ bpm

8. Repeat this procedure using the stopwatch to accurately measure 60 seconds.

    a. Does the second measurement of heart rate agree closely with the first?

    _____

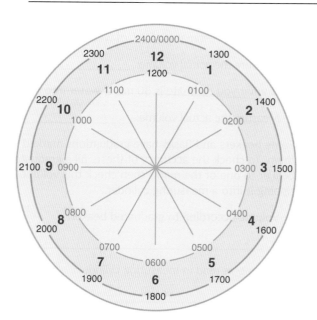

Figure 1.3 The 24-hour clock (a.m. times are in orange, p.m. times are in purple).
(*Source: Sorrentino, S. A., & Remmert, L. (2021). Mosby's Textbook for Nursing Assistants. Elsevier.*)

9. Referring to Fig.1.3, provide the following 24-hour clock times in 12-hour clock format:

   a. 15:30 _____

   b. 23:45 _____

   c. 19:12 _____

   d. 21:16 _____

   e. 13:10 _____

   f. 18:14 _____

10. Referring to Fig. 1.3, provide the following 12-hour clock times in 24-hour clock format:

    a. 2:20 pm _____

    b. 10:05 pm _____

    c. 8:45 pm _____

    d. 5:02 pm _____

    e. 4:11 pm _____

    f. 0:05 am _____

11. Is there a method for calculating 24-hour time using a 12-hour clock? Explain.

    _____

    _____

    _____

12. Using the method described above, and without referring to Fig. 1.3, provide the following 12-hour clock times in 24-hour clock format. Then check your answers by referring to Fig. 1.3:

    a. 4:21 pm _____

    b. 6:54 pm _____

    c. 1:10 pm _____

    d. 11:01 pm _____

    e. 9:45 pm _____

    f. 7:32 pm _____

13. Was the method successful?

    _____

    _____

Apply the Concepts

1. Why is the 24-hour clock sometimes referred to as the military or international clock?

   _____

   _____

2. Why is the 24-hour clock used in the clinical setting?

   _____

   _____

3. Is a 24-hour clock more accurate? Explain.

   _____

   _____

4. Is there an advantage of using a 24-hour clock over a 12-hour clock? Explain.

   _____

   _____

ACTIVITY 1.3: SCIENTIFIC NOTATION

A number that is expressed in scientific form always has the following format: $k \times 10^n$, where k is a number greater than or equal to 1 and less than 10, and n is either a positive or a negative integer. The **exponent** is equal to the number of zeros after the number one. For example, 1000 is written as 1×10^3 and 324 is written as 3.24×10^2. Exponential numbers with a negative exponent (e.g. 10^{-1}) are numbers smaller than one. This form of expressing numbers is called **scientific notation**, or **exponential notation**.

This activity illustrates the relationship between prefixes, exponents and multiplication factors in scientific notation.

1. Complete the following table:

Factor by which the unit is multiplied		Prefix	Symbol	Exponential notation
Fractional number	Decimal number			
1 000 000/1		mega	M	
	1000	kilo		10^3
10/1	10			10^1
1/1		–	–	10^0
	0.1	deci	d	
	0.01	centi	c	
1/1000		milli		10^{-3}
	0.000 001	micro		10^{-6}
1/1 000 000 000	0.000 000 001		n	

2. Complete the following table:

Exponential number	Fraction	Decimal
10^{-5}		
	1/100	
		0.001
	$1/10^4$	
		0.000 001
10^{-7}		
	1/1 000 000 000	

3. Express the following in correct scientific notation:

    a. 36 300 _____

    b. 363×10^3 _____

    c. 3.63_____

    d. 0.363 _____

    e. 0.000 363_____

    f. 255.3 _____

    g. 0.231 _____

    h. 0.007 52 _____

    i. 12 546 _____

    j. 14.235_____

4. Complete the following conversions using scientific notation:

    a. 1 km   _____m

    b. 1 m   _____cm

    c. 2.5 m   _____mm

    d. 2.5 cm   _____m

    e. 1.2 km   _____cm

    f. 480 m   _____km

5. Write the following fractions as decimal numbers and convert each to scientific notation:

	Decimal number	Scientific notation
7/10		
358/1000		
69/10 000		
3/10 000 000		

6. Convert the following to the correct form of scientific notation:

    a. 15.9×10^3 _____

    b. 561.3×10^2 _____

    c. 0.41×10^3 _____

    d. 0.0035×10^{-5} _____

    e. 361.4×10^2 _____

    f. 0.43×10^8 _____

    g. 11.901×10^{-1} _____

    h. 0.0892×10^4 _____

    i. 0.7892×10^2 _____

    j. 0.25×10^0 _____

7. Convert the following to decimal numbers:

    a. 3.5×10^2 _____

    b. 2.43×10^{-6} _____

    c. 1.54×10^{-8} _____

    d. 2.13×10^{13} _____

    e. 9.367×10^2 _____

    f. 35×10^2 _____

    g. 8.506×10^3 _____

    h. 243×10^{-6} _____

    i. 6.9×10^{-1} _____

    j. 1.54×10^{-8} _____

    k. 4.67×10^{-6} _____

    l. 0.0201×10^{-4} _____

    m. 12.34×10^2 _____

    n. 367.74×10^{-3} _____

8. Perform the following calculations and convert the answer to correct scientific notation:

    a. $(2.7 \times 10^3) + (2.3 \times 10^4)$ _____

    b. $(4.2 \times 10^7) - (5.2 \times 10^4)$ _____

    c. $(1.08 \times 10^{-1}) . (9.3 \times 10^{-1})$_____

    d. $(3.74 \times 10^4) / (1.58 \times 10^3)$ _____

Apply the Concepts

1. a. Explain why scientific notation is often used to express numbers in the science and health disciplines.

   _____

   _____

   b. Provide an example of a variable in healthcare that may be expressed in scientific notation.

   _____

2. What problems may arise if scientific notation is not used?

   _____

   _____

3. Why is scientific notation sometimes referred to as exponential notation?

   _____

   _____

4. What is an exponent?

   _____

   _____

ACTIVITY 1.4: SIGNIFICANT FIGURES

It is very important that when making measurements and performing calculations with those measurements, a figure or result is produced that shows the degree of confidence in that number. The digits that should be recorded in any measurement are all those that carry confidence plus one that is estimated. These are considered significant figures and rules apply to determining which numbers are considered significant and which are not. These rules also apply to numbers written in scientific notation.

This activity illustrates the role of significant figures and rounding in conveying confidence.

Part 1: Determining Significant Figures

Rules for counting **significant figures**:

- *All non-zero digits are significant.*
- *Zeros that precede non-zero digits are not significant and serve only to locate the decimal point.*
- *Captive zeros (located between non-zero digits) are significant.*
- *Trailing zeros (located to the right of another number) are significant only if a decimal point is present.*
- *In calculations, the answer must contain the smallest number of significant figures found in the question.*

1. Obtain an A4 sheet of paper and a ruler.

2. Measure the length of the paper with the ruler and record the length in centimetres to 2 decimal places:

    a. Length of paper: _____

    b. How many of these numbers are significant figures?

    _____

    c. Which of these numbers express confidence?

    _____

    d. Why do these numbers express confidence?

    _____

    _____

    e. Which of these numbers represents an estimation?

    _____

    _____

    f. Why does this number represent an estimation?

    _____

    _____

3. Measure the width of the paper with the ruler and record it in centimetres to 2 decimal places:

    a. Width of paper: _____

    b. How many of these numbers are significant figures?

    _____

4. Using the data collected, calculate the area of the sheet by multiplying the length and width and record the area in square centimetres exactly as it is shown on the calculator:

    a. Area of paper: _____

    b. How many of the numbers shown express confidence and can be considered significant?

    _____

    c. Explain why only those numbers are considered significant.

    _____

    _____

    _____

5. Identify the number of significant figures in each of the following:

    a. 98.46 _____

    b. 0.36 _____

    c. 79.043 _____

    d. 0.407 _____

    e. 0.02 _____

    f. 40.0 _____

    g. 0.860 _____

    h. 1056 _____

    i. 201.01 _____

    j. 0.03010 _____

6. Perform the following calculations and provide your answer in the correct number of significant figures:

    a. 25.67×0.060 _____

    b. $\dfrac{310}{140}$ _____

    c. $7.01 + 16.3 + 9.524$ _____

    d. $(5.7 \times 10^3) + (6.51 \times 10^3)$ _____

Part 2: Rounding

In many calculations, more digits are generated than the number of significant figures used. It then becomes necessary to drop excess digits by **rounding** off.

Rules for rounding:

- *If the digit to be removed is less than 5, the last digit to be retained is unchanged (e.g. 1.652 rounded off to 3 significant figures becomes 1.65).*

- *If the digit to be removed is 5 or greater, the last digit to be retained is rounded up (e.g. 7.646 rounded off to 3 significant figures becomes 7.65).*

- *Do not round off sequentially (e.g. 4.3649 becomes 4.36, and not 4.37).*

- *In a calculation with several steps, do not round off until after the final step.*

1. Round the following numbers to three significant figures:

   a. 56 184 _____

   b. 25.85 _____

   c. 0.0124463 _____

   d. 82.3995 _____

   e. 0.00061857 _____

   f. 0.0027964 _____

   g. 62.999 _____

   h. 147 300 _____

   i. 236.00 _____

   j. 1.020 _____

   k. 314 769 _____

   l. 0.036247 _____

2. Round the following numbers to two decimal places:

   a. 12.367 _____

   b. 0.245 _____

   c. 0.0789 _____

   d. 0.016 _____

   e. 12.555 _____

   f. 456.023 _____

   g. 30.263 _____

   h. 7.056 _____

   i. 145.0025 _____

   j. 79.99 _____

Apply the Concepts

1. Is a figure rounded to two decimal places the same as a figure rounded to three significant figures? Explain.

   _____

   _____

2. In a calculation with multiple steps, why is it important not to round until the end of the calculation?

   _____

   _____

ACTIVITY 1.5: SIMPLE ALGEBRA

Equations and formulae are important parts of physiology. For example, they are used in the calculations of cardiac output, renal clearance and many aspects of circulatory and pulmonary function. A mathematical equation is a statement that two quantities are equal (e.g. $3 + 5 = 8$). An **algebraic equation** is one in which symbols are used to represent one or more numbers (e.g. $y + 5 = 8$; here y represents an unknown number). To solve an algebraic equation, it is necessary to rearrange the numbers and symbols so that the unknown is on one side, and all other terms are on the other side.

This activity considers the use and manipulation of simple equations.

1. Find the value of x in each of the following:

a. $4 + 2x = 8$ _____

b. $5x - 9 = 21$ _____

c. $2x = 9 - x$ _____

d. $4x = 2(x + 9)$ _____

e. $\dfrac{2}{4} = \dfrac{x}{10}$ _____

f. $\dfrac{2}{x} = \dfrac{4}{14}$ _____

g. $\dfrac{8}{2} = \dfrac{4}{x}$ _____

h. $3(x - 1) = 21$ _____

i. $4x + 20 = x + 29$ _____

j. $3x = 170 - 5x - 10$ _____

k. $27 = 3 + 8x$ _____

l. $5(x + 2) = 15$ _____

m. $2(6 + 2x) = 3(12 + x)$ _____

n. $12x - 22 = x + 14$ _____

ACTIVITY 1.6: WORKING WITH FORMULAE

A **formula** is an equation that shows the relationship between quantities. It is a form of shorthand used frequently in science and is manipulated like any algebraic equation. An important formula commonly encountered in introductory science courses is: $F = ma$. In this formula, F stands for force, m is the mass of an object and a is the acceleration produced in the object by the force. This equation is said to be solved for force; i.e. force is isolated on the left and all other terms are on the right. If, however, the force (F) and mass (m) are known and acceleration (a) is to be calculated, the equation must be solved for acceleration, or rearranged so that a is isolated.

This activity demonstrates solving equations for a variable of interest.

1. Solve each of the following formulae for the variable indicated:

a. $a = bc$ Solve for b

_____

_____

b. $a = b + c$ Solve for c

_____

_____

c. $a = \dfrac{b+c}{d}$ Solve for b

_____

_____

d. $a = b + cd$ Solve for c

_____

_____

2. Solve each of the following formulae for the quantity stated, then use the resulting formula to find the value of that quantity from the given values of the other quantities:

a. $E = IR$ Solve for I, where $E = 6$ and $R = 10$

_____

_____

_____

b. $PV = RT$ Solve for V, where $P = 80$, $R = 20$ and $T = 120$

_____

_____

_____

c. $v = u + at$ Solve for t, where $v = 50$, $u = 10$ and $a = 8$

d. $M = mv^2$ Solve for v, where $M = 640$ and $m = 10$

Apply the Concepts

1. Cardiac output (CO) is the volume of blood pumped by the heart in mL/min. It is equal to the volume of blood pumped with each heartbeat, called stroke volume (SV) multiplied by the heart rate (HR) in beats per minute.

   Provide an equation that links these three quantities.

2. A person's cardiac output is measured as 5325 mL/min and their heart rate is 72 beats/min over the time of the measurement.

   a. Solve the equation for stroke volume.

   b. Calculate the person's stroke volume over the period of measurement.

3. Respiratory minute volume (RMV) is the volume of air breathed in and out in 1 minute. It is equal to the volume of air breathed in and out in one breath, called tidal volume (TV) multiplied by respiratory rate (RR) in breaths per minute.

   Provide an equation that links these quantities.

4. A person's respiratory minute volume is measured as 7.20 L/min while their respiratory rate is recorded as 14.0 breaths/min.

   a. Solve the equation for tidal volume.

   b. Calculate the person's tidal volume in mL.

ACTIVITY 1.7: GRAPHS

Graphs are useful ways to show trends in **data** and to present the results of experiments that demonstrate the relationships between quantities of interest (Fig. 1.4). A graph provides an overview about the data being plotted. For any graph, it is important to ask the following: What is being plotted? Why is it being plotted? What can be concluded from the data and its relationships? What cannot be concluded yet from the data? Researchers often plot data to show that there is a correlation between quantities of interest or that one quantity is having an effect on the other. These quantities are referred to as **independent** and **dependent variables**.

This activity investigates the use of graphs to demonstrate relationships between quantities of interest.

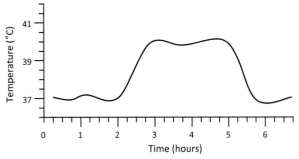

Figure 1.4 Body temperature at rest and during exercise.
(Source: Cannon, J. G. (2013). Perspective on fever: the basic science and conventional medicine. Complementary therapies in medicine, 21, S54-S60.)

1. Consider the following questions with reference to Fig. 1.4:

   a. What quantities are plotted on this graph?

   _____

   b. What is an independent variable?

   _____

   _____

   _____

   c. What is a dependent variable?

   _____

   _____

   _____

   d. Identify the axis for placement of the:

      i. Dependent variable _____

      ii. Independent variable _____

   e. In this graph, identify the:

      i. Dependent variable _____

      ii. Independent variable _____

   f. Which quantity is being affected by the other?

   _____

   g. What is the purpose of the graph?

   _____

   _____

   _____

   h. What does the graph demonstrate about the relationship between the quantities shown?

   _____

   _____

   _____

   i. Identify the time at which exercise:

      i. starts _____

      ii. finishes _____

   j. What is the person's body temperature after 5.5 hours?

   _____

2. The table below shows the speed of an athlete at different times during a 100 metre race.

Time (s)	0	1	2	3	4	5	6	7	8	9
Velocity (m/s)	0	5.4	8.8	10.6	11.4	11.9	12.2	12.2	12.2	11.3

a. In this table, identify the:

   i. dependent variable _____

   ii. independent variable _____

b. Plot these data on the graph below and connect the points with a line of best fit.

   i. Make sure axes are labelled and units shown.

c. Provide a title for the graph and write it in below. (Note: This is a statement comparing the dependent and independent variable).

d. What was the athlete's maximum velocity?

   _____

e. How long did it take the athlete to reach their maximum velocity?

   _____

f. How long did it take the athlete to reach half their maximum velocity?

   _____

g. What was the athlete's average rate of acceleration in the first 6 seconds of the race? (Note: acceleration is the rate of increase in velocity and is measured in m/s/s).

   _____

h. What was the athlete's maximum rate of acceleration during the race?

   _____

Title: _____

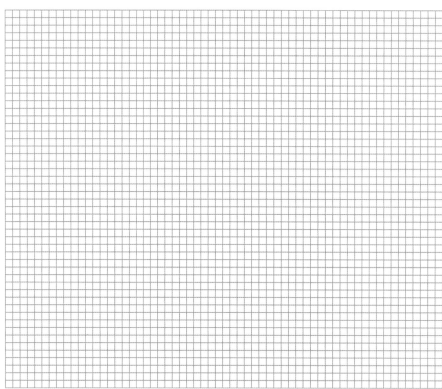

Apply the Concepts

1. What is a controlled variable?

   _____

   _____

2. What is the purpose of setting up a control in an experiment?

   _____

   _____

3. What type of data is suited to a bar or column graph?

   _____

   _____

4. What type of data is suited to a line graph?

   _____

   _____

5. What type of data is suited to a pie chart?

   _____

   _____

6. What type of data is suited to a scatter plot?

   _____

   _____

Additional Resources

BYJUS: Accuracy and Precision – The Art of Measurement
  BYJUS presents a number of content areas for educational purposes catering to a wide range of learners, from children at the start of their education to adults who are looking to upgrade their professional skills.

  byjus.com/physics/accuracy-precision-measurement/

Lumen Learning: Boundless Algebra and Introduction to Chemistry
  Lumen Learning provides a number of online courses and modules related to anatomy and physiology and a variety of biological topics, including biological molecules and enzymes. The introductory Chemistry section provides information on SI units, conversions, accuracy, precision and error.

  courses.lumenlearning.com/boundless-algebra/
  courses.lumenlearning.com/introchem/

Math is Fun: Errors in Measurement
  Math is Fun provides tools, puzzles, and worksheets in foundational maths, covering errors in measurement, algebra and the use and handling of data.

  www.mathsisfun.com/measure/error-measurement.html
  www.mathsisfun.com/algebra/index.html
  www.mathsisfun.com/data/index.html

Purplemath: Exponents – Scientific Notation
  Purplemath provides informal self-paced maths lessons that demonstrate techniques, trick questions and common student mistakes in maths testing.

  www.purplemath.com/modules/exponent3.htm

Science Notes: Unit Conversions
  Science Notes is a repository of chemistry, physics, and maths projects and homework, and provides worked problems with answers in a number of content areas.

  sciencenotes.org/unit-conversion-example-problems/
  sciencenotes.org/systematic-vs-random-error-differences-and-examples/

Sciencing: Systematic/Random Errors and Independent/Dependent Variables
  Sciencing provides educational and explanatory articles and projects on science and maths-related topics for all students.

  sciencing.com/difference-between-systematic-random-errors-8254711.html
  sciencing.com/independent-dependent-variables/

ThoughtCo: Math
  ThoughtCo is a reference site focusing on expert-created education content and provides a core section on science, tech and maths.

  www.thoughtco.com/math-4133545

CHAPTER 2
Physical Quantities in Physiology

Scientific terms are often used with an incomplete understanding of their meaning, and are sometimes used interchangeably with terms that are inaccurate. Terms such as mass, weight, force, pressure, heat, temperature, energy and work, all signify physical quantities that are fundamental to physiological understanding and need to be both understood and used correctly. The concepts behind these terms are also fundamental to our understanding of chemical processes in the body. (Refer to Chapter 3: Basic Chemistry, for further information on chemical bonding and compounds, and Chapter 4: Biological Chemistry, for further information on organic and biological molecules.)

Blood pressure, pulse rate, body weight and body temperature are routinely measured in clinical settings using specific units of measurement. (Refer to Chapter 1: Measurement and Scientific Mathematics, for further information on measurement and SI units.) The mechanisms underpinning physiological functions such as blood flow, respiration, thermoregulation, metabolic rate, body mechanics, vision and hearing, however, require an understanding of the physical factors involved in order that appropriate monitoring and care can be delivered. In addition, clinical diagnosis, treatment and therapies often involve not only chemical testing, but also radiology, sonography, laser procedures and radiation therapy, which require an understanding of the physical concepts involved.

LEARNING OUTCOMES

On completion of these activities the student should be able to:

1. define mass, weight, force and acceleration and describe their relationships
2. explain the importance of centre of gravity to stability
3. measure the density of objects and relate density to specific gravity
4. explain pressure in fluids as the result of the application of a force
5. distinguish the importance of pressure gradients, viscosity and resistance as determinants of fluid dynamics
6. discuss the relationship between work and energy
7. explain the electromagnetic spectrum and the different types of energy

LEARNING OUTCOMES—cont'd

8. distinguish between heat and temperature and assign to each their correct units
9. define heat capacity and explain its importance to living things
10. relate electromagnetic radiation to therapeutic procedures
11. explain radioactivity and its clinical importance
12. discuss electricity in terms of its biological importance and therapeutic uses.

KEY TERMS

Acceleration	Force	Radioisotope
Alpha particle	Frequency (v)	Radionuclide
Amplitude (A)	Friction	Reflection
Atmospheric pressure	Gamma ray	Refraction
Base of support	Gravity	Resistance
Beta ray	Half-life	Specific gravity
Centre of gravity	Heat	Static electricity
Conduction	Heat capacity	Temperature
Conductor	Insulator	Translucent
Convection	Mass	Transparent
Current	Opaque	Velocity
Density	Optics	Viscosity
Dynamic electricity	Pressure	Volume
Electricity	Pressure gradient	Wavelength (λ)
Electromagnetic radiation (EMR)	Radiation	Weight
Energy	Radioactivity	Work

ACTIVITY 2.1: MASS, WEIGHT AND FORCE

The **mass** of a body is the amount of matter in it, and as long as the body remains unchanged its mass is unchanged. Mass could be measured in terms of the number and types of atoms in the body, but because this is impractical it is measured in kilograms (kg). Wherever a body is found, whether in the weightlessness of space, on Earth, or on the moon, it will have the same mass. An average human male will have a mass of about 70 kg irrespective of location. A 70 kg human, however, will not have the same **weight** everywhere in the universe. A body only has weight in a gravitational field. The stronger the gravitational force, the greater the weight of the body. Weight is the downward **force** exerted by a mass in a gravitational field. The unit of force is the newton (N).

On Earth, every kilogram of mass exerts a force of about 9.8 newtons on the surface of the earth due to **gravity**. The gravitational force on the surface of the Earth therefore is 9.8 N/kg^{-1}, thus a mass of 1.0 kg has a weight of 9.8 N. Strictly speaking, weight is a force and should be given in newtons. A 70 kg man has a weight of about 686 N on Earth, but on the moon would weigh only about 114 N due to the moon's lower gravity. By convention, weight is given not in newtons but in kilograms because the gravitational force varies very little over the surface of the Earth.

This activity explores the relationship between the physical quantities of mass, weight and force.

Part 1: Mass, Weight and Force

A force can be defined as a push or pull on an object and also includes **friction**. A force applied to an object causes it to accelerate (change **velocity**) in the direction of the force. The rate of **acceleration** (*a*) is proportional to the size of the force (*F*) and the mass (*m*) of the object. Those three quantities are linked by the following equation:

$$F = ma$$

A force of 1.0 N causes a mass of 1.0 kg to accelerate by 1.0 m/s^{-2}. Note that in the SI system, the unit of velocity is metre per second (m/s^{-1}), but acceleration is the rate of change of velocity, so its unit is metre per second per second (m/s^{-2}).

1. Identify how much each of the following masses will weigh on the surface of the Earth:

   a. 64 kg _____

   b. 10 000 kg _____

   c. 150 g _____

   d. 2.5 g _____

   e. 17 mg _____

2. Consider the following questions:

   a. A patient steps onto the scales and records a weight of 1070 N. What is their mass?

   _____

   _____

   _____

   b. An astronaut who weighs 75 kg experiences an acceleration of 40 m/s^{-2} during a rocket test. What force produced that acceleration?

   _____

   _____

   _____

   c. A nurse applies a force of 55 N to a patient in a wheelchair with a total mass of 110 kg. Assuming no friction, how fast will the wheelchair accelerate?

   _____

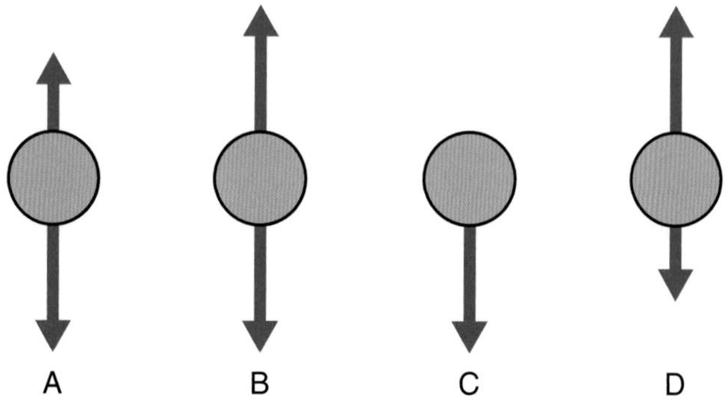

   _____

Figure 2.1 Possible forces acting on a ball thrown upwards.

3. Examine Fig. 2.1, which shows a ball that has just been thrown into the air and is moving upwards, away from the hand that threw it. The arrows represent the sizes and directions of forces that may or may not be acting on the ball.

   a. Assuming no friction, identify whether A, B, C or D correctly shows the force(s) acting on the ball.

   _____

   b. Provide an explanation for your answer.

   _____

   _____

   _____

4. Ensure your hands are dry and rub the palms of your hands together for 30 seconds.

5. Note the resulting effect on your hands.

   a. How did your hands feel?

   _____

   _____

b. Which force was experienced?

_____

c. How can this force be defined?

_____

_____

_____

d. Identify the products resulting from this force.

_____

_____

e. Explain how friction may be advantageous in certain circumstances.

_____

_____

_____

f. Explain how friction may be disadvantageous in certain circumstances.

_____

_____

_____

g. Explain how friction can be reduced.

_____

_____

_____

h. Provide two examples of natural lubricating substances found within the body.

_____

_____

_____

i. Explain what would happen if these substances were absent.

_____

_____

_____

6. Obtain a chair or trolley with wheels and give it a push with as much force as possible over a flat smooth surface, such as linoleum.

a. Which forces acting on the chair cause it to stop?

_____

_____

7. Repeat the process on a flat, carpet-covered surface.

a. How did the distance travelled by the chair differ from that on the linoleum-covered surface?

_____

b. What property provided by the carpet was responsible?

_____

c. If this force was not present, what would have happened to the movement of the chair?

_____

_____

_____

d. Is this phenomenon affected by mass or gravity? Explain.

_____

_____

_____

e. Describe an activity which requires a high level of friction.

_____

_____

f. How can the friction of a surface be increased?

_____

g. Identify one process in the body that is affected by the force of gravity.

_____

h. When pushing a wheelchair containing a patient, which forces will act to move the wheelchair and which forces will act to impede movement of the wheelchair?

_____

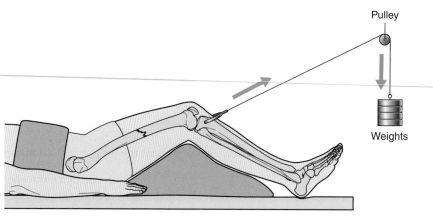

Figure 2.2 Perkins traction.
(Source: Browner, B. D. (2009). Skeletal trauma: basic science, management, and reconstruction (Vol. 1). Elsevier.)

8. Examine Fig. 2.2, which shows the use of Perkins traction in the treatment of a broken femur.

   a. What is represented by the green arrows?

   _____

   b. Explain why the pulley has been placed in that position.

   _____

   _____

   c. If the weights have a total mass of 4 kg, what force is being applied to the patient's leg?

   _____

   _____

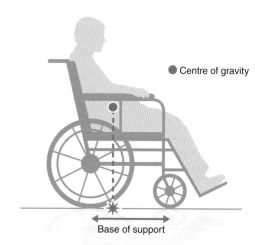

A

Part 2: Centre of Gravity and Base of Support

The **centre of gravity** of an object is the point through which the entire weight of the object can be seen to be acting. An object is stable if a vertical line drawn from the centre of gravity falls within the **base of support** of the object.

1. Explain what has occurred to the centre of gravity in Fig. 2.3B to cause the wheelchair and its occupant to become unstable.

   _____

   _____

   _____

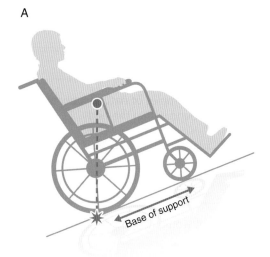

B

Figure 2.3 Centre of gravity and base of support. **A** Stable use of a wheelchair. **B** Unstable use of a wheelchair.
(Source: Kerr, A., & Rowe, P. (Eds.). (2019). An Introduction to Human Movement and Biomechanics. Elsevier.)

2. Stand upright with your normal posture and feet slightly apart.

3. Note that your feet are your base of support and your centre of gravity is directly over the centre of your base of support.

    a. Do you feel stable? _____

4. Maintain the same position, but lean forward.

    a. Do you feel stable? _____

    b. What has happened to your centre of gravity?

    _____

    _____

5. Stand balanced on one leg.

    a. Do you feel stable? _____

    b. What has happened to your base of support?

    _____

    _____

6. Sit upright in a chair.

    a. Where is your centre of gravity in relation to the base of support (your feet and the legs of the chair)?

    _____

    _____

7. Attempt to leave the chair without changing your body shape.

    a. Is this difficult to achieve? _____

    b. Explain your observation.

    _____

    _____

8. Now rise from the chair normally.

    a. How did you adjust your centre of gravity to make this possible?

    _____

    _____

9. Explain, in terms of centre of gravity and stability, why you should carry a heavy weight as close as possible to your body.

    _____

    _____

    _____

Apply the Concepts

1. Provide two examples where application of a lubricant may be employed during nursing care.

    _____

    _____

2. Provide two examples of nursing care that utilise the force of gravity.

    _____

    _____

3. What is involved in traction and what is its purpose?

    _____

    _____

4. How do pulleys assist the application of traction?

    _____

    _____

5. What precautions must be observed when caring for a patient in traction? Explain why.

_____

_____

6. Why is it necessary to keep the centre of gravity inside the base of support?

_____

_____

7. How could the centre of gravity of a book be determined?

_____

_____

ACTIVITY 2.2: MEASUREMENT OF DENSITY

The **density** (d) of an object is the mass (m) of the object per unit **volume** (V) and is given by the equation:

$$d = \frac{m}{V}$$

The derived SI unit for density is kg/m³, but in clinical settings more commonly used units are g/cm³ or g/mL. The density of water at 4°C is 1.0g/cm³. **Specific gravity** is a measure of the density of a substance relative to the density of water and is a dimensionless number. A substance denser than water will have a specific gravity greater than 1.0, whereas a substance less dense than water will have a specific gravity less than 1.0. Whole blood has a specific gravity of about 1.05 and urine is normally from 1.005 to 1.030.

This activity explores methods of measuring density, behaviours of liquids and solids of different densities, and estimates of specific gravity.

Part 1: Density of a Solid of Irregular Shape

Many objects have a volume that is difficult to measure because they are irregular in shape. As such, their volume may be measured by water displacement and can then be used to calculate their density.

1. This activity is best conducted in groups of two or three.

2. Obtain an electronic balance, 100 mL measuring cylinder, water, paper clip and five solid objects small enough to fit into the cylinder (e.g. marble, bolt, pebble, cork, rubber stopper).

3. Measure the mass of each object with the electronic balance, recording it in the table provided.

4. Fill the measuring cylinder with water to 50 mL.

5. Record the initial volume of water, ensuring that the volume is read from the bottom of the meniscus.

6. Carefully place the first object into the measuring cylinder.

7. Record the final volume of water.

8. Repeat the process for each of the remaining objects, recording the results in the table provided.

9. If the object floats, unfold the paperclip and use this to push the object completely under the water.

10. Calculate the volume of each of the objects, recording your results in the table.

11. Calculate the density of each of the objects, recording your results in the table.

Object	Description	Mass (g)	Initial volume (mL)	Final volume (mL)	Volume of object (cm³)[1]	Density of object (g/cm³)[2]
1						
2						
3						
4						
5						

Notes:
1. Volume of object (cm^3) = Final volume (mL) − Initial volume (mL). (Remember 1.0 mL = 1.0 cm^3).
2. Density of object (g/cm^3) = Mass of object (g) ÷ Volume of object (cm^3).

12. Undertake the following tasks:

   a. List the objects in order of decreasing density.

   _____

   _____

   b. Identify the objects that have a specific gravity:

   i. less than 1.0 _____

   ii. greater than 1.0 _____

   c. List three possible sources of error in this experiment.

   _____

   _____

   _____

   d. Explain why water was used to determine the volume of the given objects.

   _____

   _____

   _____

   e. Describe how the volume of a regular-shaped object, such as a cube, can be determined.

   _____

   _____

   _____

Part 2: Densities of Liquids and Solids

Liquids of different densities tend to separate into layers when undisturbed. Solid objects tend to be trapped in different layers according to their densities.

1. This activity is best conducted in groups of two or three.

2. Obtain a 250 mL measuring cylinder, two 100 mL beakers, honey (or corn syrup), dishwashing liquid (preferably coloured), water, vegetable oil, ethanol (or methylated spirit), food colouring, a variety of solid objects (e.g. marble, bolt, pebble, cork, rubber stopper, pasta, grape, Lego block, sultana, etc).

3. Pour 50 mL honey into the measuring cylinder (this should come up to the first large graduation).

4. Gently pour 50 mL dishwashing liquid down the side of the measuring cylinder, ensuring that the honey is not disturbed (this should come up to the second large graduation).

5. Pour 50 mL water into a beaker and add 2 drops of food colouring, ensuring that the colour differs from that of the dishwashing liquid and the vegetable oil. Mix well.

6. Gently pour the coloured water down the side of the measuring cylinder, ensuring that the dishwashing liquid is not disturbed (this should come up to the third large graduation).

7. Gently pour 50 mL vegetable oil down the side of the measuring cylinder, ensuring that the water is not disturbed (this should come up to the fourth large graduation).

8. Pour 50 mL ethanol into a beaker and add 2 drops food colouring, ensuring that the colour differs from that of the vegetable oil. Mix well.

9. Gently pour the coloured ethanol down the side of the measuring cylinder, ensuring that the vegetable oil is not disturbed (it should come up to the fifth large graduation).

10. Allow the contents of the measuring cylinder to settle.

11. In the space below, draw a labelled sketch of the measuring cylinder and the various liquid layers.

12. Gently lower each of the small solid objects into the measuring cylinder, one at a time.

13. Record on your diagram where each object settles.

14. Consider the following questions:

    a. List the liquids used in order from least dense to most dense.

    _____

    _____

    _____

b. Identify the liquids that have a specific gravity:

    i. greater than one _____

    ii. less than one _____

c. List the solids tested in order from least dense to most dense.

    _____

    _____

    _____

d. Explain why the objects sink to different levels.

    _____

    _____

    _____

e. Explain why some objects do not sink in water but float.

    _____

    _____

    _____

f. Is there a distinction between floating and buoyancy? Explain.

    _____

    _____

    _____

15. Ensure all items are disposed of as instructed.

Apply the Concepts

1. Is it easier to float in salt water or fresh water? Explain.

    _____

    _____

2. Explain whether the density of water would be greater on a hot day or a cold day.

    _____

    _____

ACTIVITY 2.3: PRESSURE

Pressures of various kinds affect physiological processes and are routinely monitored. These include arterial and central venous blood pressures, partial pressures of respiratory gases, gases dissolved in the blood, and pressure changes involved in ventilation of the lungs. **Pressure gradients** drive the flow of all liquids and gases in the body.

This activity focuses on the nature of pressure and its importance to body functions.

Part 1: The Nature of Pressure

Pressure is exerted when a force is applied over an area. For a given force, the smaller the area over which it is exerted, the greater the pressure experienced. As the area over which the force is exerted increases, the pressure decreases. Pressure (p) is thus defined as force (F) per unit area (A):

$$p = \frac{F}{A}$$

The SI unit of pressure is the pascal (Pa), which is a force of 1 N per square metre (1 Pa = 1 N/m^2). In practice, a pressure of 1 Pa is a very small amount of pressure, thus the unit kilopascals (kPa) is commonly used.

1. What pressure is exerted on a surface when a 2000 kg elephant stands on it, if its feet have a total area of 1.6 square metres?

   _____

   _____

   _____

2. What pressure is exerted on a surface when a 60 kg woman stands on it in high heels with a total area of 0.04 square metres?

   _____

   _____

   _____

3. Every square metre of the surface of Earth has a mass of about 10 340 kg of air above it.

   a. What force does this mass exert on each square metre of Earth's surface?

      _____

      _____

      _____

b. Calculate the pressure of the atmosphere at the Earth's surface in:

   i. kilopascals _____

   ii. hectopascals _____

c. Do your results broadly agree with published

   values? _____

d. Explain why your body does not collapse under such pressure.

   _____

   _____

   _____

4. Water has a density of about 1000 kg/m^3. If a diver descends to a depth of 10 m, what pressure will they experience at that depth? (Hint: Consider air pressure at the surface of the water.)

   _____

   _____

   _____

5. Several non-SI units of pressure are used in the clinical setting:

   • Millimetres of mercury (mmHg)

   • Centimetres of water (cmH$_2$O)

   • Atmospheres (atm)

   • Bars (bar)

   Complete the conversions below.

   a. 1.0 kPa = _____ mmHg

   b. 1.0 kPa = _____ cmH$_2$O

   c. 1.0 atm = _____ kPa

   d. 1.0 bar = _____ kPa

6. In a clinical setting, identify what is likely to be recorded in:

   a. mmHg _____

   b. cmH$_2$O _____

   c. atm _____

Part 2: Atmospheric Pressure

Since air has mass, and therefore weight, every object on Earth experiences the pressure caused by the weight force of the air above it. When moving to higher altitudes, the weight of the air above decreases, and so does the pressure it causes. This pressure is referred to as **atmospheric pressure**. At sea level it is approximately 1 atm (standard atmosphere), 101 325 Pa (pascals) or 760 mmHg.

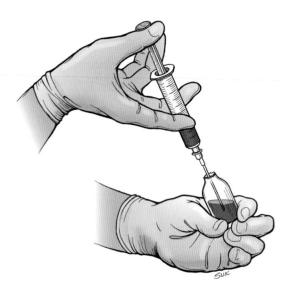

Figure 2.4 Removal of fluid from an ampoule.
(Source: Burchum, J., & Rosenthal, L. (2022). Lehne's Pharmacology for Nursing Care. Elsevier.)

1. Refer to Fig. 2.4, which shows a fluid being drawn into a syringe from an opened ampoule.

   a. What is causing the fluid to flow?

   _____

   b. What is the practitioner doing to establish a pressure gradient?

   _____

   _____

   c. Where is the high-pressure end of the gradient?

   _____

   d. What is the source of the pressure pushing the liquid into the syringe?

   _____

2. Obtain a 250 mL beaker and a 25 mL syringe.

3. Pour 100 mL water into the beaker and draw approximately 15 mL into the syringe.

4. Note the force that was applied to the plunger to draw the water from the beaker.

   a. Which component contains water at a higher pressure and which at a lower pressure?

   _____

   _____

5. Dispense the water in the syringe back into the beaker.

6. Note the force that was applied to the plunger to expel the water back into the beaker.

   a. Which component contains water at a higher pressure and which at a lower pressure?

   _____

   _____

Part 3: Applications of Pressure (The Siphon)

A siphon works on the principle that there is a pressure gradient between liquids at two different levels. A continuous column of liquid can be made to rise above its initial level and fall to a lower level by a combination of gravitational force and atmospheric pressure pushing on the liquid surface.

1. This activity is best conducted in pairs.

2. Obtain two 500 mL beakers, water, 1 m of PVC tubing, two rubber stoppers and measuring tape.

3. Fill the PVC tube with water and place a stopper in each end.

4. Fill one beaker with 500 mL water and place one end of the tubing into the water in the beaker. This is beaker 1.

5. Place the other end of the tube into the empty beaker. This is beaker 2.

6. Place Beaker 1 on a table and place beaker 2 approximately 10 cm below beaker 1, measuring the distance with the measuring tape.

7. Remove the stopper from the tube in beaker 1 while keeping the end of the tube underwater.

8. Remove the stopper from the end of the tube in beaker 2.

9. Note the flow of water into beaker 2.

10. Place beaker 2 approximately 25 cm below beaker 1, measuring the distance with the measuring tape.

11. Fill and stopper the tube as before, and repeat steps 7 and 8.

12. Note the flow of water into beaker 2.

    a. Is there a notable change in the flow of water from a height difference of 10 cm to 25 cm? Explain any change observed.

    _____

    _____

    _____

13. Place beaker 2 approximately 50 cm below beaker 1, measuring the distance with the measuring tape.

14. Fill and stopper the tube as before, and repeat steps 7 and 8.

15. Note the flow of water into beaker 2.

    a. Is there a notable change in the flow of water from a height difference of 25 cm to 50 cm? Explain.

    _____

    _____

    _____

    b. Explain how a siphon works.

    _____

    _____

    _____

    c. Apart from changing the elevation of beaker 2, how could the flow rate in the tube be varied?

    _____

    _____

    _____

Apply the Concepts

1. Explain why placing a patient on an air cushion can assist in preventing pressure injuries.

   _____

   _____

2. Explain the mechanism which causes ears to 'pop' when altitude is altered.

   _____

   _____

3. Explain why guidelines for the height placement of an enema bag should be followed closely.

   _____

   _____

ACTIVITY 2.4: FLUID DYNAMICS

Pressure differences drive the flow of fluids such as blood through hollow vessels such as arteries and veins. **Resistance** is the tendency to reduce this flow; it depends on three factors: the **viscosity** of the fluid, the length of the vessel and the diameter of the vessel.

This activity explores the factors determining flow rates in fluids.

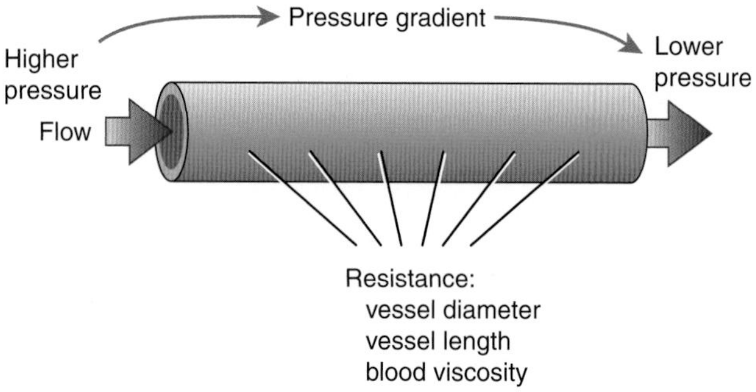

Figure 2.5 Factors affecting blood flow in an artery.
(Source: Patton, K. T., Bell, F. B., Matusiak, D. J., & Wood, S. R. (2021). Anatomy & Physiology Laboratory Manual. Elsevier.)

1. Consider the following questions with reference to Fig. 2.5:

   a. Explain what is causing the high pressure at the left end of the artery.

   _____

   _____

   _____

   b. Given that the artery diameter and the viscosity of the blood are both constant, explain why the blood pressure drops.

   _____

   _____

   _____

   c. Explain the effect of vessel length on the resistance to blood flow.

   _____

   _____

   _____

   d. Explain whether blood would flow through the artery if the pressure was the same at both ends.

   _____

   _____

   _____

   e. Explain the term viscosity.

   _____

   _____

   _____

   f. Identify two factors that could cause the viscosity of blood to change.

   _____

   _____

   _____

2. Consider the following questions with reference to Fig. 2.6, which shows the effect of changing a blood vessel's diameter on the rate of blood flow through the vessel. (Note that each vessel has twice the diameter of the one below it.)

   a. For a given driving pressure, how does blood flow change when a vessel reduces its diameter?

   _____

   _____

   b. When a vessel doubles its diameter, identify:

   i. by how much blood flow increases.

   _____

   ii. by how much its resistance decreases.

   _____

   c. Explain why a small reduction in the diameter of a vessel can markedly increase its resistance.

   _____

   _____

   _____

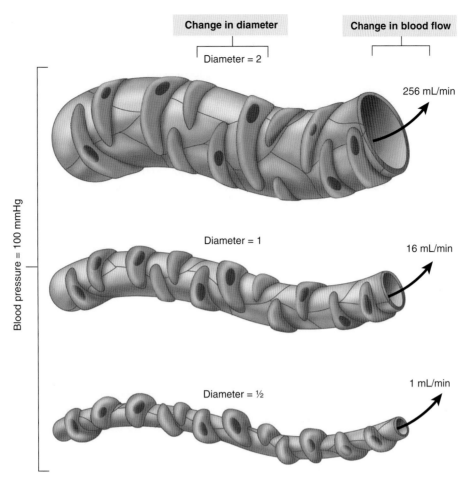

Figure 2.6 Effect of changing blood vessel diameter on blood flow.
(Source: Washington, C. M., & Leaver, D. T. (2015). Principles and Practice of Radiation Therapy. Elsevier.)

Apply the Concepts

1. Is there a distinction between resistance and friction? Explain.

   _____

   _____

2. A fluid loses pressure as it moves through a tube.

   a. Explain the effect of friction on pressure.

   _____

   _____

   b. Explain the effect of viscosity on pressure.

   _____

   _____

ACTIVITY 2.5: WORK AND ENERGY

Another quantity related to force is **work**. This term is often used loosely in connection with function, but scientifically work is done whenever force is applied to an object over a distance. For example, force must be applied to a pen to make it write; the heavier the pen and the more text that is written, the more work is done. Thus, work (W) is a function of both force (F) and distance (d), and is given by:

$$W = Fd$$

The unit of work is the newton metre (Nm), where 1 Nm is called a joule (J); therefore, 1 joule of work is done when a force of 1 N is applied over a distance of 1 m. This is a very small amount of work, so the term kilojoule (kJ) is more commonly used.

This activity explores the relationship between work and energy.

Part 1: Work and Energy

Energy is simply the capacity to do work and is also measured in joules or kilojoules. Occasionally the non-SI units, calories (cal) or kilocalories (kcal) are used. Work is essentially the product of an unbalanced force and the distance through which the force moves.

1. How much work is done when a mass of 3 kg is lifted vertically through 6 m?

_____

_____

_____

2. A 50 kg hiker climbs a hill 200 m high. How much work does he do in lifting his body to that height?

_____

_____

_____

3. A student picks up a bag full of books. This requires a force of 200 N and the expenditure of 124 J of work. Through what distance is the bag moved?

_____

_____

_____

4. Obtain a book and place it on the palm of your open hand.

   a. Are you doing any work while holding the book? Explain.

   _____

   _____

   _____

   b. Are you expending energy? Explain.

   _____

   _____

   _____

5. The work done by the heart in pumping blood through the body is 0.50 J per heartbeat. If a student's average heart rate is 65 beats/min:

   a. How much work is done by the heart per day?

   _____

   _____

   _____

   b. What proportion of the body's daily work is done by the heart? (Hint: assume a total daily expenditure of 670 kJ.)

   _____

   _____

   _____

6. What is the source of the energy the body uses for doing work?

   _____

   _____

   _____

Part 2: Forms of Energy

The law of conservation of energy states that energy cannot be created or destroyed, but only converted from one form to another. Thus, the total energy of a system remains constant over time. The various forms of energy all have the ability to do work on an object. In addition, some forms of energy are gravity-dependent while others are not.

1. For each of the following forms of energy, provide a definition and an example:

   a. Thermal energy

      i. Definition: _____

      _____

      ii. Example: _____

   b. Nuclear energy

      i. Definition: _____

      _____

      ii. Example: _____

   c. Magnetic energy

      i. Definition: _____

      _____

      ii. Example: _____

   d. Electrical energy

      i. Definition: _____

      _____

      ii. Example: _____

   e. Sound energy

      i. Definition: _____

      _____

      ii. Example: _____

   f. Chemical energy

      i. Definition: _____

      _____

      ii. Example: _____

   g. Elastic energy

      i. Definition: _____

      _____

      ii. Example: _____

   h. Light energy

      i. Definition: _____

      _____

      ii. Example: _____

2. Identify the form(s) of energy involved in each of the following situations (Note: Some energy forms may be used once or more than once):

   a. A firecracker exploding

      _____

   b. An elastic band being stretched

      _____

   c. Lightning strike

      _____

   d. Atomic bomb explosion

      _____

   e. Sunlight warming a room

      _____

   f. Burning of wood to heat a room

      _____

   g. Iron filings attracted to a magnet

      _____

   h. Vibration of fabric covering a radio speaker

      _____

   i. Light emission from a lightbulb

      _____

   j. Natural gas used to fuel a gas stove

      _____

   k. A metallic spring recoiling

      _____

l. A kettle boiling to produce steam

_____

m. A dog barking

_____

n. A jet plane overhead

_____

o. A balloon being inflated.

_____

3. Define the following basic types of energy:

a. Potential energy: _____

_____

b. Kinetic energy: _____

_____

4. An apple is attached to a tree by its stem. It then falls to the ground where it comes to rest.

a. Which force pulled the apple to the ground?

_____

b. How fast did the apple accelerate based on this force?

_____

c. When did the apple experience maximum potential energy?

_____

d. When did the apple experience maximum kinetic energy?

_____

e. If the apple experienced both potential and kinetic energy, what does this indicate about the nature of energy?

_____

_____

_____

Apply the Concepts

The Mifflin–St Jeor equation was derived in the 1990s as a tool for estimating daily energy expenditure and energy requirements. A person's daily energy expenditure at rest in kcal is given by the equation:

$$E = 10.0\,m + 6.25\,h - 5.0\,a + s$$

where:
- m is body mass in kg
- h is height in cm
- a is age in years
- s = 5 for males and –161 for females.

(Multiply the result by 4.2 to convert to kJ).

1. Using the Mifflin–St Jeor equation, calculate your own expected daily energy expenditure at rest.

_____

_____

2. Average adults need a daily energy intake of 8000 to 11 000 kJ. Why is this so much greater than their daily energy expenditure?

_____

_____

ACTIVITY 2.6: HEAT AND TEMPERATURE

Heat is a form of energy possessed by every object in the universe, to a greater or lesser extent, and is simply a measure of how fast the atoms and molecules of an object are moving or vibrating. The greater the heat content of a substance, the greater the kinetic energy of its particles. The amount of heat a body contains depends on two factors – the number of particles in the body (i.e. the mass of the body) and how much individual kinetic energy those particles have. As with all forms of energy, heat is measured in joules (J).

This activity demonstrates the relationship between heat and temperature.

Part 1: Heat and Temperature Principles

Temperature is not dependent on mass. Temperature is a measure of the average kinetic **energies** of the particles in a substance (i.e. the intensity of the heat). The SI unit of temperature is the kelvin (K), but a more convenient unit is the degree Celsius (°C). There is more heat in a bathtub of warm water than in a cup of boiling water, even though the boiling water is at a higher temperature. Heat energy is transferred by three mechanisms – **conduction**, **convection** and **radiation**.

1. Explain why a cup of boiling water and a jug of warm water might both have the same heat content, even though they have different temperatures.

   _____

   _____

   _____

2. The heat capacity of a substance is the amount of heat energy required to raise the temperature of 1.0 g of the substance by 1.0°C.

   a. If the heat capacity of water is 4.2 J/g/°C, calculate the amount of heat required to raise the temperature of 50 kg water by 2°C.

   _____

   _____

   _____

3. Water has a relatively high heat capacity compared to most substances.

   a. Explain how this might assist the body to stabilise internal temperature.

   _____

   _____

   _____

4. For each of the following heat transfer processes, define the process and give an example of that type of transfer associated with the human body:

   a. Conduction

   i. Definition: _____

   _____

   ii. Example: _____

   b. Convection

   i. Definition: _____

   _____

   ii. Example: _____

   c. Radiation

   i. Definition: _____

   _____

   ii. Example: _____

5. Explain why a piece of iron will often feel colder than a piece of plastic, even though they are both at the same temperature.

   _____

   _____

   _____

6. Explain why a window should be opened at the top and the bottom to enhance the flow of air in a room.

   _____

   _____

   _____

7. What type of energy is involved in radiative heat transfer?

_____

8. Evaporative heat loss occurs when people sweat. Each gram of water draws 2.26 J of heat from the body as it evaporates (the latent heat of vaporisation).

   a. What is the total heat loss by vaporisation from a person who sweats 0.85 kg of water?

   _____

   _____

   _____

Part 2: Heat and Temperature Relationships

Heat and temperature are closely related, but should not be confused. **Temperature** is a measure of the average kinetic energies of the particles in a substance, whereas heat is the thermal energy that is transferred from one object to another, which can then be measured in the form of temperature change. A rise in heat content usually results in a higher temperature.

⚠ To conduct this activity, it is important to ensure the following safety precautions:

- *Wear safety glasses when using the hotplate as heated liquids may superheat and splutter, causing permanent eye damage.*
- *Take care when handling and working around hotplates as they heat quickly and retain heat, causing skin burns.*

1. This activity is best conducted in pairs.

2. Obtain two 250 mL beakers, electronic balance, heatproof mat, water, hotplate, tongs, 5 cent coin, 50 cent coin, two thermometers, stopwatch and safety glasses.

3. Use the electronic balance to measure the mass of each coin.

   a. Mass of 5 cent coin: _____

   b. Mass of 50 cent coin: _____

4. Pour 100 mL water into each beaker and place onto the heatproof mat.

5. Insert a thermometer into each beaker, recording the initial water temperature.

   a. Beaker 1 initial temperature: _____

   b. Beaker 2 initial temperature: _____

6. Turn the hotplate to the highest setting and place the two coins onto the hotplate.

7. Allow the 50 cent coin to heat for 2 minutes, measuring the time with a stopwatch.

8. Allow the 5 cent coin to heat for 10 minutes, measuring the time with a stopwatch.

9. Remove each coin from the hotplate with the tongs after the specified heating times and place the 5 cent coin into beaker 1 and the 50 cent coin into beaker 2.

10. Note any temperature changes in the water over a period of 30 minutes, recording the final water temperature in each.

    a. Beaker 1 final temperature:_____

    b. Beaker 2 final temperature:_____

11. Consider the following questions:

    a. Suggest a reason for the difference in final temperatures in the beakers with regard to the mass of the coins.

    _____

    _____

    _____

    b. Explain why the temperature of the water increased in both beakers.

    _____

    _____

    _____

    c. Is there a distinction between thermal energy and heat? Explain.

    _____

    _____

    _____

Apply the Concepts

1. a. What is latent heat?

    _____

    _____

    b. Explain why salt may be sprinkled onto an ice pack to delay the melting process.

    _____

    _____

2. a. What is humidity?

    _____

    _____

    b. Relate high humidity to cooling effect and the need for ventilation.

    _____

    _____

    c. Explain how insensible and sensible perspiration are affected by humidity.

    _____

    _____

3. Explain why a burn caused by steam is often much worse than a burn caused by boiling water.

    _____

    _____

4. a. Explain why patients should be kept out of draughts when being bathed.

    _____

    _____

    b. Suggest a reason why only small areas of a patient are washed at one time.

    _____

    _____

5. Predict the effect of extreme heat and extreme cold on body tissues.

    _____

    _____

Additional Activities

For additional activities visit Activity 2A: Comparing Heat Capacities on Evolve®.

ACTIVITY 2.7: ELECTROMAGNETIC RADIATION

Electromagnetic radiation (EMR) is a form of energy emitted by matter and transmitted as waves, whose properties are determined by their length and frequency. EMR emitted by the sun can be transmitted through empty space and is the main source of energy in the solar system. High energy EMR is generally hazardous to living organisms, but properly controlled, can be used to provide quality health care.

This activity explores the different types of radiation that comprise the electromagnetic spectrum.

Part 1: The Electromagnetic Spectrum

Energy transmitted as waves travels through materials based on the vibrations in the source and the receiving material. Energy waves occurring in cycles can be analysed to provide information about the nature of the energy transmitted. **Frequency (𝑣)** refers to the number of wave cycles per second and is measured in hertz (Hz) or kilohertz (kHz). **Wavelength (λ)** is the distance between identical points in a wave cycle, such as peak to peak, and is measured in metres (m), millimetres (mm), or nanometres (nm). **Amplitude (A)** refers to the height of the wave above the centre line and is measured in metres (m).

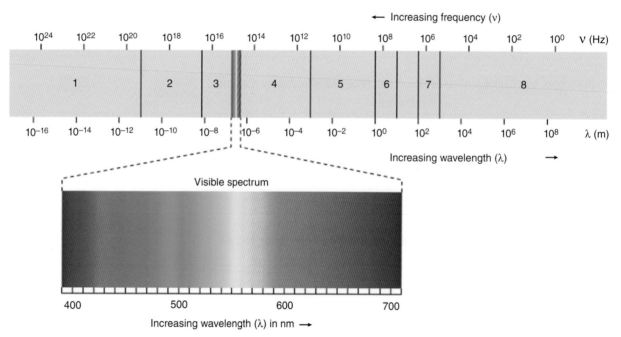

Figure 2.7 The electromagnetic spectrum. (High frequency radiation is on the left, low frequency radiation is on the right).
(Source: Nagelhout, J. J., Elisha, S., & Plaus, K. (2023). Nurse anesthesia. Elsevier.)

1. Fig. 2.7 shows the electromagnetic spectrum with the names of the various types of EMR removed. Assign each of the following terms to the various types of radiation within the labelled regions of the spectrum.

AM radio	Microwave
Long-wave radio	X-rays
Gamma rays	FM radio
Ultraviolet	Infrared

Region of the electromagnetic spectrum:

a. 1:_____   e. 5:_____

b. 2:_____   f. 6:_____

c. 3:_____   g. 7:_____

d. 4:_____   h. 8:_____

2. Consider the following questions with reference to Fig. 2.7:

    a. What relationship can be seen between the frequency of EMR and its wavelength?

    _____

    _____

    _____

    b. What is the range of wavelengths that can be seen by the human eye?

    _____

    c. What colour is the highest frequency of visible light?

    _____

    d. What colour is the lowest frequency of visible light?

    _____

    e. What features do all electromagnetic waves have in common?

    _____

    _____

3. Gamma rays and X-rays are harmful to living tissues, while radio waves pass harmlessly through them. Suggest a reason for this phenomenon.

    _____

    _____

    _____

4. What properties do X-rays have that make them particularly useful?

    _____

    _____

    _____

Part 2: Properties of Light

The behaviour and properties of light, or the portion of the electromagnetic spectrum (EMR) visible with the human eye, is referred to as **optics**. White light, or normal sunlight, can be separated to reveal its constituent wavelengths (λ) in the form of colour. Since light travels in waves it can interact with and bounce off matter (**reflection**), be transmitted in varying degrees by materials which can be **transparent** or **translucent** or **opaque**, or be transmitted from one transparent medium to another (**refraction**).

1. Obtain a 250 mL beaker and fill it with 100 mL water.

2. Place a pencil in the water and lean it against the side of the beaker.

3. View the pencil in the water from the side of the beaker.

    a. How does the pencil appear?

    _____

    b. What term can be used to describe this observation?

    _____

    c. Explain how this phenomenon is caused.

    _____

    _____

    _____

    d. This phenomenon can also occur in the eyes and affect vision. Explain how this can be adjusted artificially.

    _____

    _____

    _____

4. Consider the appearance of an object in a mirror.

    a. What term can be used to describe the image in the mirror?

    _____

    b. Explain how this phenomenon is caused.

    _____

    _____

    _____

    c. Is a real image produced? Explain.

    _____

    _____

    _____

5. Obtain a piece of card, a single layer of tissue paper and a glass slide.

6. Hold the piece of card up to the light.

   a. Has any light been transmitted through the object?

   _____

   b. What term can be used to describe this material?

   _____

   c. Explain the interaction between the material and the light.

   _____

   _____

7. Hold the tissue paper up to the light.

   a. Has any light been transmitted through the object?

   _____

   b. What term can be used to describe this material?

   _____

   c. Explain the interaction between the material and the light.

   _____

   _____

8. Hold the glass slide up to the light.

   a. Has any light been transmitted through the object?

   _____

   b. What term can be used to describe this material?

   _____

   c. Describe the interaction between the material and the light.

   _____

   _____

9. Describe what happens to light waves coming in contact with dark surfaces.

   _____

   _____

   _____

10. Obtain a piece of white paper and a glass or plastic prism.

11. Place the white paper on the ground under direct sunlight.

12. Place the prism onto the centre of the paper.

13. Rotate and move the prism around on the paper until rainbow colours can be seen on the paper (this is best conducted in a dark room with access to bright sunlight coming in through the window).

    a. What do the results suggest about the composition of white light?

    _____

    _____

    _____

    b. List the colours that can be seen, from lowest frequency to highest frequency.

    _____

    _____

    c. With reference to the movement of electrons, explain what causes the emission of white light.

    _____

    _____

    _____

14. If white light were to fall onto a red object, all colours except one would be absorbed.

    a. Which colour would not be absorbed?

    _____

    b. Based on this principle, what causes colour?

    _____

    _____

    _____

    c. Explain how black objects interact with light.

    _____

    _____

    _____

Part 3: Properties of Sound

Amplitude (A) indicates the energy of a wave and, in the case of sound waves, provides a measure of loudness; however, sound energy is often a function of hertz (Hz) or kilohertz (kHz), which refers to the frequency (v) of the waves, or of decibels (dB), which is used in acoustics to denote the pressure level of sound in air.

1. Obtain a tuning fork (128 Hz, 256 Hz or 512 Hz) and a rubber stopper.

2. Holding the fork at the base of the prongs, strike it firmly on the rubber stopper and hold it next to your ear without touching the outer ear.

   a. How discernible was the sound produced?

   _____

3. Repeat the process, placing the end of the tuning fork handle on the top of the table.

   a. Was the sound more or less pronounced?

   _____

   b. What do your observations indicate about the transmission of sound?

   _____

   _____

4. Consider the following:

   a. Explain how sound and light are similar in terms of transmission.

   _____

   _____

   _____

   b. Explain how sound and light differ in terms of transmission.

   _____

   _____

   _____

   c. Explain what is meant by pitch.

   _____

   _____

   _____

   d. Explain what is meant by sound intensity.

   _____

   _____

   _____

   e. Explain what is meant by loudness.

   _____

   _____

   _____

   f. Explain what occurs when sound is reflected.

   _____

   _____

   _____

Apply the Concepts

1. Electromagnetic radiation is used for many purposes in the clinical setting. Provide a brief description of each of the following applications:

   a. Laser surgery:

   _____

   b. UVC sterilisation:

   _____

   c. Thermography:

_____

   d. Phototherapy:

_____

   e. Magnetic resonance imaging:

_____

2. What precautions must technicians take when performing an X-ray and why?

_____

_____

3. Explain why exposure to ultraviolet radiation has been linked to skin cancer.

_____

_____

4. Explain why exposure to adequate lighting is important in the hospital environment to both nurses and patients.

_____

_____

5. Explain how sunglass lenses interact with light to allow vision, yet filter out unnecessary light.

_____

_____

6. Identify and explain two methods that can be used to reduce noise in a healthcare setting.

_____

_____

7. What is the Doppler effect?

_____

_____

8. Identify and describe two applications of sound waves in medicine.

_____

_____

ACTIVITY 2.8: RADIOACTIVITY

Radioactivity is the spontaneous emission of particles and electromagnetic radiation from the nucleus of unstable isotopes. Isotopes that are unstable are often referred to as **radioisotopes** or **radionuclides**, and decay to produce **alpha particles**, **beta rays** and **gamma rays**. Nuclear radiation produced in this way is often called ionising radiation because of its ability to strip electrons from atoms. From the moment it is formed, the activity of a radioisotope starts to decay. The time it takes for half the sample to decay to a stable isotope is termed its **half-life**. Half-lives can vary from a fraction of a second to billions of years.

This activity highlights the different types of nuclear radiation, their behaviours and clinical applications.

1. Consider the following, with reference to Fig. 2.8:

   a. Describe the composition of alpha particles.

   _____

   b. Why are alpha particles easily stopped?

   _____

   _____

   c. Describe the composition of beta rays.

   _____

   d. Why are beta rays able to penetrate further than alpha particles?

   _____

   _____

   e. Describe the composition of gamma rays.

   _____

   f. Why are gamma rays able to penetrate further than beta rays?

   _____

   _____

   _____

   g. In what way are gamma and X-rays different from other types of nuclear radiation?

   _____

   _____

   _____

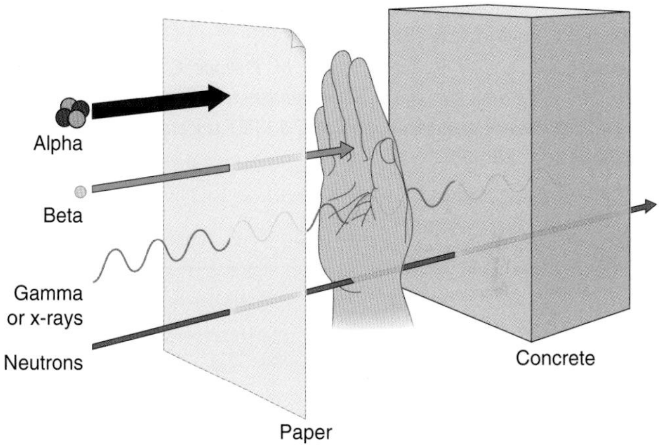

Figure 2.8 Penetrating powers of four types of radiation - alpha particles, beta rays, gamma and X-rays, and neutrons. *(Source: Goldman, L., & Schafer, A. I. (2015). Goldman's Cecil Medicine (Vol. 1). Elsevier.)*

   h. Which type of radiation is the most dangerous? Explain why.

   _____

   _____

   _____

2. Based on Fig. 2.9, which shows the decay rates of four isotopes, identify the approximate half-life of:

   a. N-13: _____

   b. C-11: _____

   c. Ga-68: _____

   d. F-18: _____

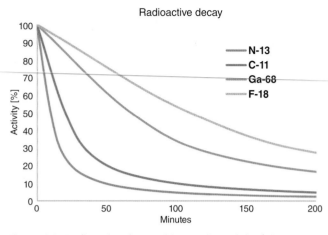

Figure 2.9 Radioactive decay of four radionuclides (nitrogen-13, carbon-11, gallium-68, fluorine-18).
(Source: Nics, L., Steiner, B., Klebermass, E. M., Philippe, C., Mitterhauser, M., Hacker, M., & Wadsak, W. (2018). Speed matters to raise molar radioactivity: fast HPLC shortens the quality control of C-11 PET-tracers. Nuclear Medicine and Biology, 57, 28-33.)

3. Radioisotopes are normally considered to have fully decayed after 10 half-lives.

    a. Have any of the isotopes in Fig. 2.9 fully decayed?

    _____

4. Iodine-125 has a half-life of 60 days and is widely used in the treatment of prostate and brain cancer.

    a. Once implanted, how long will it take for the activity of I-125 to decline to one-eighth of its original activity?

    _____

    _____

5. What is the SI unit of radioactivity?

    _____

Apply the Concepts

1. Is there a distinction between ionising and non-ionising radiation? Explain.

    _____

    _____

2. Most radioisotopes commonly used for diagnostic and therapeutic purposes have half-lives measured in days rather than hours or years.

    a. Why are isotopes with much longer or shorter half-lives avoided?

    _____

    _____

3. Radiation has its greatest effect on tissues which are dividing rapidly.

    a. Why does this make it suitable for the treatment of cancerous tumours?

    _____

    _____

    b. What other tissues in the body are likely to be especially susceptible to radiation damage?

    _____

    _____

4. Give two examples of the use of radioisotopes in diagnostic tests.

    _____

    _____

Additional Activities

For additional activities visit Activity 2B: Electricity on Evolve*.

Additional Resources

BYJUS: Physics

BYJUS presents a number of content areas for educational purposes, catering to a wide range of learners, from children at the start of their education to adults who are looking to upgrade their professional skills.

byjus.com/physics/

HyperPhysics

HyperPhysics is an exploration environment for concepts in physics which employs concept maps and other linking strategies to facilitate smooth navigation.

hyperphysics.phy-astr.gsu.edu/hbase/hframe.html

JavaLab: Physics

An online animation resource that allows users to interact with the interface and adjust the factors that affect simulations on a variety of physics topics.

javalab.org/en/category/electricity_en/
javalab.org/en/category/mechanics_en/
javalab.org/en/category/light_wave_en/
javalab.org/en/category/energy_en/

LabXchange

LabXchange is an online community for learning, sharing and collaboration in a variety of science-related topic areas and also provides simulations and digital content.

www.labxchange.org/library

PhET Interactive Simulations: Physics

The PhET Interactive Simulations project at the University of Colorado Boulder creates free interactive maths and science simulations based on research, exploration and discovery.

https://phet.colorado.edu/

Physclips

Physclips is a multi-level, multimedia resource provided by the School of Physics at the University of New South Wales and provides clips, animations and diagrams as part of educational modules on mechanics, waves and sound and light.

www.animations.physics.unsw.edu.au/

Science Notes: Physics Problems and Solutions

Science Notes is a repository of chemistry, physics and maths projects, and provides worked problems with answers in a number of content areas.

sciencenotes.org/physics-problems-solutions/

Sciencing: Physics

Sciencing provides educational and explanatory articles and projects on science and maths-related topics for all students.

sciencing.com/physics/

The Physics Classroom

The Physics Classroom is an online, free to use physics website developed primarily for beginning physics students and provides tutorials, videos and interactive materials.

https://www.physicsclassroom.com/

ThoughtCo: Physics

ThoughtCo is a reference site focussing on expert-created education content and provides a core section on science, tech and maths.

www.thoughtco.com/physics-4133571

CHAPTER 3
Basic Chemistry

Living things are composed entirely of chemicals. Thousands of chemical compounds are needed for normal body function and all living processes involve the constant movement of, formation of, and breaking down of these substances. Chemical reactions are at the heart of all physiological processes: digestion and metabolism, respiration, circulatory function, nerve impulses and even consciousness. It is impossible to understand anatomy and physiology without an understanding of chemical structure and function at all levels, from cellular components to organ systems. (Refer to Chapter 6: Cells and Metabolism for further information on cell structure, and Chapter 7: Tissues and Organs for further information on organs and organ systems.)

To properly understand the chemical basis of life, it is important to recognise and explore the structural hierarchy of organisation in living things. For this reason, it is fundamental to commence with the lowest level of biological organisation, that is, the ordering of atoms into molecules, the behaviour of some simple compounds, and the characteristics of solutions. (Refer to Chapter 4: Biological Chemistry for further information on biological molecules, and Chapter 21: The Urinary System and Electrolyte Balance for further information on electrolytes and electrolyte balance.)

LEARNING OUTCOMES

On completion of these activities the student should be able to:

1. describe the structure of atoms and explain the arrangement of elements in the Periodic Table

2. explain the formation of ions, ionic compounds and molecules, and deduce the chemical formulae of ionic and covalent compounds

3. recognise physical and chemical changes and explain their differences

4. write balanced chemical equations for simple chemical reactions

5. work with SI and non-SI units of concentration of substances in solution

6. describe the properties of the different types of aqueous mixtures: solutions, suspensions, emulsions and colloids

7. discuss the properties of electrolytes and distinguish between acids, bases and salts

LEARNING OUTCOMES—cont'd

8. explain the concept of pH and its role in measuring levels of acidity in the body

9. describe the nature and functions of buffers in stabilising pH in aqueous mixtures, including body fluids

10. conduct a series of experiments to illustrate the nature of acid–base balance.

KEY TERMS

Acid	Element	Orbital
Anion	Emulsion	Periodic Table
Aqueous solution	Formula mass	pH
Atom	Hydrogen bond	pH scale
Atomic mass	Indicator	Physical change
Atomic number	Ion	Polar
Avogadro's number	Ionic bond	Polarity
Base	Isotope	Polyatomic ion
Buffer	Matter	Product
Cation	Metal	Proton
Chemical change	Molar mass	Radioisotope
Chemical equation	Molarity	Reactant
Chemical formula	Mole	Salt
Chemical reaction	Molecular mass	Solute
Colloid	Molecule	Solution
Compound	Neutralisation	Solvent
Concentration	Neutron	Surfactant
Covalent bond	Non-electrolyte	Suspension
Electrolyte	Non-metal	Valency
Electron	Non-polar	
Electron configuration	Nucleus	

ACTIVITY 3.1: ATOMIC STRUCTURE AND THE PERIODIC TABLE

According to the atomic theory, all **matter** is composed of tiny particles called atoms which cannot be created or destroyed in a **chemical reaction**. Most of the mass of an atom is found in a dense central region called the **nucleus**, packed with **protons** and **neutrons** (Figs 3.1 and 3.2). When the number of protons and the number of neutrons in an atom's nucleus are added together, the **atomic mass** of the atom is determined. Atoms that have different numbers of neutrons but the same number of protons are called **isotopes**, and if these become unstable and decay to a stable form by emitting sub-atomic particles, they are referred to as **radioisotopes**, which are useful for scientific and clinical purposes. The space of an atom is almost empty, traversed only by charged particles called **electrons** (Fig. 3.3). Electrons are not scattered randomly about the nucleus but are arranged in **orbitals**, or levels, according to a strict pattern (Fig. 3.4). The **electron configuration** of an atom shows the number of electrons at each level around the nucleus of the atom.

This activity examines the structure and organisation of the atom and the properties of the periodic table.

Part 1: Atomic Structure

Helium

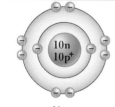

Neon

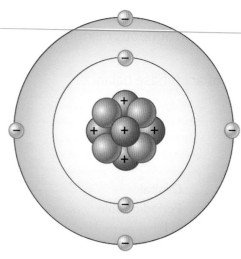

Figure 3.1 An atom of carbon.
(Source: Patton, K. T., Thibodeau, G. A., & Douglas, M. M. (2012). Essentials of anatomy & physiology. Elsevier.)

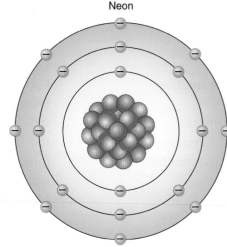

Argon

 18 protons   22 neutrons   18 electrons

Figure 3.3 Atoms of helium, neon and argon.
(Source: Patton, K. T., Thibodeau, G. A., & Douglas, M. M. (2012). Essentials of anatomy & physiology. Elsevier.)

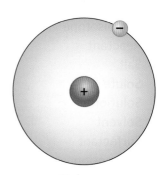

Hydrogen

Figure 3.2 An atom of hydrogen.
(Source: Patton, K. T., Thibodeau, G. A., & Douglas, M. M. (2012). Essentials of anatomy & physiology. Elsevier.)

1. Identify the charges and locations of the following sub-atomic particles:

   a. Proton

      i. Charge: _____

      ii. Location: _____

   b. Neutron

      i. Charge: _____

      ii. Location: _____

   c. Electron

      i. Charge: _____

      ii. Location: _____

2. Compare Fig. 3.1 with Fig. 3.2.

   a. What particles are present in a carbon atom but not in a hydrogen atom?

      _____

   b. Will this affect the electrical charge on the nucleus? Explain.

      _____

      _____

      _____

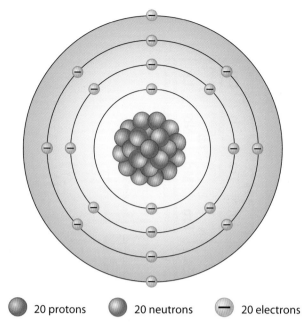

20 protons	20 neutrons	20 electrons

Figure 3.4 A calcium atom.

3. Use the atomic structures shown in Fig. 3.1, Fig. 3.3 and Fig. 3.4 to derive the electron configurations of the following elements:

a. Carbon _____

b. Helium _____

c. Neon _____

d. Argon_____

e. Calcium_____

4. Which of these elements would be expected to have similar chemical properties? Explain.

_____

_____

_____

Part 2: The Periodic Table

Elements are pure substances that cannot be broken down to simpler substances by ordinary means. There are 118 known elements, which are usually arranged into a **periodic table** in order of their **atomic number**, which is unique to each element (Fig. 3.5). In the periodic table, the vertical columns are called groups and are numbered I to VIII from left to right, and the horizontal rows are called periods.

Each element is represented by a shorthand symbol. The symbol for an element is often its first letter or the first two letters, or the first letter and some other letter from the element's name. In a few cases, the symbols are letters from the element's Latin or German name (e.g. Na for sodium or *natrium* in Latin, and Pb for lead or *plumbum* in Latin).

1. Identify the language of origin and full name of the following chemical symbols:

a. Hg

   i. Language origin: _____

   ii. Full name: _____

b. K

   i. Language origin: _____

   ii. Full name: _____

c. Fe

   i. Language origin: _____

   ii. Full name: _____

d. Cu

   i. Language origin: _____

   ii. Full name: _____

e. Au

   i. Language origin: _____

   ii. Full name: _____

f. Ag

   i. Language origin: _____

   ii. Full name: _____

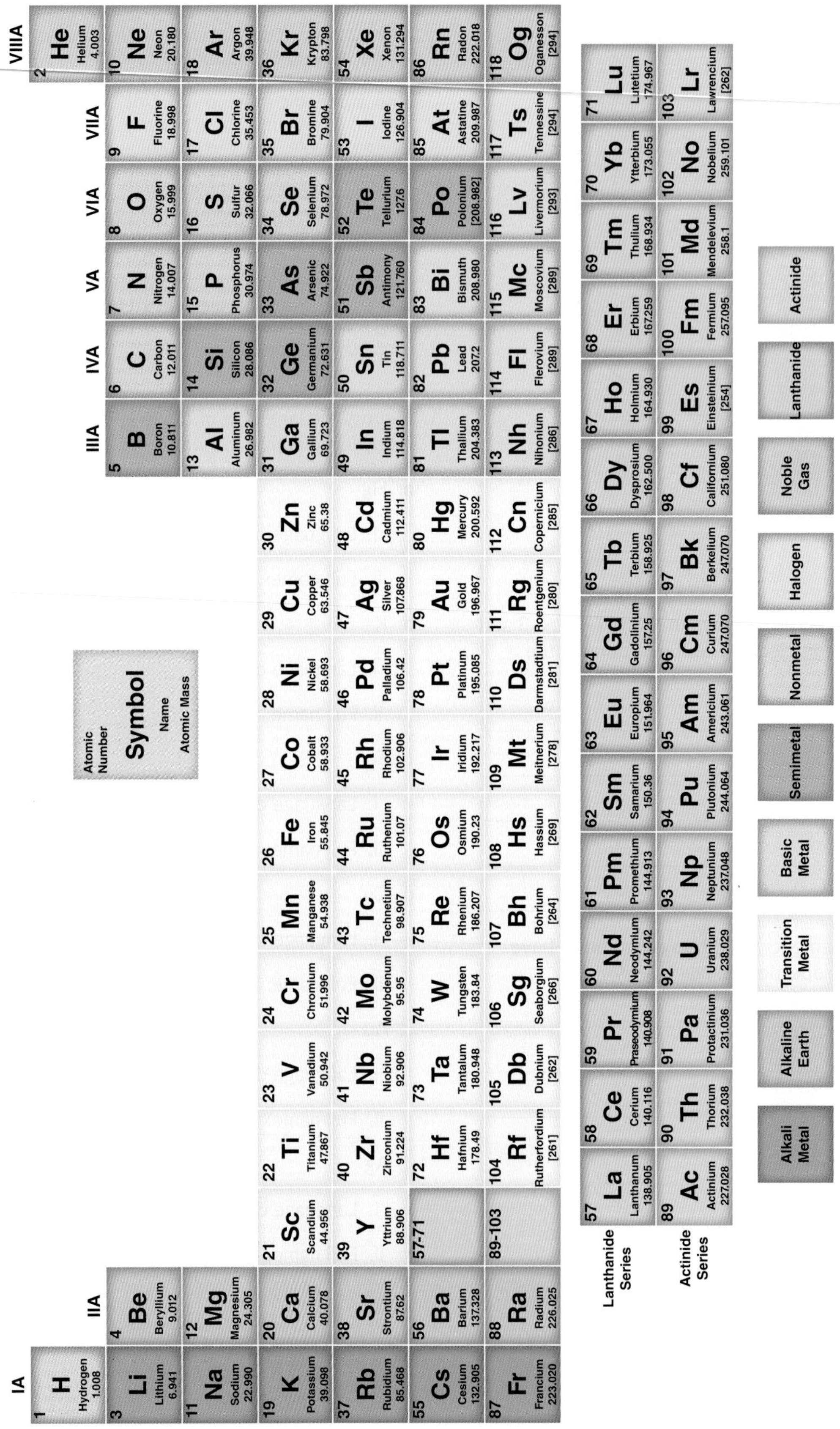

Figure 3.5 The periodic table of elements.
(Source: O'Malley, J. P., & Ziessman, H. A. (2020). Nuclear medicine and molecular imaging: the requisites. Elsevier.)

2. Refer to Fig. 3.5 to complete the table:

(Note: Number of protons = Number of electrons = Atomic number; Number of neutrons = Atomic mass – Atomic number).

Atom	Protons	Neutrons	Electrons
Oxygen			
	20		
		0	
			13
	80		
Iodine			

3. What important characteristics do the members of Group VIII have in common?

_____

_____

_____

4. Helium and neon have never been known to form compounds. Explain why.

_____

_____

_____

5. Explain why the atomic mass of each element in the periodic table is presented as a decimal number.

_____

_____

_____

6. Refer to Fig. 3.5 and complete the table for each isotope:

Isotope	Number of protons	Number of electrons	Number of neutrons
Barium – 132			
Hydrogen – 3			
Argon – 40			
Caesium – 135			
Oxygen – 13			

7. Refer to Fig. 3.5 to complete the table for each element:

Element	Atomic number	Electron configuration
Lithium		
Nitrogen		
Sodium		
Chlorine		
Argon		
Potassium		

8. Refer to Fig. 3.5 to complete the table for each electron configuration:

Electron configuration	Name of element	Metal or non-metal	Reactive or inert
2			
2.8.5			
2.7			
2.8.8.2			
2.8			

Part 3: Ions

Electron transfer from one **atom** to another causes electrical imbalance in those atoms because protons remain in the nucleus. **Metal** atoms are located to the left of the table and with few electrons in their outer orbital tend to lose electrons and develop a positive charge (electron donors), whereas **non-metal** atoms are located to the right of the table and with more electrons in their outer orbital tend to gain electrons and develop a negative charge (electron acceptors). In both cases, an **ion** is formed (Fig. 3.6). Ions are charged particles, the charge being caused by gain or loss of electrons to achieve electronic stability. The names of non-metal ions always end in -*ide*. Group VIII elements are electronically stable and do not form ions.

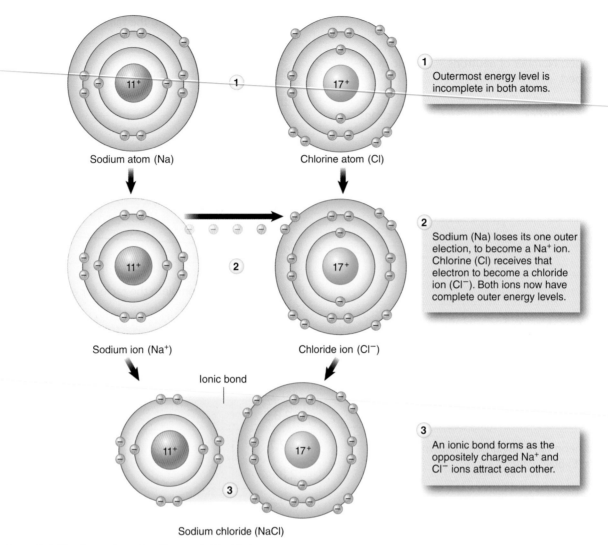

Figure 3.6 The formation of sodium and chloride ions.
(Source: Patton, K. T., Thibodeau, G. A., & Douglas, M. M. (2012). Essentials of anatomy & physiology. Elsevier.)

1. Refer to Fig. 3.5 to complete the table for each atom. (The first line has been provided as an example.)

Element	Symbol	Charge on ion	Formula of ion	Name of ion
Sodium	Na	+	Na⁺	Sodium
Magnesium				
Zinc				
Nitrogen				
Iron				
Chlorine				
Sulphur				
Oxygen				
Carbon				

2. Refer to Fig. 3.5 to complete the table for each atom. (The first line has been provided as an example.)

Atom	Formula of atom	Electron configuration of atom	Electron configuration of ion	Formula of ion	Number of electrons lost or gained
Magnesium	Mg	2.8.2	2.8	Mg^{2+}	2e lost
Potassium					
Oxygen					
Fluorine					
Phosphorus					
Lithium					
Aluminium					

3. In the process of ionisation seen in Fig. 3.6, identify the element that has the same electron configuration as a:

   a. Sodium ion _____

   b. Chloride ion_____

   c. Sulphide ion_____

   d. Nitride ion _____

4. In Fig. 3.6, compare the sizes of the sodium and chlorine atoms and the sizes of the sodium and chloride ions.

   a. Why has the size of the sodium changed but not the size of the chloride?

   _____

   _____

   _____

Apply the Concepts

1. Which sub-atomic particles are responsible for the chemical properties of elements?

   _____

2. Why do metals always form positive ions?

   _____

   _____

3. Why are elements arranged as they are in the periodic table?

   _____

   _____

4. Provide a general statement about the position in the periodic table of:

a. Metallic elements _____

_____

b. Non-metallic elements _____

_____

5. Although there are 118 known elements, just four elements make up more than 95% of the mass of the human body.

Identify these four elements.

_____

ACTIVITY 3.2: IONIC AND COVALENT BONDING AND COMPOUNDS

A **compound** is a substance consisting of two or more elements chemically bonded together in a way which is largely determined by the electron configurations of their atoms. There are two kinds of bonds in compounds. An **ionic bond** is the force of electrostatic attraction between a positive and a negative ion (Fig. 3.6). Ionic compounds are formed when electrons are transferred between metal and non-metal ions. A **covalent bond** occurs when electrons are shared between non-metal atoms; atoms of the same element may form covalent bonds (Fig. 3.7). A covalent bond may be single, double or triple, depending on how many pairs of electrons are shared. The number of electrons that can be lost, gained or shared by an element is that element's **valency**, or combining power. The valency of an element corresponds to its position in the periodic table.

This activity examines the formation of ionic and covalent bonds and their compounds.

Part 1: Ionic and Covalent Bonding

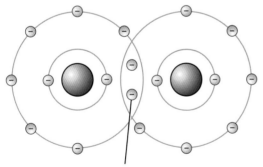

Shared electrons

Figure 3.7 Formation of a covalent bond.
(Source: Shen, C., Rawls, H. R., & Esquivel-Upshaw, J. F. (Eds.). (2022). Phillips' Science of Dental Materials. Elsevier.)

1. Consider the following questions, with reference to Fig. 3.6:

a. Which two atoms have come together to form an ionic bond?

_____

b. What name is given to the structure formed by ionic bonds such as this?

_____

c. What is the formula of this new compound?

_____

d. What evidence suggests that an ionic bond has been formed?

_____

_____

_____

2. Consider the following questions, with reference to Fig. 3.7:

   a. Which two atoms have come together to form a covalent bond?

   _____

   b. What name is given to the structure formed by this covalent bond?

   _____

   c. What is the formula of this new structure?

   _____

   d. What evidence suggests that a covalent bond has been formed?

   _____

   _____

   _____

3. Provide the chemical formulae for the following compounds and state whether each is ionic or covalent:

Compound name	Chemical formula	Ionic or covalent
Calcium chloride		
Beryllium oxide		

Compound name	Chemical formula	Ionic or covalent
Oxygen fluoride		
Carbon chloride		
Sodium bromide		
Aluminium sulphide		

4. Provide the names of the following compounds and state whether each is ionic or covalent:

Chemical formula	Compound name	Ionic or covalent
HCl		
PbO		
ZnF_2		
Ba_3N_2		
MgS		
$MnCl_2$		
FeO		
$HgCl_2$		

Apply the Concepts

1. What is a pure substance and how does it differ from a mixture?

   _____

   _____

2. What is a mixture?

   _____

   _____

3. Is a mixture easily separated? Explain.

   _____

   _____

4. How does the composition of a mixture differ from that of a compound?

   _____

   _____

5. Identify which of the following are mixtures and which are compounds:

a. Air _____

b. Carbon dioxide _____

c. Iron ore _____

d. Carbonated water_____

e. Iron oxide _____

f. Urine _____

g. Alcohol_____

ACTIVITY 3.3: POLYATOMIC IONS AND THEIR COMPOUNDS

Many compounds are formed by the combination of more than two elements. For example, washing powder contains sodium, carbon and oxygen, while chalk contains calcium, carbon and oxygen. It is possible to identify the number of each type of atom present in these compounds as chemists have identified groups of atoms that commonly occur together. In both washing powder and chalk there is the carbonate group, which consists of one carbon atom and three oxygen atoms and has the formula CO_3^{2-}. Such a group of atoms is electrically charged and is called a **polyatomic ion**. There are nine common polyatomic ions that are important to living organisms; eight of these are negatively charged while one is positively charged (Table 3.1).

This activity provides practice in deriving the formulae and names of compounds of polyatomic ions.

Table 3.1 Common polyatomic ions

Valency 1		Valency 2		Valency 3	
Hydroxide	OH^-	Carbonate	CO_3^{2-}	Phosphate	PO_4^{3-}
Nitrate	NO_3^-	Sulphate	SO_4^{2-}		
Bicarbonate (hydrogencarbonate)	HCO_3^-				
Acetate (ethanoate)	CH_3COO^-				
Cyanide	CN^-				
Ammonium	NH_4^+				

1. For each ion, provide the ion symbol and identify whether it is an anion or cation:

Ion	Ion symbol	Anion or cation
Bicarbonate		
Lithium		
Beryllium		
Sulphate		
Magnesium		
Sodium		
Barium		
Chloride		
Sulphide		
Fluoride		

2. Provide the formula for the following compounds, referring to Table 3.1 for assistance:

   a. Sodium carbonate _____

   b. Calcium sulphate _____

   c. Beryllium hydroxide _____

   d. Ammonium sulphate _____

3. Name the compounds with the following formulae, referring to Table 3.1 for assistance:

   a. KOH _____

   b. $Mg_3(PO_4)_2$ _____

   c. CH_3COONa _____

   d. $BaSO_4$ _____

   e. NH_4NO_3 _____

   f. $Al(OH)_3$ _____

   g. $MgSO_4$ _____

   h. $KHCO_3$ _____

   i. $AlPO_4$ _____

   j. $CuCO_3$ _____

4. Referring to Fig. 3.5 and Table 3.1 for valencies, derive the formula of each of the following compounds, and state whether it is ionic or covalent:

Compound	Formula	Ionic or covalent
Nitrogen hydride		
Magnesium sulphide		
Calcium fluoride		
Silicon oxide		
Phosphorus chloride		
Sodium sulphate		
Ammonium chloride		
Ammonium phosphate		
Potassium bicarbonate		
Aluminium hydroxide		

Apply the Concepts

In many clinical and laboratory work settings, material safety data sheets (MSDS) can be found.

1. What is a material safety data sheet (MSDS)?

   _____

   _____

2. Explain the importance of providing and displaying MSDS in these settings.

   _____

   _____

ACTIVITY 3.4: PHYSICAL AND CHEMICAL CHANGES

Whenever a change takes place in which a new substance is formed, a **chemical change** is said to have occurred. Chemical changes are not easily reversed as bonds have been broken to form new compounds. If a change does not result in the production of a new substance it is said to be a **physical change**. Physical changes are often easily reversed as the chemical identity of the original substances is unchanged.

This activity distinguishes between physical and chemical changes.

Part 1: Identifying Physical and Chemical Changes

1. Identify whether each of the following results in a physical or chemical change:

   a. Lighting a match_____

   b. Burning gas in a stove _____

   c. Digesting bread_____

   d. Dissolving salt in water _____

   e. Chopping wood _____

   f. Making H_2O from O_2 and H_2 _____

   g. Mixing sand and H_2O _____

   h. Dissolving an antacid tablet_____

   i. Cutting bread _____

   j. Growing from a child into an adult _____

Part 2: Observing Physical and Chemical Change

⚠️ To conduct these activities, it is important to ensure the following safety precautions:

- *Demonstrators should carry out these activities for demonstration purposes only in accordance with safety procedures.*

1. Observe the demonstration of the procedures described in the table provided.

2. Decide which are physical and which are chemical changes, recording your observations in the table.

Substance	Treatment	Observed result	Type of change
Sodium metal	Piece dropped onto water under safe conditions		
Zinc oxide	Heated in test tube, then cooled		
Fluorescein	Sprinkled onto water		
Sugar	Concentrated sulphuric acid added		
Potassium iodide	Added to mixture of hydrogen peroxide and detergent		

Part 3: The Effect of Time on Physical and Chemical Change

⚠️ To conduct these activities, it is important to ensure the following safety precautions:

- *Ensure disposable gloves are worn when handling chemicals to avoid skin irritation.*

- *Ensure safety glasses are worn at all times.*

- *Ensure all chemicals and compounds are disposed of as instructed.*

1. Collect six test tubes and number them 1 to 6.

2. Into each tube place a small amount of the substance indicated in the table below.

3. Carry out the procedures described in the table and note any changes that occur immediately and after 30 minutes.

4. Record your observations in the table.

5. If a change has occurred, decide whether it is physical or chemical.

Tube number	Substance	Instruction	Change (immediate)	Change (after 30 mins)	Type of change
1	Ice	Do nothing			
2	Lead nitrate solution	Add a piece of zinc			
3	Potassium permanganate	Gently run water down inside of tube			
4	Copper oxide	Gently run water down inside of tube			
5	Copper oxide	Add a little dilute sulphuric acid			
6	Calcium	Gently run water down inside of tube			

Apply the Concepts

1. Is a colour change always indicative of a chemical change? Explain.

   _____

   _____

2. Is a substance dissolving always indicative of a chemical change? Explain.

   _____

   _____

3. Is the generation of heat always indicative of a chemical change? Explain.

   _____

   _____

ACTIVITY 3.5: CHEMICAL REACTIONS

When one or more substances react or change to form a new substance, a chemical reaction has occurred. This can be represented in the form of a **chemical equation**:

Reactant(s) → Product(s)

The Law of Conservation of Mass states that matter cannot be created or destroyed in a chemical change, so the numbers and types of atoms on the left-hand side of the equation must always be the same as on the right-hand side. If they are not, the equation is unbalanced. To balance the equation, balancing coefficients must be used – large numbers placed to the left of the **chemical formula** which multiply all the atoms in that formula by that number. Once the atoms of the **reactants** and the **products** are made the same, the equation is balanced.

This activity demonstrates the reactions that are typical of classes of reactions encountered in chemistry.

⚠ To conduct these activities, it is important to ensure the following safety precautions:

- *Ensure disposable gloves are worn when handling calcium hydroxide and hydrochloric acid to avoid skin irritation and burns.*
- *Ensure safety glasses are worn at all times.*
- *When heating liquids in test tubes over Bunsen burners, ensure test tubes point away from individuals to avoid scalding.*
- *Ensure matches and tapers are handled and disposed of appropriately.*
- *Ensure all chemicals are disposed of as instructed.*

Part 1: Reaction Between Hydrogen and Oxygen

1. Observe the demonstration of the reaction between hydrogen and oxygen.

2. Complete the following for the reaction provided:

   Reactants: Hydrogen and oxygen
   Products: Water

   a. Word equation:

   _____

   b. Chemical equation (unbalanced):

   _____

   c. Chemical equation (balanced):

   _____

Part 2: Decomposition of Copper Carbonate

1. Place a spatula of copper carbonate into a large test tube and fit the test tube with a stopper and delivery tube.

2. Heat the test tube with a Bunsen burner and pass any gas evolved through a few mL of lime water (calcium hydroxide solution) in another test tube. Lime water turns milky in the presence of carbon dioxide.

3. Complete the following for the reaction provided:

   Reactant: Copper carbonate (copper has a valency of 2)
   Products: Copper oxide and carbon dioxide

   a. Word equation:

   _____

   b. Chemical equation (unbalanced):

   _____

   c. Chemical equation (balanced):

   _____

Part 3: Reaction Between Magnesium and Hydrochloric Acid

1. Place a 3 cm strip of magnesium in a test tube.

2. Take another test tube and fill it to a depth of 3 cm with dilute hydrochloric acid (HCl).

3. Tip the magnesium strip into the HCl and keep the empty tube inverted over the reaction tube to collect the gas evolved.

4. Test the gas evolved by placing a lighted taper in the inverted test tube.

5. Complete the following for the reaction provided:

   Reactants: Magnesium and hydrochloric acid
   Products: Magnesium chloride and hydrogen

   a. Word equation:

   _____

   b. Chemical equation (unbalanced):

   _____

   c. Chemical equation (balanced):

   _____

Part 4: Word Equations

1. Provide word equations for the following reactions:

   a. $Mg(OH)_2 + 2HCl \rightarrow MgCl_2 + 2H_2O$

   _____

   b. $CaSO_4 + CuCl_2 \rightarrow CuSO_4 + CaCl_2$

   _____

   c. $Hg(OH)_2 + 2H_3PO_4 \rightarrow Hg_3(PO_4)_2 + 6H_2O$

   _____

   d. $3CaCl_2 + 2Na_3PO_4 \rightarrow Ca_3(PO_4)_2 + 6NaCl$

   _____

   e. $2AgI + Na_2S \rightarrow Ag_2S + 2NaI$

   _____

Part 5: Balancing Equations

1. Balance the following chemical equations:

   a. $K + Cl_2 \rightarrow KCl$

   b. $H_2 + O_2 \rightarrow H_2O$

   c. $Mg + HCl \rightarrow MgCl_2 + H_2$

   d. $Fe + O_2 \rightarrow Fe_2O_3$

e. $Zn + H_2SO_4 \rightarrow ZnSO_4 + H_2$

f. $CuCO_3 \rightarrow CuO + CO_2$

g. $Al + Br_2 \rightarrow AlBr_3$

h. $P_4 + O_2 \rightarrow P_2O_5$

i. $C_3H_6 + O_2 \rightarrow CO_2 + H_2O$

j. $Sb_2S_3 + HCl \rightarrow SbCl_3 + H_2S$

2. For each of the chemical equations in question 1, name at least one compound in the reaction.

_____

_____

_____

_____

Part 6: Completing and Balancing Equations

1. Complete the following reactions and balance the final equation:

   a. $CuSO_4 + NaOH \rightarrow$ _____

   b. $SnO_2 + H_2 \rightarrow$ _____

   c. $Na + O_2 \rightarrow$ _____

   d. $Fe + O_2 \rightarrow$ _____

   e. $H_2O_2 \rightarrow$ _____

   f. $MgSO_4 + HCl \rightarrow$ _____

Apply the Concepts

1. Ferrous sulphate is sometimes prescribed for anaemia.

   a. Which metallic element does this compound contain?

   _____

   b. Assuming the metal has a valency of 2, what is the formula of ferrous sulphate?

   _____

2. Chemical reactions can be classified as synthesis reactions, decomposition reactions or exchange reactions. Classify the following reactions based on those terms:

   a. $2Fe_2O_3 \rightarrow 4Fe + 3O_2$

   _____

   b. $HCl + NaOH \rightarrow NaCl + H_2O$

   _____

   c. $4CO_2 + 4H_2O \rightarrow C_4H_8 + 6O_2$

   _____

ACTIVITY 3.6: CALCULATING FORMULA MASS

As atoms have atomic mass, so all chemical substances have a relative **formula mass** (Mr). The formula mass is obtained by adding the atomic masses of all atoms present in the formula of the substance. When dealing with molecular substances such as oxygen and water, the term **molecular mass** is often used instead of formula mass.

This activity addresses naming chemical compounds, deriving their formulae, and calculating their formula mass.

1. Complete the following table:

Formula name	Chemical formula	Formula mass (Mr)	Formula name	Chemical formula	Formula mass (Mr)
Potassium chloride				OF_2	
Calcium sulphate			Ammonium sulphate		
	NaCN			$Pb(CH_3COO)_2$	
	NH_4NO_3			CaC_2	
Sodium carbonate			Barium nitride		
Sulphur dioxide			Magnesium bicarbonate		

2. Define the following terms:

   a. Formula mass _____

   _____

   b. Molecular mass _____

   _____

   c. Molar mass_____

   _____

3. How are these terms the same, and how are they different?

   _____

   _____

   _____

Apply the Concepts

1. Explain how formula mass, for example of acetaminophen ($C_8H_9NO_2$), relates to the action of a medication.

   _____

   _____

   _____

ACTIVITY 3.7: MOLES AND MOLARITY

A **mole** of a substance is the quantity which is the formula mass of the substance expressed in grams. This mass is called the **molar mass** of the substance. The molar mass is the mass of one mole (6.02×10^{23} particles) of a substance. Moles of different substances will have different masses but they all contain the same number of particles. It is now known that there are 6.02×10^{23} particles per mole, a number called **Avogadro's number**. Since the mole is an SI unit, it has the shorthand designation mol and the usual prefixes apply. For example, 1 millimole (mmol) = 1×10^{-3} mol.

This activity demonstrates working with moles, molarity and related quantities.

Part 1: Moles and Molar Mass

1. Examine and compare the molar masses of carbon, sulphur, copper, zinc, iron, aluminium, sodium chloride, water and calcium chloride, which have been provided.

   a. Is there a relationship between the molar masses and the volumes of the substances provided? Explain.

   _____

   _____

   _____

   b. Is there a relationship between the number of moles and the volumes of the substances provided? Explain.

   _____

   _____

   _____

2. Identify how many moles (mol) are present in each of the following:

   a. 54 g of water _____

   b. 9 g of water_____

   c. 3.55 g of NaCl _____

   d. 161 g of ethanol (C_2H_5OH)_____

   e. 1.8 g of glucose ($C_6H_{12}O_6$) _____

3. Calculate the mass of the following:

   a. 0.5 mol of carbon dioxide _____

   b. 2.5 mol of potassium carbonate _____

   c. 0.1 mol of calcium hydroxide _____

   d. 0.01 mol of silver nitrate ($AgNO_3$)_____

   e. 20 mol of oxygen gas _____

4. Identify how many particles are present in the following:

   a. 1 mole of copper _____

   b. 3 moles of sodium _____

   c. 0.2 moles of carbon _____

   d. 7 moles of O_2 _____

   e. 16 moles of NH_3 _____

   f. 0.5 moles of H_2S _____

b. How many moles of Na_2CO_3 are in 10.0 mL of a 2.0 M solution?

   _____

   _____

c. What volume (mL) of 12.0 M HCl is needed to obtain 3.00 mol of HCl?

   _____

   _____

Part 2: Moles and Molarity

The **concentration** of a substance dissolved in water can be expressed most conveniently in terms of the number of moles of that substance dissolved per litre of **solution**. When 1 mole of a substance is present in 1 litre of solution, it is said to be a 1 molar (1.00 M) solution. It is also said to have a **molarity** of 1.00. For example, a sodium chloride (saline) solution containing 58.5 g of NaCl per litre of solution is a 1.00 M NaCl solution. Molarity can be calculated in the following way:

$$\text{Molarity (mol/L)} = \frac{\text{Number of moles (mol)}}{\text{Volume in litres (L)}}$$

1. Make up a 1.0 L of a 1.0 mol.L^{-1} solution of sodium chloride using the volumetric equipment supplied.

   a. What mass of NaCl was used? _____

   b. If half the quantity of NaCl had been used, what would be the molarity of the resulting solution?

   _____

   c. Explain how a 1 molar solution of sodium chloride could be made in just 500 mL of solution.

   _____

   _____

   d. Explain how the 1 mol.L^{-1} NaCl solution could be used to prepare a 0.1 mol.L^{-1} solution.

   _____

   _____

2. Consider the following questions:

   a. How many moles of Na_2CO_3 are in 10.0 L of a 2.0 M solution?

   _____

   _____

Part 3: Solution Concentration

In most clinical settings, concentrations are expressed in SI units. However, in some situations, non-SI units may be used, such as the concentration of a solution based on the weight (w) of **solute** per volume (v) of solution. This gives rise to the following units:

% (w/w) = g/100 g

% (w/v) = g/100 mL

% (v/v) = mL/100 mL

1. Explain what is meant by a 10% (w/v) NaCl solution.

   _____

   _____

2. Describe how 50 mL of a 10% (w/v) NaCl solution could be made.

   _____

   _____

3. Physiological saline has a concentration of 0.9% (w/v) NaCl and is safe to inject when prepared under sterile conditions.

   a. Make up 100 mL of physiological saline and explain how this was achieved.

   _____

   _____

4. A sore throat spray contains 0.35 g phenol dissolved in 25 mL of solution.

   a. What is the weight/volume concentration of phenol?

   _____

   _____

b. What is the percent weight/volume concentration of phenol?

_____

_____

5. A 750 mL bottle of wine contains 101 mL ethanol.

a. What is the volume/volume concentration of ethanol?

_____

_____

b. What is the percent volume/volume concentration of ethanol?

_____

_____

6. Some medicated items, such as toothpaste, state the active ingredient in parts per million (ppm). Explain what this means.

a. _____

_____

_____

b. Does parts per million (ppm) bear a relationship to % (w/v) concentration or to molarity? Explain.

_____

_____

_____

Apply the Concepts

1. Glucose is oxidised in the body's cells to produce carbon dioxide, water and energy. The balanced equation for this is as follows:

$$C_6H_{12}O_6 + 6O_2 \rightarrow 6CO_2 + 6H_2O$$
(Glucose)

a. How many moles of oxygen are required to completely break down 1 mole of glucose?

_____

b. How many moles of carbon dioxide would be produced by the complete oxidation of 0.1 mole of glucose?

_____

c. What is the mass (g) of 1 mole of glucose?

_____

d. What mass (g) of oxygen is required to completely oxidise 1 mole of glucose?

_____

2. In clinical reports, the concentrations of many substances in body fluids are given in mmol/L. For example, it is considered desirable for blood triglyceride (fat) levels to be below 1.7 mmol/L and for cholesterol to be below 5 mmol/L.

a. Explain what 5 mmol/L means.

_____

_____

b. A mole of cholesterol weighs 386.7 grams. How much does 5 mmol of cholesterol weigh?

_____

_____

Additional Activities

For additional activities visit Activity 3A: Electrolysis of Water on Evolve˙.

For additional activities visit Activity 3B: Solubility on Evolve˙.

ACTIVITY 3.8: EMULSIONS AND COLLOIDS

An emulsion is said to be temporary if the component liquids separate into layers on standing for a short time. This occurs because the dispersed droplets gradually merge together, or coalesce, and eventually form a separate layer. A permanent or stable emulsion does not separate so readily. This type of emulsion is composed of colloidal-sized droplets of one liquid dispersed in another. The droplets are prevented from coalescing, usually by the use of an emulsifying agent (also called a **surfactant**). These act by coating the surface of the dispersed droplets with a film that attracts the molecules of the suspending liquid and so prevent the droplets from contacting one another.

Colloids are mixtures of particles bigger than those in a solution, but smaller than those in a suspension, dispersed in another substance. Colloidal particles are too small to be separated by filtration as they pass through the holes in the filter paper. However, they are large enough to scatter light passing through the mixture. This explains why colloids are usually cloudy or opaque in contrast to transparent solutions. The white colour of milk is due to this property. If a beam of light is shone through most colloidal mixtures, the path of the beam can be seen like a ray of sunshine in a dusty room. This is called the Tyndall Effect.

This activity demonstrates the composition and properties of emulsions and colloids.

Part 1: Emulsions and Emulsification

Mayonnaise is a common permanent emulsion in which oil droplets are dispersed in vinegar and stabilised by the emulsifying action of egg yolk. Other common emulsions are hand lotions and other cosmetic creams. Soaps and detergents exert their cleaning effect on oily or greasy objects by acting as emulsifiers, forming a stable oil-in-water emulsion. This can be easily rinsed away from the original dirty object. Fatty food substances are emulsified by bile salts in the digestive tract in order to aid the process of digestion.

1. Label two test tubes A and B.

2. Half-fill both test tubes with water, then add 5 mL cooking oil to each.

3. Add 1 mL detergent to tube B.

4. Stopper both tubes and shake vigorously then leave to stand for 5 minutes.

5. Describe the changes observed in both tubes.

   a. Tube A (oil + water)

   _____

   _____

   b. Tube B (oil + water + detergent)

   _____

   _____

   c. Explain the effect of the detergent in tube B.

   _____

   _____

   _____

Part 2: Colloids

Toothpaste, smoke, gelatine desserts, butter and blood plasma are examples of colloids. Colloidal particles are also too large to pass through the fine pores of cell membranes or those in dialysis tubing. Dialysis tubing is used in artificial kidney machines to remove wastes from the blood without depleting the body of vital colloidal substances, such as plasma proteins.

1. Obtain two short lengths (about 20 cm) of dialysis tubing and soak them in water.

2. Tie off one end of each tube with a knot and rub the other end between your fingers to open it.

3. Dispense 5 mL of copper sulphate solution into one tube and 5 mL of skimmed milk into the second tube.

4. Tie off the open end of each tube to keep the liquid inside.

5. Rinse both bags with water and place them in separate 250 mL beakers of clean water for 30 minutes.

   a. How do the pores in dialysis tubing compare to those in filter paper?

   _____

   _____

   _____

   b. What evidence suggests that some substances are smaller than the pores in dialysis tubing?

   _____

   _____

   c. What are these substances?

   _____

d. What evidence suggests that some substances are larger than the pores in dialysis tubing?

_____

_____

e. What are these substances?

_____

6. Blood can be described as a complex aqueous mixture containing particles in solution, suspension and colloidal form.

a. Based on the composition of blood, list some of these substances in the table provided.

Constituents of blood		
In solution	*In suspension*	*In colloidal form*

7. Determine whether the following are suspensions, emulsions or colloids:

a. Mayonnaise _____

b. Salad dressing _____

c. Blood _____

d. Sand and water _____

e. Muddy water _____

f. Milk _____

g. Smoke _____

h. Face cream _____

Apply the Concepts

1. A dishwashing detergent is claimed by its manufacturers to 'dissolve grease and dirt in seconds'.

a. Explain why this claim cannot be true.

_____

_____

2. Colloidal silver is a popular dietary supplement favoured by practitioners of alternative medicine, but it has doubtful health benefits and can cause serious side effects. It is a mixture of solid silver particles and a liquid.

a. Is colloidal sliver likely to be a true colloid? Explain.

_____

_____

b. What type of mixture is it most likely to be?

_____

3. The shape of most of the body's cells is important to their function and the colloidal effect of proteins found within cells can help them maintain their shape. Explain this relationship.

_____

_____

ACTIVITY 3.9: ACIDS, BASES AND SALTS

Acids may be defined as compounds that yield hydrogen ions (H^+) in **aqueous solution**. Since a hydrogen ion is a proton, acids are also called proton donors. It is the hydrogen ions that are responsible for the properties of acids. **Bases** may be defined as compounds that accept H^+ in aqueous solution (proton acceptors). Many yield hydroxide (OH^-) ions in an aqueous solution. A **salt** may be defined as a compound formed by a metal and an acid radical, and which usually does not yield or accept H^+ or OH^- in aqueous solution. The **pH** of a solution is measured using the **pH scale**, which is based on hydrogen ion concentration on a range of 0 to 14 (Fig. 3.8).

This activity examines the chemical composition and characteristics of acids, bases and salts.

Part 1: Acids and Bases

1. The pH is often referred to as the negative logarithm of hydrogen ion concentration. Explain this statement.

_____

_____

_____

2. What do the square brackets around $[H^+]$ indicate?

_____

3. Identify whether each of the following is acidic, basic, or neutral, with reference to Fig. 3.8.

a. $[H^+] = 10^{-4}$ _____

b. $[OH^-] = 10^{-5}$ _____

c. $[OH^-] = 10^{-1}$ _____

d. $[H^+] = 10^{-11}$ _____

e. $[H^+] = 10^{-7}$ _____

f. $[OH^-] = 10^{-12}$ _____

g. $[OH^-] = 10^{-7}$ _____

h. $[H^+] = 10^{-13}$ _____

4. What is the magnitude of change in the $[H^+]$ for an increase of 1 pH unit?

_____

5. What is the magnitude of change in the $[H^+]$ for a decrease in 1 pH unit?

_____

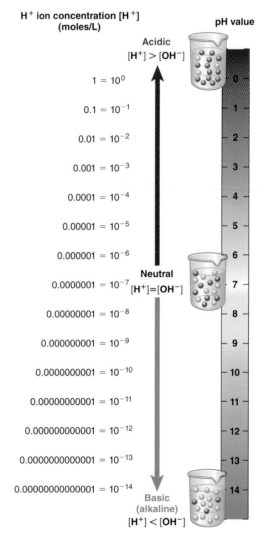

Figure 3.8 The pH scale.
(Source: Patton, K. T., Bell, F. B., Matusiak, D. J., & Wood, S. R. (2016). *Anatomy & Physiology Laboratory Manual*. Elsevier.)

6. If the pH of a solution changes from pH 7 to pH 6, identify what would happen to the:

   a. $[H^+]$ _____

   b. $[OH^-]$ _____

7. Identify each of the following compounds and categorise it as an acid, base or salt:

Compound	Compound name	Acid, base, salt
NaCl		
$Ca(OH)_2$		
KNO_3		
HNO_3		
$KHCO_3$		
H_2SO_4		
$MgSO_4$		
CH_3COOH		
CH_3COONa		
HCl		
$Mg(OH)_2$		
NH_4OH		

8. Complete the following equations involving acids:

   Example: HCl $\rightarrow$ H^+ + Cl^-
   Hydrochloric acid

   a. H_2SO_4 $\rightarrow$ $2H^+$ + ____
   Sulphuric acid

   b. HNO_3 $\rightarrow$ ____ + ____
   Nitric acid

   c. HCN $\rightarrow$ ____ + ____
   Cyanic acid

   d. H_2CO_3 $\rightarrow$ ____ + ____
   Carbonic acid

9. Complete the following equations involving bases:

   Example: NaOH $\rightarrow$ Na^+ + OH^-
   Sodium hydroxide

   a. KOH $\rightarrow$ ____ + ____
   Potassium hydroxide

   b. NH_4OH $\rightarrow$ ____ + ____
   Ammonium hydroxide

   c. $Ca(OH)_2$ $\rightarrow$ ____ + ____
   Calcium hydroxide

   d. $Al(OH)_3$ $\rightarrow$ ____ + ____
   Aluminium hydroxide

10. Explain what is meant by the following terms:

    a. Strong acid _____

    _____

    b. Weak acid _____

    _____

    c. Concentrated acid _____

    _____

    d. Dilute acid _____

    _____

11. Using a combination of the terms strong, weak, concentrated, and dilute, describe the following solutions.

    Example: 0.1 M HCl   This is a dilute solution of a strong acid

    a. 5.0 M H_2SO_4

    _____

    b. 0.1 M NaOH

    _____

    c. 5.0 M H_2CO_3

    _____

    d. 0.1 M HNO_3

    _____

12. Determine whether the following are characteristics of acids or bases based on the description provided:

    a. Has a sour taste_____

    b. Conducts an electrical current _____

    c. Has a slippery feel _____

    d. Produces H^+ in water _____

    e. Is named barium hydroxide _____

    f. Neutralises H^+ _____

    g. Is an electrolyte_____

    h. Is named hydrogen sulphate_____

Part 2: Neutralisation Reactions

The reaction of an acid with a base is called **neutralisation**. Acids react with bases to form a salt and water only.

1. Complete and balance the following neutralisation equations:

Example:	$2HCl$	$+$	$Ca(OH)_2$	$\rightarrow$	$CaCl_2$	$+$	$2H_2O$
a.	HNO_3	$+$	KOH	$\rightarrow$	_____	$+$	_____
b.	H_2SO_4	$+$	$Ba(OH)_2$	$\rightarrow$	_____	$+$	_____
c.	HCN	$+$	$Mg(OH)_2$	$\rightarrow$	_____	$+$	_____
d.	H_3PO_4	$+$	$LiOH$	$\rightarrow$	_____	$+$	_____

Part 3: Neutralisation Reaction – Taste Test

⚠️ To conduct these activities, it is important to ensure the following safety precautions:

- *Ensure that only solutions labelled for tasting are sampled.*

- *Ensure all chemicals and compounds are disposed of as instructed.*

1. Dispense exactly 5 mL of 0.1 M HCl and 5 mL of 0.1 M NaOH into a disposable cup.

2. Mix thoroughly and taste the resulting solution.

   a. What taste does it have?

   _____

   b. Write a balanced chemical equation for this neutralisation reaction:

   HCl + NaOH → _____ + _____

Part 4: Acid–Base Indicators

Substances that change colour in the presence of acids are called **indicators**. One of the most common indicators for acid is litmus. Blue litmus turns red in the presence of an acid (i.e. in the presence of hydrogen ions). Another common indicator, phenolphthalein, turns from pink to colourless in the presence of an acid.

1. Using a white tile, place a drop of 0.1 M HCl onto pieces of red and blue litmus paper.

2. Repeat using 0.1 M NaOH.

3. Note and record any colour changes.

	Acid	Base
a. Effect on red litmus	_____	_____
b. Effect on blue litmus	_____	_____

4. Place a few drops of 0.1 M HCl into each of three dimples on a dimple tile.

5. Add a drop of methyl orange to the first dimple, bromothymol blue to the second dimple, and phenolphthalein to the third dimple.

6. On a clean dimple tile, repeat using 0.1 M NaOH instead of HCl.

7. Note and record your observations in the table provided.

Indicator	Colour in acid	Colour in alkali
Methyl orange		
Bromothymol blue		
Phenolphthalein		

Apply the Concepts

1. The following salts are commonly used in clinical practice. Provide an example of the use of each:

   a. Sodium chloride _____

   _____

   b. Calcium chloride _____

   _____

   c. Barium sulphate _____

   _____

   d. Magnesium sulphate _____

   _____

2. Explain why antacids containing $Mg(OH)_2$ and $Al(OH)_3$ are used to relieve indigestion and heartburn caused by stomach hyperacidity.

   _____

   _____

   _____

Additional Activities

For additional activities visit Activity 3C: Measuring pH on Evolve˚.

For additional activities visit Activity 3D: A Buffer System in Action on Evolve˚.

For additional activities visit Activity 3E: Electrolytes on Evolve˚.

Additional Resources

ChemCollective
ChemCollective is a collection of virtual labs, scenario-based learning activities, tutorials and concept tests with each module including worked examples and scaffolded practice problems.

chemcollective.org/home

goREACT: Virtual Chemical Reactions
goREACT allows users to experiment virtually with chemistry by means of an interactive drag-and-drop periodic table.

www.msichicago.org/science-at-home/games/goreact/

JavaLab: Chemistry
An online animation resource that allows users to interact with the interface and adjust the factors that affect the simulation, on a variety of chemistry topics.

javalab.org/en/category/chemistry_en/

LabXchange
LabXchange is an online community for learning, sharing and collaboration in a variety of science-related topic areas, and also provides simulations and digital content.

www.labxchange.org/library

Merlot: Chemistry Community Portal
The Merlot Chemistry Portal provides access to teaching and learning chemistry resources which also allow users to submit and create materials for community use.

www.merlot.org/merlot/Chemistry.htm

Molecular Workbench
Molecular Workbench is a modelling tool for designing and conducting computational experiments in science and delivers an interactive learning environment that supports science inquiry.

mw.concord.org/modeler/

KEY TERMS

Activation energy (Ea)

Amino acid

Carbohydrate

Catalyst

Cistron

Codon

Concentration gradient

Dehydration synthesis

Denaturation

Diffusion

DNA

DNA replication

Double helix

Emulsion

Enzyme

Fatty acid

Gene

Glycerol

Glycogen

Hexose

Hydrogen bond

Hydrolysis

Kinetic energy

Kinetic theory

Lipid

Messenger RNA

Monomer

Monosaccharide

Nitrogenous base

Non-polar

Nucleic acid

Nucleotide

Osmosis

Pentose

Peptide

Polar

Polymer

Polysaccharide

Protein

Ribosome

RNA

Saturated

Semipermeable

Soluble

Surfactant

Transcription

Transfer RNA

Translation

Triglyceride

Unsaturated

ACTIVITY 4.1: BROWNIAN MOTION

The **kinetic theory** of matter states that the particles that make up solids, liquids and gases are in constant motion. It also states that the speed at which these particles move is lowest in solids, greater in liquids and greatest in gases. The particles of a gas move faster than those of liquids and solids because they have more **kinetic energy**. The fact that the particles comprising solids, liquids and gases are in constant motion can be demonstrated by a series of simple experiments.

Robert Brown first observed the continuous movement of liquid molecules while viewing pollen grains through a microscope. He noticed that the pollen grains appeared to be rolling and turning all the time and he concluded correctly that they were being continuously bumped by smaller particles, the water molecules in which the pollen grains were suspended. The easiest way to see this Brownian motion is not with pollen grains but with a very small amount of carmine dye suspended in a drop of water.

Carmine dye consists of a suspension of tiny red solid particles in water. The particles are invisible to the naked eye, but can be easily seen under the light microscope. The smallest particles are so small that they are visibly bumped about by molecules of water that collide with them.

This activity demonstrates Brownian motion.

1. View a suspension of carmine dye on a preset microscope, being careful to make adjustments only to the fine focus.

2. Look very carefully at the smallest particles you can see (they are only just visible). They will be jerking about in a random fashion.

   a. Is the movement of the carmine particles observed due to the kinetic energies of the carmine particles?

   _____

   b. If not, explain why the carmine particles are in motion.

   _____

   _____

ACTIVITY 4.2: DIFFUSION IN A LIQUID

Kinetic theory predicts that particles that are free to move, such as those in liquids and gases, will eventually occupy the entire volume or shape of a space available to them in the absence of any mixing force. This activity tests this prediction by allowing crystals of lead nitrate and potassium iodide to dissolve in water on opposite sides of a petri dish. The movement of the dissolved ions in water can be detected by observing the reaction that occurs between them (Fig. 4.1). These two **soluble** salts are ideal for demonstrating **diffusion** because they react to produce a yellow insoluble solid, lead iodide.

This activity investigates the diffusion of two soluble solids in a liquid.

 To conduct this activity, it is important to ensure the following safety precaution:

- *Ensure disposable gloves are worn when handling lead nitrate as it is a toxic compound.*

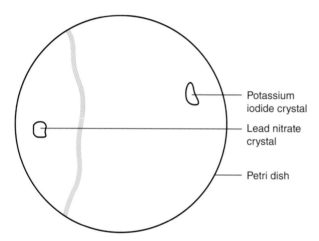

Figure 4.1 Diffusion of ions in a liquid.
(Source: Reproduced by permission of Royal Society of Chemistry, edu.rsc. org/experiments/diffusion-in-liquids/685.article)

1. Place a petri dish on a white tile or piece of paper.

2. Fill it nearly to the top with distilled water and place it where it will not be disturbed.

3. Wearing safety glasses and using a pair of forceps, place a few crystals of potassium iodide (KI) in the water at one side of the petri dish and a few crystals of lead nitrate [$Pb(NO_3)_2$] at the other.

4. Place the lid on the petri dish and mark it with the letters 'K' and 'Pb' to show the locations of the crystals.

5. Note the time and observe the salts dissolving.

6. Check the dish every 10 minutes and note any changes seen in the water over a period of 1 hour.

7. Dispose of the fluid in the container provided.

   a. What was observed?

   _____

   _____

   b. The dish was sealed and protected from movement and disturbance. Suggest a reason for the changes you observed.

   _____

   _____

   _____

   c. A yellow precipitate may have formed closer to the lead nitrate than to the potassium iodide. Explain this observation in terms of the kinetic theory.

   _____

   _____

   _____

   d. What difference would have been observed if hot water had been used?

   _____

   e. How would kinetic theory explain this difference?

   _____

   _____

   _____

Apply the Concepts

1. a. Using your knowledge of Kinetic Theory, explain how effervescent tablets are able to form a solution.

    _____

    _____

    _____

    b. Which gas is liberated as a result?

    _____

ACTIVITY 4.3: OSMOSIS – A SPECIAL KIND OF DIFFUSION

Cell membranes allow most ions in solution and small molecules like oxygen to freely enter and leave cells by simple diffusion. These substances move along their **concentration gradient**, from regions of their high concentration to low concentration. However, these membranes are said to be selectively permeable or **semipermeable**, because larger molecules such as glucose and **proteins** cannot cross the membrane. These larger molecules will have an effect on the diffusion of smaller particles. The membrane is permeable to the smaller particles. This is referred to as **osmosis** and the effect produced is an osmotic effect (Fig. 4.2).

This activity investigates the effect of a semipermeable membrane on water movement.

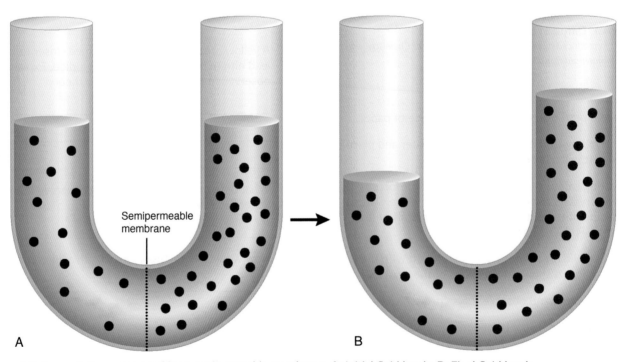

Figure 4.2 Two solutions separated by a semipermeable membrane. **A:** Initial fluid levels. **B:** Final fluid levels.
(Source: Mulroney, S. E., & Myers, A. K. (2016). Netter's Essential Physiology. Elsevier.)

1. Consider the following questions, based on Fig. 4.2:

   a. Describe the composition and concentration of the solutions in the compartments.

   _____

   _____

   _____

   b. The membrane is permeable to which substance?

   _____

   c. The membrane is impermeable to which substance?

   _____

   d. What is occurring at time zero (Fig. 4.2A)?

   _____

   _____

   e. What has occurred after an hour (Fig. 4.2B)?

   _____

   _____

2. Place an arrow on the diagram on Fig. 4.2A to show the nett movement of water that will initially take place across the membrane.

   a. What process will cause water to move across the membrane?

   _____

3. As water moves, explain what happens to the concentration of solute on:

   a. The left side of the tube

   _____

   b. The right side of the tube

   _____

4. What causes the fluid levels to change?

   _____

5. What causes the fluid levels to eventually stabilise?

   _____

6. Place arrows on Fig. 4.2B to show the nett movement of water across the membrane when the levels are stable.

   a. Are the fluid pressures on each side of the membrane equal in Fig. 4.2B?

   _____

   b. What name is given to the process that produced this result?

   _____

   c. Does this process require energy input?

   _____

   d. What is the significance of this process to cells?

   _____

7. Consider the following questions:

   a. Define the term osmotic pressure.

   _____

   _____

   _____

   b. Define the term hydrostatic pressure.

   _____

   _____

   c. Explain how osmosis relates to the tonicity of the cellular environment.

   _____

   _____

   _____

Apply the Concepts

1. Carefully describe the difference between simple diffusion and osmosis.

   _____

   _____

   _____

2. Apart from ventilating the lungs, the body expends no energy in the exchange of carbon dioxide and oxygen in the respiratory exchange surfaces.

   a. What process must be involved in the exchange of these gases?

   _____

3. What is osmolarity and how is it measured?

   _____

   _____

   _____

4. What is osmolality and how is it measured?

   _____

   _____

   _____

5. Why is the osmotic concentration of body fluids often expressed as mOsmol/L and not Osmol/L?

   _____

   _____

6. Pseudoephedrine is often administered in tablet form referred to as an osmotic-controlled release oral delivery system.

   a. Explain how the outer coating of these tablets operates, based on the principles of osmosis.

   _____

   _____

ACTIVITY 4.4: BIOLOGICALLY IMPORTANT MOLECULES

It is important to become familiar with the structural, functional and chemical differences between **carbohydrates**, **lipids**, proteins and **nucleic acids** (Fig. 4.3), as well as the processes by which they are constructed through **dehydration synthesis,** or condensation, and deconstructed through the process of **hydrolysis**. The basic building blocks of biological molecules are **monomers**, which are bonded to form **polymers**, increasing the structural complexity of the molecule.

This activity investigates the structural and functional differences of biologically important molecules.

1. Decide whether the following properties are more typical of organic or inorganic compounds:

    a. Insoluble in water

    _____

    b. High melting point

    _____

    c. Burns in air

    _____

2. Carefully define the following terms:

    a. Dehydration synthesis _____

    _____

    b. Hydrolysis_____

    _____

    c. Saturated fatty acid _____

    _____

    d. Monosaccharide_____

    _____

    e. Peptide _____

    _____

    f. Nucleotide _____

    _____

3. Identify the structures in Fig. 4.3, by writing the letters that correspond to the following descriptions. (Note: letters may be used once, more than once, or not at all. There may be more than one correct answer.)

    a. Is a component of a protein _____

    b. Contains only carbon, hydrogen and oxygen _____

    c. Is formed by dehydration synthesis _____

    d. Is a disaccharide _____

    e. Is a component of a lipid _____

    f. Is an acid _____

    g. Is a pentose _____

    h. Consists of nucleotides _____

    i. Is a monosaccharide _____

4. Name a biological structure containing:

    a. Lipid molecules

    _____

    b. Protein molecules

    _____

    c. Polysaccharide molecules

    _____

    d. Nucleotides

    _____

5. Identify one location of each of the following in the body and state its function in this location.

    a. Glycogen

        i. Location _____

        ii. Function_____

    b. Glucose

        i. Location _____

        ii. Function_____

    c. Nucleotides containing uracil

        i. Location _____

        ii. Function_____

    d. A protein that combines reversibly with oxygen

        i. Location _____

        ii. Function_____

    e. Triglyceride molecules

        i. Location _____

        ii. Function_____

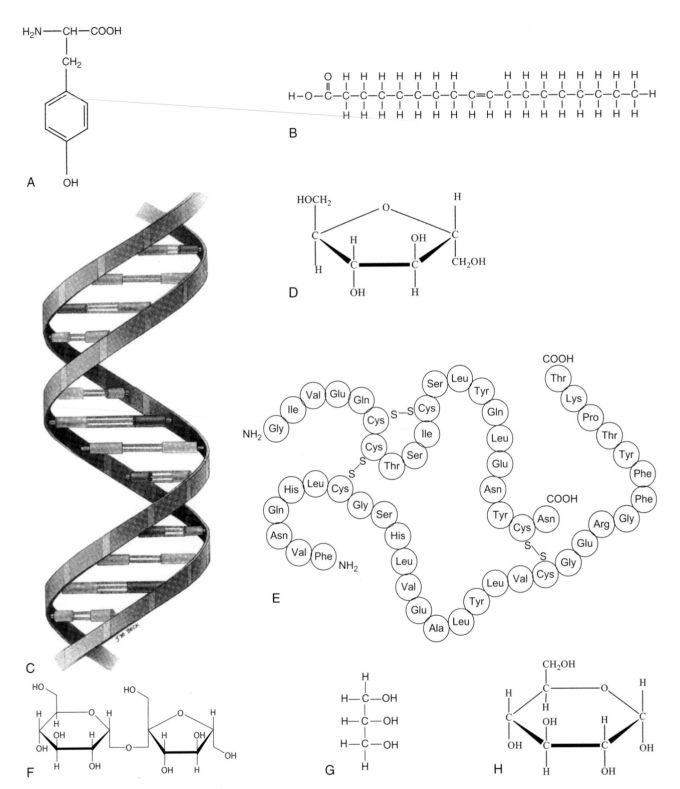

Figure 4.3 Biologically important molecules.
(Source: A Koutsopoulos, S., & Dalas, E. (2000). Hydroxyapatite crystallization in the presence of serine, tyrosine and hydroxyproline amino acids with polar side groups. Journal of crystal growth, 216(1-4), 443-449. B Caballero, B., Finglas, P., & Toldrá, F. (2015). Encyclopedia of food and health. Academic Press. C Gerdin, J. (2023). Workbook for Health Careers Today. Elsevier. D, H Nayak, A. K., Dhara, A. K., & Pal, D. (Eds.). (2021). Biological Macromolecules: Bioactivity and Biomedical Applications. Academic Press. E Feher, J. J. (2017). Quantitative human physiology: an introduction. Academic press. F Lord, R. (2021). Clinical Herbalism-E-Book: Plant Wisdom from East and West. Elsevier. G Litwack, G. (2017). Human biochemistry. Academic Press.)

6. The table below lists the properties of biologically important compounds. Place a tick in each column to which the property can be assigned. (Note: More than one column may be selected.)

Property	Carbohydrates	Lipids	Proteins	Nucleic acids
Contain carbon, oxygen and hydrogen				
Contain only carbon, oxygen and hydrogen				
Units are linked by peptide bonds				
Strongly hydrophobic				
Include enzymes				
Include molecules that contain genetic material				
Include the triglycerides				
The main sources of energy in cells				
Contain nitrogen				
Transport oxygen in the body				
Consist of saccharides				
Formed by dehydration synthesis reactions				
Include fats and oils				
Have a primary, secondary and tertiary structure				
All contain a 5-carbon sugar				

7. Complete the following sentences by filling in the blanks with the key terms provided at the beginning of this chapter. (Note: Key terms may be modified to fit the sentence.)

   a. Carbohydrates can be hydrolysed to form simple sugars called _____.

   b. Excess carbohydrates in the diet can be converted to _____ and stored in the liver, or _____ and stored in adipose tissue.

   c. DNA and RNA are examples of _____ and contain five-carbon sugars called _____.

   d. About 20 different types of _____ _____ make up protein molecules, linked together by _____ bonds.

   e. Enzymes are _____ molecules that are able to _____ chemical reactions.

   f. Steroids and triglycerides are examples of _____ molecules.

   g. Triglycerides are synthesised from _____ and _____.

   h. Strands of DNA are twisted around each other to form a _____ _____ structure, and the strands are held together by _____ bonds.

8. Explain what is meant by the following terms in relation to proteins:

    a. Primary structure _____

    _____

    b. Secondary structure_____

    _____

c. Tertiary structure _____

    _____

9. What types of bonds hold a protein molecule in shape?

    _____

    _____

Apply the Concepts

1. Explain why carbon is particularly suited to forming the backbone of organic compounds.

    _____

    _____

2. A diet consisting only of carbohydrates and lipids would be very hard to sustain. Explain why.

    _____

    _____

3. What is a hydrogel and why is it beneficial as a wound dressing component?

    _____

    _____

    _____

ACTIVITY 4.5: PHYSICAL PROPERTIES OF CARBOHYDRATES

Carbohydrates are organic compounds of great importance in living organisms and are composed of 5-carbon (**pentose**) or 6-carbon (**hexose**) rings. The simplest are the **monosaccharides**, or simple sugars, such as glucose and fructose. Cells of both plants and animals use monosaccharides as their main source of energy, glucose being the most vital for this purpose. Dehydration synthesis of two monosaccharides yields disaccharide sugars, such as sucrose or maltose, while the addition of further monosaccharides to the structure forms a **polysaccharide** or complex carbohydrate, such as starch.

This activity investigates some of the physical properties of carbohydrates.

To conduct this activity, it is important to ensure the following safety precautions:

- *Ensure appropriate hygiene practices are in place when tasting samples and disposing of contaminated test materials.*
- *Ensure safety glasses are worn at all times.*
- *When heating liquids in test tubes over Bunsen burners, ensure test tubes point away from individuals to avoid scalding.*
- *Ensure kerosene is used only within a fume cupboard or well-ventilated area due to volatile fumes, and dispose of it appropriately after use.*

Part 1: Taste

1. Obtain solid samples of several carbohydrates and set aside for tasting.

2. Taste a few grains of each and record their relative sweetness on a 0–5 scale in the table provided. (Note: Pay special attention to hygiene when tasting the samples.)

Carbohydrate	Sweetness (0 = not sweet; 5 = very sweet)
Glucose	
Fructose	
Galactose	
Sucrose	
Maltose	
Lactose	
Starch	

3. Identify the sugars tasted that are:

    a. Monosaccharides _____

    b. Disaccharides _____

    c. Polysaccharides _____

4. Was a relationship between sweetness and structure identified?

    _____

5. Are the simple sugars (monosaccharides) any more or less sweet than the disaccharides or the polysaccharide? Explain.

    _____

    _____

Part 2: Solubility

1. Obtain solid samples of several carbohydrates to examine.

2. Test the solubility of a small amount of each carbohydrate in water, a very polar solvent, and in kerosene, a solvent which is not polar.

3. Mix thoroughly by shaking and observe whether a solution has been formed.

4. Record your results in the table provided.

Carbohydrate	Solubility (0 = insoluble; 5 = very soluble)	
	Cold water	Kerosene
Glucose		
Fructose		
Galactose		
Sucrose		
Maltose		
Lactose		
Starch		

5. Consider the following questions:

    a. Which of the carbohydrates is or are the most strongly polar?

    _____

    b. Are any of these substances soluble in the non-polar solvent?

    _____

    c. Explain the result obtained for starch.

    _____

6. Heat a small amount of starch in a test tube half-filled with water, shaking the tube gently while heating.

    a. Describe the resulting mixture.

    _____

    _____

    b. Is this a solution or a colloid?

    _____

    c. How can this be confirmed?

    _____

    _____

Apply the Concepts

Explain why a meal consisting of a chocolate bar is less likely to satisfy hunger than a meal consisting of pasta.

_____

_____

_____

ACTIVITY 4.6: CHEMICAL PROPERTIES OF CARBOHYDRATES

Larger carbohydrate molecules, such as starch, glycogen and cellulose, can be formed by the dehydration synthesis of many monosaccharides. These macromolecules act as short-term energy storage compounds in cells or have a structural role, as is the case with cellulose in plants.

This activity demonstrates some of the tests commonly used to detect different carbohydrates based on their chemical properties.

Part 1: Iodine Test

The iodine test identifies the presence of starch, which reacts with iodine to form a blue–black complex.

1. Obtain a dimple tile and place a little of each of the following carbohydrate solids in order on the tile:

   - Glucose
   - Fructose
   - Sucrose
   - Starch
   - Cellulose

2. Add 2 drops of water to each of the carbohydrates.

3. Add 2 drops of iodine solution to each of the carbohydrates and note any colour changes in the table provided below.

Part 2: Benedict's Test

Benedict's test identifies those carbohydrates possessing an available alkanal or alkanone group, which will react with the reagent to give a coloured precipitate of copper (I) oxide. The colour of the precipitate varies from green to yellow to orange-red depending on the concentration of the test sugar. The test is positive for all monosaccharides and certain disaccharides.

1. Place a small amount of each carbohydrate in separate test tubes and add about 2 mL of Benedict's solution to each tube.

2. Mix thoroughly and bring to the boil over a low Bunsen flame.

3. Note any colour changes in the table provided below.

Part 3: Schultz's Test

Schultz's test identifies the presence of cellulose, an insoluble polysaccharide, which gives a purple colour with this reagent.

1. Place a small amount of each carbohydrate on a dimple tile and add a few drops of Schultz's solution to each carbohydrate.

2. Note any colour change that occurs within 30 seconds in the table provided.

Carbohydrate	Iodine test	Benedict's test	Schultz's test
Glucose			
Fructose			
Sucrose			
Starch			
Cellulose			

Part 4: Sugar Test Sticks and Strips

1. Observe the demonstration of commercially prepared sticks and strips, which enable rapid determinations of the glucose concentration in body fluids, such as urine.

2. Note that these are specific for glucose.

   a. Explain why these are useful in detecting glucose in body fluids such as urine.

   _____

   _____

   _____

Apply the Concepts

1. Explain why disaccharides, such as sucrose, are soluble in water, yet polysaccharides, such as starch, are not.

   _____

   _____

   _____

   a. If they are not soluble, how are starches able to be digested and absorbed in the human body?

   _____

   _____

2. People who are lactose-intolerant lack the enzyme lactase and are unable to digest the disaccharide lactose, so cannot drink milk. They can, however, eat cheese and yoghurt. Explain why.

   _____

   _____

ACTIVITY 4.7: PHYSICAL PROPERTIES OF PROTEINS

Proteins are large molecules containing about 20 different types of **amino acids** linked together by **peptide** bonds in a multitude of sequences and lengths, resulting in a vast number of different proteins. Living organisms are dependent on proteins to provide their main structural components and major regulatory substances.

This activity investigates the physical properties of proteins.

Part 1: Protein Structure

1. Identify the components comprising an amino acid.

   _____

   _____

   _____

2. Explain the structural arrangement of each of the following levels of protein structure:

   a. Primary structure: _____

   _____

   b. Secondary structure: _____

   _____

c. Tertiary structure: _____

_____

d. Quaternary structure: _____

_____

3. Consider the following questions:

a. Identify the term used to describe the process whereby protein structure is lost.

_____

b. Is this process reversible? Explain.

_____

_____

c. Which level of protein structure is retained following this process?

_____

d. Identify the term used to describe the resulting material following loss of protein structure.

_____

Part 2: Solubility

1. Examine the dry samples of the proteins provided.

2. Test the solubility of the proteins in water and in kerosene.

3. Place a small amount of each dry protein in a labelled test tube, add 5 mL of water, shake well and leave to stand.

4. Repeat, using 5 mL of kerosene. It may take a while for the proteins to become dispersed in the solvent.

5. Record your results in the table provided.

Protein	Solubility in	
	Water	Kerosene
Gelatine		
Casein		
Egg albumin		

6. Consider the following questions:

a. What can be deduced about the polarity of proteins?

_____

b. Since proteins are large molecules that are not hydrolysed when mixed with water, do they form a true solution? Explain.

_____

_____

_____

Part 3: Sensitivity of Protein Structure

The complexity of protein structure makes it uniquely sensitive to alteration by a wide variety of factors. Structural alteration, or **denaturation**, even if very slight, usually results in loss of function, and can be caused by many factors that affect protein structure.

1. Collect 10 test tubes and label them 1–10 with a glass marker.

2. Into tubes 1–5 dispense 2 mL egg albumin, and into tubes 6–10 dispense 2 mL skim milk.

3. Take tubes 1 and 6 and heat to boiling, noting the effect in the table provided below.

4. Take tubes 2 and 7 and add 5 mL 2.0 M HCl to each, mixing after addition. Note the effect.

5. Take tubes 3 and 8 and add 5 mL 2.0 M NaOH to each, mixing after addition. Note the effect.

6. Take tubes 4 and 9 and add 5 mL ethanol to each, mixing after addition. Note the effect.

7. Take tubes 5 and 10 and add 5 mL 0.1 M mercuric chloride (a heavy metal salt) to each, mixing after addition. Note the effect.

Treatment	Egg albumin	Skim milk
Heat		
HCl (strong acid)		
NaOH (strong base)		
Ethanol		
Mercuric chloride (heavy metal)		

8. Consider the following questions:

a. What general change have these agents brought about in the protein molecules?

_____

_____

b. Why is heat sterilisation effective in killing most bacteria?

_____

_____

c. What might occur if a strong acid or base were spilt on the skin?

_____

_____

d. Why is acid–base homeostasis important in the body?

_____

_____

e. Why are heavy metal ions often toxic in the body?

_____

_____

9. For each of the following items containing proteins, explain whether denaturation will occur by the addition of the substance in brackets:

a. Raw egg (by water)

_____

b. Meat (by lemon juice)

_____

c. Milk (by bacteria)

_____

d. Butter (by heating)

_____

e. Meat (by oil)

_____

f. Bacteria (by alcohol)

_____

g. Milk (by egg)

_____

h. Stomach (by lead)

_____

Apply the Concepts

1. Egg albumin can be used as a first aid measure in cases of accidental swallowing of heavy metal salts or solutions. Explain why this is beneficial.

_____

_____

2. After protein-rich food is eaten, which chemical processes must occur if the amino acids in the food are to be incorporated into proteins of the body cells?

_____

_____

ACTIVITY 4.8: CHEMICAL PROPERTIES OF PROTEINS

The biuret test gives a positive result with most proteins. A blue copper sulphate solution yields a pink-to-violet colour when mixed with protein in solution, because copper (II) ions bind to the nitrogen present in the peptide bonds of proteins, forming a coloured complex in an alkaline solution.

This activity demonstrates the chemical properties of proteins through the biuret test.

1. Into a test tube, dispense 2 mL egg albumin and add 2 mL concentrated NaOH, mixing thoroughly.

2. Slowly add 1 mL CuSO$_4$ solution with continuous mixing until a permanent colour is obtained in the solution.

3. In another test tube, pour 2 mL gelatine solution and add 2 mL concentrated NaOH, mixing thoroughly.

4. Slowly add 1 mL CuSO$_4$ solution with continuous mixing until a permanent colour is obtained in the solution.

   a. What colour changes were observed?

   _____

   _____

b. Although proteins are made up of amino acids, this test does not give a positive result for amino acid solutions. Explain why.

_____

_____

_____

Apply the Concepts

1. The hormone insulin, a protein, cannot be taken orally by diabetics, but instead must be injected subcutaneously. Explain why.

   _____

   _____

2. Why is alcohol used as a skin disinfectant prior to a hypodermic injection?

   _____

   _____

ACTIVITY 4.9: PROPERTIES OF LIPIDS

The organic compounds known as lipids include fats and oils, steroids, prostaglandins and several more complex types of substances such as the phospholipids of all membranes. Their molecular structure is variable, but generally consists of a **glycerol** backbone attached to three **fatty acid** groups to form a **triglyceride**. Fatty acids are composed of carbon chains and exhibit **saturated** and **unsaturated** structures based on the amount of hydrogen attached to the carbon backbone and the prevalence of single or double bonds between adjacent carbon atoms. All lipids share the ability to dissolve in **non-polar** solvents. In the body, they are important as long-term energy storage materials, as structural materials, particularly in cell membranes, and as a variety of regulatory substances such as steroid hormones.

This activity investigates the physical and chemical properties of lipids.

Part 1: Appearance and Feel

1. Examine the oil, fat and steroid (cholesterol) samples provided.

2. Rub a little of each substance between the fingers to determine how they feel.

3. Record your observations in the table provided.

Lipid	Appearance	Feel
Oil		
Fat		
Cholesterol		

Part 2: Spot Test

1. Rub a small piece of fat onto a piece of paper or let 1 drop of oil fall onto the paper.

2. Note the translucent spot.

Part 3: Solubility

1. Test the solubility of a small sample of each lipid in water and kerosene.

2. Record your observations in the table provided.

Lipid	Solubility in water	Solubility in kerosene
Oil		
Fat		
Cholesterol		

3. What do the results indicate about the polarity of lipid molecules?

_____

_____

Part 4: Emulsification of Fats

Fats and oils can be dispersed in water if they are broken up into small droplets and coated with something to make the surface of the droplet water-attracting. The resulting **emulsion** is cloudy like a colloid, but stable if an effective emulsifying agent is used. Emulsifying agents, also called **surfactants**, are used to emulsify lipids for digestion, for transport in the blood and for cleaning.

1. Mix 2 drops of vegetable oil with 2 mL of each of the solutions in the table provided.

2. Shake well and note how long it takes for the solution to become clear or for a definite oil layer to form.

Solution	Time taken to separate (seconds)
Water	
Egg albumin	
Bile salts	
Household detergent	
Lecithin solution	

3. Consider the following questions:

   a. Which substance is the most effective emulsifying agent?

   _____

   b. Which is the least effective?

   _____

   c. What is the function of lecithins in the blood?

   _____

   _____

   d. What is the function of bile salts in the human body?

   _____

   _____

Part 5: A Test for Lipids

Dyes that are soluble in lipids can be used to identify the presence of lipids, as both are non-polar.

1. Pour a little oil into a test tube.

2. Add an equal amount of water, then add a few drops of scarlet R dye.

3. Shake vigorously then observe what happens to the dye when the tube has been left to stand for a short while.

4. Identify whether the dye is soluble in:

   a. Water_____

   b. Lipids _____

Apply the Concepts

1. What is rancidification?

   _____

   _____

   a. What is produced as a result of rancidification?

   _____

2. What is oxidation and why are lipids prone to this process?

   _____

   _____

   _____

   a. How do antioxidants reduce lipid oxidation?

   _____

   _____

3. What are ketones and why can they present a problem in the blood?

   _____

   _____

   _____

4. Why should inducing vomiting be avoided if a hydrocarbon such as kerosene has been swallowed?

   _____

   _____

5. Gallstones have the effect of blocking the flow of bile into the duodenum. People suffering from this condition may experience increased pain after eating fatty food and produce faeces with a high fat content.

   a. Explain why this happens.

   _____

   _____

   _____

   b. What is the composition of gallstones?

   _____

   _____

6. Explain why medications such as atenolol stay within the bloodstream to exert their effects and do not enter the tissue cells.

   _____

   _____

7. Explain why medications such as propranolol enter tissue cells rapidly to exert their effect rather than remain within the bloodstream.

_____

_____

_____

8. What is a liposome and how is it beneficial as a drug delivery vehicle?

_____

_____

_____

ACTIVITY 4.10: *DNA STRUCTURE AND PROTEIN SYNTHESIS*

Deoxyribonucleic acid, or **DNA**, is the genetic material for the vast majority of organisms (Fig. 4.4). This means that it is the chemical substance that transmits the characteristics of parents to their offspring in the form of **genes**. To understand how a chemical compound can achieve this, it is necessary to examine the chemical composition of DNA, as well as its overall structure. DNA consists of two strands that form a symmetrical structure called a double helix (Fig. 4.5) and is composed of monomers, referred to as **nucleotides**, which contain **nitrogenous bases**. In addition, DNA contains information that is important for the synthesis of structural and functional proteins (Fig. 4.6), which occurs through the processes of **transcription** and **translation**. Although DNA can create copies of itself through **DNA replication**, protein synthesis requires a DNA copy in the form of **messenger RNA**, which is translated by **transfer RNA** and **ribosomes**, which are also composed of **RNA**.

This activity explores the structure of DNA and the process of converting genetic information to protein structure in cells.

1. Examine Fig. 4.4, showing the overall structure of DNA and its nucleotide components, and Fig. 4.5, which shows the arrangement of nucleotides in a small section of a DNA molecule.

2. Consider the following questions:

   a. How many nucleotides are present on each strand in Fig. 4.5?

   _____

   b. What is the maximum number of amino acids that could be coded for here?

   _____

   c. What is represented by the dotted lines connecting the two strands?

   _____

   d. The backbone of each strand consists of phosphate groups and which 5-carbon sugar?

   _____

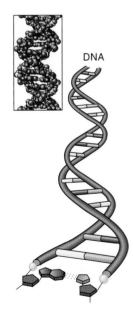

Figure 4.4 The DNA molecule.
(Source: Gerdin, J. (2023). Workbook for Health Careers Today. Elsevier.)

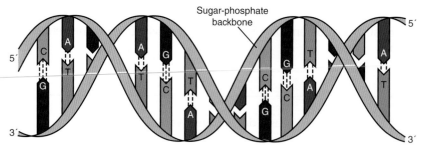

Sugar-phosphate backbone

Figure 4.5 DNA structure.
(Source: Turgeon, M. L. (2020). Immunology & Serology in Laboratory Medicine. Elsevier.)

e. What is represented by the letters A, T, C and G?

_____

3. Based on Fig. 4.4 and Fig. 4.5, construct a model of DNA using adhesive labels and a large piece of card.

   a. Using different shapes of labels (one for phosphates, one for sugars and four for nitrogenous bases), construct a model based on Fig. 4.4 and Fig. 4.5, but with a different sequence of nitrogenous bases.

   b. Draw solid lines to connect the components of the nucleotides and dotted lines in the appropriate place to connect the two strands.

   c. Construct a key to identify the differently shaped labels with the components of the nucleotides.

4. Consider the model you have just constructed, which suggests how DNA might replicate.

   a. Since A always pairs with T, and G always pairs with C, explain how DNA strands form the template for DNA replication.

   _____

   _____

   _____

5. Complete the following sentences by filling in the blanks with the terms provided. (Note: Some terms are used more than once.)

Amino acid	Hydrogen	Polyribosome
Cistron	Identical	Protein
Codon	Messenger	Ribosome
Cytoplasm	Mirror	Separate
Cytosine	Nitrogenous bases	Thymine
Deoxyribose	Nucleotides	Transcription
Gene	Nucleus	Transfer RNA
Guanine	Phosphate	Translation

   a. A DNA molecule is made up of structural units called _____, each of which consists of three

components: the sugar _____, a _____ group and one of four _____.

   b. A DNA double helix is held together by _____ bonds that form between _____ on opposite strands.

   c. In this arrangement, adenine is always paired with _____ and _____ is always paired with _____. Thus, the two strands are _____ images of each other.

   d. Genetic information is found in the sequences of _____ along a DNA strand.

   e. The genetic code is a code for the structure of protein molecules, and a sequence of three nucleotide bases, called a _____, codes for a single _____.

   f. The part of a DNA molecule that codes for a complete protein molecule is called a _____. When DNA replicates itself, the two strands _____, exposing the _____ of each strand.

   g. A new strand is assembled on each old strand and the two new DNA molecules are _____ to each other and to the original molecule. The genetic DNA of a cell always remains in the cell's _____.

   h. In protein synthesis, when a gene is 'read', its information is used to assemble a _____ RNA molecule by a process known as _____. This molecule moves from the nucleus to the _____ of the cell, where it becomes attached to a _____. Here the process of _____ begins.

i. Amino acids are brought to the ribosome by _____ molecules and are joined in sequence to form a complete _____ molecule.

j. Several ribosomes moving along the same mRNA molecule are collectively called a _____.

6. Identify three ways in which RNA differs from DNA.

_____

_____

_____

7. Consider Fig. 4.6, which shows the mechanism of protein synthesis and identify the labelled structures.

a. Structure A: _____

b. Structure B: _____

c. Structure C: _____

d. Structure D: _____

e. Structure E: _____

f. Structure F: _____

g. Structure G: _____

h. Structure H: _____

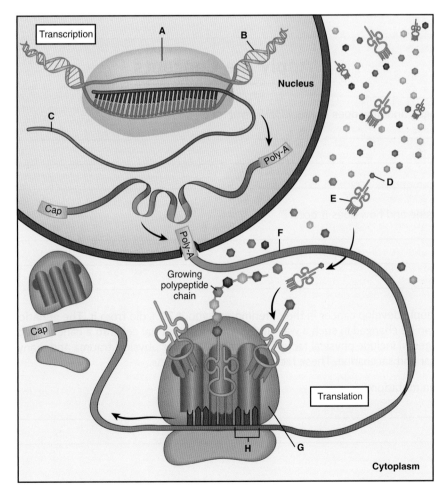

Figure 4.6 Protein synthesis.
(Source: Power-Kean, K., Zettel, S., El-Hussein, M. T., Huether, S. E., & McCance, K. L. (2022). Huether and McCance's Understanding Pathophysiology, Canadian Edition. Elsevier.)

8. The following events occur during protein synthesis. Place the corresponding letters in their correct sequence.

   A. tRNA carries an amino acid to the ribosome

   B. The ribosome attaches to a mRNA

   C. Amino acids are linked to form a peptide chain

   D. Two strands of DNA separate

   E. Ribosome moves along the mRNA

   F. mRNA moves into the cytoplasm

   G. mRNA is synthesised from a DNA strand

   H. Ribosome receives an amino acid from the tRNA

   I. Ribosome becomes detached from mRNA

   J. tRNA becomes detached from the ribosome

   K. Protein molecule detaches from ribosome

   L. tRNA attaches to an amino acid

Correct sequence:

_____

_____

9. Explain what determines the primary structure of a protein molecule.

   _____

   _____

10. Why is the primary structure of a protein important to the shape of the molecule?

   _____

   _____

Apply the Concepts

1. What is a carcinogen and how does it affect DNA structure?

   _____

   _____

   _____

2. What is an oncogene and how does it occur?

   _____

   _____

   _____

3. Almost 50% of people develop cancer in their lifetime and about 20% die from it. The genetic code carried on DNA molecules can be changed in such a way that it converts a normal cell into a cancerous cell. Carcinogens (cancer-causing agents) include physical factors such as radiation or physical trauma and many chemical agents such as tobacco tar and saccharine. These factors all cause mutations.

   a. Define the term mutation.

   _____

   _____

4. In a point mutation, a single nucleotide in a DNA strand is replaced by a different nucleotide.

   a. What effect will this have on the protein molecule produced from that DNA template?

   _____

   _____

   _____

5. In a deletion mutation, one or more nucleotides are deleted from a DNA strand.

   a. What effect will this have on the protein produced from that DNA template?

   _____

   _____

   _____

6. What is gel electrophoresis and how is it conducted?

   _____

   _____

   _____

   a. How can gel electrophoresis assist with forensic investigations?

   _____

   _____

   _____

ACTIVITY 4.11: ENZYME STRUCTURE AND FUNCTION

Genes, or **cistrons**, control body structure and function by coding for proteins. Proteins are remarkable molecules that carry out many different functions within the human body. For example, some hormones, such as insulin, are proteins; some proteins, such as haemoglobin, transport or store oxygen; structural proteins, such as keratin, are found in hair and fingernails; proteins such as albumin have storage or transport functions; contractile proteins are found in muscle cells; and the immune system utilises proteins as antibodies. Most importantly, all **enzymes** are proteins, and genes are able to control cellular activities by producing, or ceasing production of, enzymes which **catalyse** specific reactions. Catalysis is achieved by lowering the **activation energy (Ea)** of the reaction. Almost all metabolic activity is catalysed by enzymes and would effectively cease if enzyme production ceased.

This activity explores the structure and function of enzymes.

1. Using the terms listed below, complete the following sentences.

Activation
Active site
Amino acids

Changed
Protein
Specificity

Substrate
Tertiary

a. Enzymes are _____ molecules whose function depends on their three-dimensional shape, or _____ structure. This, in turn, depends on their primary structure, which is their sequence of _____.

b. An enzyme will usually catalyse just one particular reaction, a property referred to as enzyme _____. This is because of the shape of the enzyme's _____, which will allow attachment to just one _____.

c. Enzymes speed up reactions by lowering the energy barrier to the reaction, known as the energy of _____. Catalysts like enzymes speed up chemical reactions without being _____ by the reaction.

2. Explain each of the following with reference to enzyme function:

a. Optimum temperature _____

_____

b. Optimum pH _____

_____

c. Competitive inhibition _____

_____

d. Non-competitive inhibition _____

_____

e. Lock-and-key mechanism _____

_____

3. Consider the following questions:

a. What is the function of an enzyme?

_____

_____

b. In what way are enzymes and other catalysts the same?

_____

_____

c. In what way do enzymes and other catalysts differ?

_____

_____

d. In an enzyme-catalysed reaction, what is the active site and what occurs there?

_____

_____

e. In an enzyme-catalysed reaction, what is the substrate?

_____

_____

f. What effect do enzymes have on activation energy?

_____

_____

g. Are enzymes affected by the reactions in which they participate? Explain.

_____

_____

Apply the Concepts

1. Explain what is meant by the induced fit model, with reference to enzyme activity.

_____

_____

_____

2. A system contains an enzyme, a substrate and a competitive inhibitor.

   Predict whether the reaction will proceed quickly or slowly, and explain why.

_____

_____

_____

Additional Activities

For additional activities visit Activity 4A: Enzyme Activity on Evolve˚.

Additional Resources

American Society for Biochemistry and Molecular Biology: Structure and Function
The American Society for Biochemistry and Molecular Biology is a scientific and educational organisation that publishes journals, and also provides online educational resources for students.

www.asbmb.org/education/core-concept-teaching-strategies/foundational-concepts/structure-function

BioNinja: Molecular Biology and Nucleic Acids
BioNinja is an online biology resource that provides interactive learning modules arranged according to difficulty, with summary and additional resources options available.

ib.bioninja.com.au/standard-level/topic-2-molecular-biology/
ib.bioninja.com.au/higher-level/topic-7-nucleic-acids/

Learn-Biology: Biochemistry Tutorials
Learn-Biology is an interactive resource providing background learning modules for biology students with a focus on guidance, practice, feedback and motivation.

learn-biology.com/ap-biology/module-6-menu-biochemistry/

Learn Genetics: Virtual Labs
Learn Genetics is an online genetic science learning centre provided by the University of Utah, and offers virtual labs covering DNA extraction, gel electrophoresis, PCR testing and DNA microarray.

learn.genetics.utah.edu/content/labs/

Lumen Learning: Biology for Majors
Lumen Learning provides a number of online courses and modules related to anatomy and physiology on a variety of biological topics, including biological molecules and enzymes.

courses.lumenlearning.com/wm-biology1/part/important-biomolecules/
courses.lumenlearning.com/wm-biology1/chapter/reading-enzymes/

Sumanas Inc: Animated Tutorials – Molecular Biology
Sumanas Inc. provides a range of animated tutorials in molecular biology, covering topics such as proteins, ribosomes, mRNA, enzyme assays and DNA structure.

www.sumanasinc.com/webcontent/animations/molecularbiology.html

Visible Body: DNA and RNA Basics – Replication, Transcription and Translation
Visible Body provides interactive and highly accurate visualisations and apps for learning and teaching anatomy and physiology for students and healthcare professionals, including biological topics such as DNA basics.

www.visiblebody.com/blog/dna-and-rna-basics-replication-transcription-and-translation

Your Genome: What Is DNA?
Your Genome is a website provided by the Wellcome Trust UK, that provides information about genetics and genomics, allowing users to explore topics, facts and stories relating to DNA structure, replication, discoveries and the human genome.

www.yourgenome.org/facts/what-is-dna

CHAPTER 5
Microscopy

A microscope is an instrument used to examine objects that are too small to be seen by the naked eye. Microscopy is the science of investigating small objects and structures using a microscope. Microscopes come in several different types; however, the most commonly used in the study of cells and tissues is the optical microscope.

Simple optical microscopes using a single lens were invented in the 17th century, but the compound microscope, which uses a system of lenses to generate magnified images of small objects, is now in common use in laboratories. Compound microscopes can achieve magnifications of up to $\times 1000$ before the properties of visible light become limiting. Beyond this, an electron microscope is needed to resolve objects such as cell membranes and bacterial cell structures. Good microscope skills are essential for studying the morphology of cells, tissues and microorganisms. (Refer to Chapter 3: Cells and Metabolism for further information on cell structure and Chapter 7: Tissues and Organs for further information on tissue structure)

LEARNING OUTCOMES

On completion of these activities the student should be able to:

1. discuss the nature of microscopy and the uses and limitations of the light microscope
2. describe the component parts of the compound microscope
3. practise the correct procedures for setting up and using the compound microscope
4. determine the diameters of the fields of view at different magnifications
5. prepare and examine stained and unstained wet mount slides
6. estimate the true sizes of microscopic objects
7. estimate the magnifications of diagrams
8. demonstrate good techniques for drawing and labelling microscopic objects
9. demonstrate skills for troubleshooting technical problems that occur in microscopy.

KEY TERMS

Arm	Inverted image	Parfocal
Base	Iris diaphragm	Resolution
Coarse focus	Magnification	Resolving power
Compound microscope	Micrometre	Slide
Condenser	Microscope	Slide holder
Coverslip	Microscopy	Stage
Eyepiece	Objective lens	Voltage control
Field of view	Ocular lens	Wet mount
Fine focus	Oil immersion	Working distance

ACTIVITY 5.1: INTRODUCTION TO THE MICROSCOPE

The **microscope** is a sophisticated, sensitive and accurate piece of equipment which will provide the best performance if it is given reasonable care and maintenance (Fig. 5.1). In particular, it is important to avoid any abrupt motion or impact, to keep the microscope covered when not in use, to keep the lenses clean and to use only the correct lens tissue for this purpose. Keep the microscope in an upright position and use both hands to carry it if it must be moved, using one hand to hold the **arm** and the other to support the **base**. Ensure **voltage control** of the lamp is at a minimum before and after use. **Compound microscopes** are **parfocal**, so that focus is maintained when changing between **magnifications**. High power magnification, such as ×1000, of very small objects should only be conducted via **oil immersion**, which requires knowledge of the correct technique.

This activity introduces the parts of the microscope and their functions.

1. Remove the cover from the microscope.

2. Locate and identify the components labelled in Fig. 5.1.

3. Become familiar with the function of each of these components:

   - The light source is a *lamp*, whose intensity can be varied by controls on the *base* of the microscope. Light passes directly upwards through the *condenser*, through a hole in the stage and through the specimen itself before entering the lenses.

   - The *condenser* focuses the light onto the specimen being observed and is controlled by the *condenser height adjustment knob*. The condenser is generally used in the fully raised position, but when using low power, it may be necessary to lower the condenser in order to evenly illuminate the field.

   - The aperture *iris diaphragm lever* is located on the side of the condenser. This controls depth of focus, image contrast and resolution. It will need to be adjusted every time the magnification is changed. The intensity of illumination should only be adjusted by using the

   voltage control on the base of the microscope, and never by adjusting the iris diaphragm or condenser height.

   - The *ocular lenses* are the lenses through which the observer looks into the microscope. They usually have a *power* (magnification) of ×10.

   - As well as ocular lenses, most microscopes are equipped with three colour-coded *objective lenses* – a red ×4 magnification (extra low power) objective, a yellow ×10 magnification (low power) objective, and a blue ×40 magnification (high power) objective. Some microscopes also have a white ×100 magnification (*oil immersion*) objective.

   - The objective lenses of modern microscopes are parfocal. This means that having focused correctly at lower power, the lens will not touch the stage and the object will nearly be in focus on changing to a higher power. All that is needed is a small adjustment of the *fine focusing knob*. It is imperative that objective lenses are kept very clean. The smallest mark on a lens will result in a fuzzy image. (Note: Whenever the high power objective is in

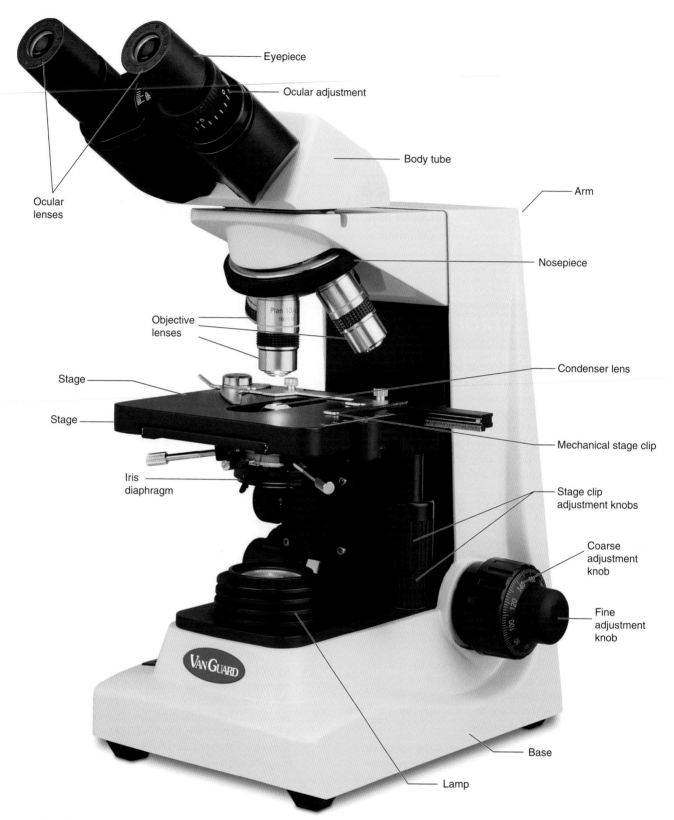

Figure 5.1 The compound microscope.
(*Source: Patton, K. T., Bell, F. B., Matusiak, D. J., & Wood, S. R. (2019). Anatomy and physiology laboratory manual. Elsevier.*)

place, all focusing must be done with the fine focus only.)

- The *stage* is the platform on which a *slide* rests while it is being examined. It is equipped with a *slide holder*, allowing a slide to be held in place using spring clips or some other clamping device.

4. Swing the *objective lenses* round and note that each 'clicks' into place. Rotate the lowest power objective into position.

5. Turn the *coarse focus knob* about 180° and note how far the stage moves in response. Now turn the *fine focus knob* about 180° and again note how far the stage moves. Lower the stage fully using the coarse focus.

6. Place a prepared slide on the stage and observe the distance between the top of the coverslip and the objective lens as you carefully move from the ×4 to the ×10, then ×40 objectives. (Note: Never allow an objective lens to make contact with the slide.)

   a. What trend can be observed?

   _____

   _____

   b. Explain why the coarse focus control should never be used when examining an object under high power.

   _____

   _____

7. In the compound microscope, magnification is achieved by the combination of the ocular lenses and objective lenses. The total magnification of the microscope is given by the product of the magnification of the ocular (usually ×10) and the magnification of the objective.

a. Complete the table below based on this information.

Ocular lens	Objective lens	Total magnification
×10	× 4	
×10	×10	
×10	×40	
×10	×100	

8. The magnification of objective and ocular lenses is always written on them.

   a. What is the magnification of the ocular lenses on your microscope?

   _____

   b. What are the magnifications of the objective lenses on your microscope?

   _____

9. In the table provided, list all combinations of the ocular and objective lenses for your microscope and calculate the total magnification for each.

Ocular lens	Objective lens	Total magnification

Apply the Concepts

1. What is a stereo microscope?

   _____

   _____

2. How does a stereo microscope differ from a compound microscope, in terms of the image that is viewed?

   _____

   _____

3. Is there a distinction between a transmission electron microscope and a scanning electron microscope? Explain.

_____

_____

4. Explain why viruses cannot be visualised with a compound microscope.

_____

_____

ACTIVITY 5.2: SETTING UP AND USING THE MICROSCOPE

A compound microscope will deliver good results only if care is taken to set it up correctly prior to each use. As part of general **microscopy**, steps 1–7 should be followed whenever the microscope is used, so it is important to become familiar with the locations and functions of the **ocular lenses (eyepieces)**, **objective lenses**, voltage control, **condenser** and **iris diaphragm** (Fig. 5.2). Once this has been achieved, a specimen can be placed on the **stage** and held in position via the **slide holder** for observation, first using the **coarse focus** and then using the **fine focus**. The **working distance** can be determined once the objective lens is in place and the specimen is in focus.

This activity demonstrates setting up and using the compound microscope.

1. Check that all exposed lens surfaces are clean. If necessary, clean carefully by wiping with a lens tissue and cleaning fluid.

2. Check that the voltage adjustment is at the minimum, then switch on the lamp and adjust the light intensity to about half its maximum.

3. Raise the condenser to its highest position.

4. Place the ×4 objective in position over the stage.

5. Remove one of the ocular lenses and look down the exposed tube. Adjust the iris diaphragm lever until the diaphragm obscures about one-third of the field of view, as shown in Fig. 5.2.

6. Replace the ocular lens quickly to avoid dust accumulation in the tube.

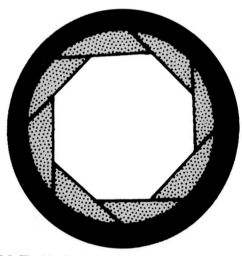

Figure 5.2 The iris diaphragm partially closed.

Good Microscope Technique

- To avoid eyestrain when looking through the microscope, always keep both eyes open.
- Even if the microscope has only one ocular lens, aim to keep both eyes open and concentrate only on what the active eye is seeing.

7. Make sure the microscope is in a position which is comfortable to use. Look through the ocular lenses and slide them apart or together to give good binocular vision, or until just one circle can be seen.

8. Place a prepared slide in the slide holder on the stage with the coverslip facing upwards and carefully raise the stage with the coarse focus adjustment until the slide is just below the objective lens.

9. Looking through the eyepieces, slowly lower the stage with the coarse focus adjustment until the specimen is correctly focused. Adjust light intensity if necessary.

10. Use a ruler to measure the distance in millimetres between the bottom of the objective lens and the specimen on the slide. This the *working distance* of the objective.

11. Record the working distance in the table below.

Objective	Working distance (mm)
×4	
×10	
×40	

12. Place an object of interest in the centre of the field and swing the ×10 (low power) objective into place.

13. The microscope should have a mechanical stage that enables the specimen to be smoothly moved sideways, forwards or backwards by use of the two special control knobs at the side of the stage. In addition, there are scales for precisely locating any part of a specimen, if required.

14. Adjust focus by using the coarse and fine focusing knobs.

15. Adjust the light intensity until the detail of the image is at its clearest.

16. Measure the working distance and record it in the table provided.

17. Place an object of interest in the centre of the field and swing the ×40 (high power) objective into place. (Note: If the specimen has been correctly focused under low power, the high power objective will not touch the slide.)

18. Re-focus the object using the fine focus knob only. (Note: Never adjust the coarse focus under high power. If focus is lost under high power, return to the low power objective and re-focus.)

19. Adjust the light intensity and the iris diaphragm until the image detail and contrast are optimal.

20. Measure the working distance and record it in the table provided.

   a. What is the relationship between the power of the objective and the working distance?

   _____

   b. Why must the coarse focus never be adjusted under high power?

   _____

   _____

   c. The area that can be seen through the microscope is called the field of view. What happens to the field of view as magnification is increased?

   _____

   d. Why is it necessary to place the object of interest in the centre of the field each time magnification is increased?

   _____

   _____

Good Microscope Technique

- Always examine a specimen first under low or extra low power and then, if required, under high power.
- Never examine a specimen without a coverslip unless instructed to do so.
- Before removing a slide from the stage, swing the high power objective away from the slide.
- Most specimens are too thick for all parts to be in focus simultaneously under high power. Experienced microscopists continually use the fine focus to obtain a 3-dimensional view.

Fault Finding and Troubleshooting

- Use only the special lens tissue provided to clean lenses.
- If an image cannot be seen, check that:
  o the lamp is on
  o the iris diaphragm is open
  o the objective has 'clicked' into place
  o the specimen is centred on the stage.
- A blurred image may be caused by:
  o dirty or wet lenses, especially the objectives
  o a wet or dirty coverslip or slide
  o poor adjustment of the iris diaphragm or condenser.
- If it is impossible to focus a specimen under high power, check that the slide is the right way up. The coverslip should always face upwards.

Apply the Concepts

1. What is the nosepiece?

   _____

2. What is the function of the condenser?

   _____

   _____

3. What is the function of the iris diaphragm?

   _____

   _____

4. Explain why the ×4 objective lens is also referred to as the scanning lens.

   _____

   _____

5. Why is oil immersion required for objective lenses with higher magnification power, such as the ×100 lens?

   _____

   _____

ACTIVITY 5.3: PREPARING A WET MOUNT SLIDE

When observing living tissues or cells, it is usually necessary to prepare a **wet mount**, consisting of cells immersed in a clear fluid that will keep them alive (Fig. 5.3). In addition to the ocular lenses and objective lenses, compound microscopes contain of a series of mirrors. This results in an inverted image rather than a true image of the specimen being viewed.

This activity demonstrates the technique involved in preparing a wet mount slide.

1. Observe the demonstration of how to prepare a wet mount slide.

2. Collect all the necessary equipment before starting and thoroughly clean the slide and coverslip.

3. Using a Pasteur pipette place a small drop of water on the centre of the slide.

4. On a piece of newspaper find and cut out a small letter 'e'.

5. Using forceps, place the piece of paper in the water on the slide.

6. Place the coverslip over the water and paper. An easy way of doing this without trapping too many air bubbles is to rest the coverslip on a dissecting needle after bringing one edge up to the water, then lowering it gently over the specimen (Fig. 5.3).

7. If there is excess fluid around the coverslip, carefully remove it with a tissue or piece of filter paper.

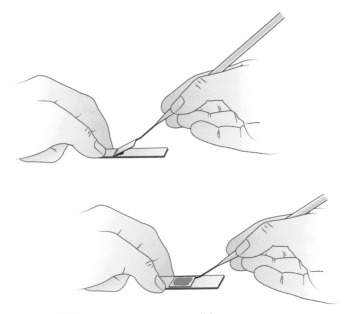

10. Draw a diagram of what you can see in the space below.

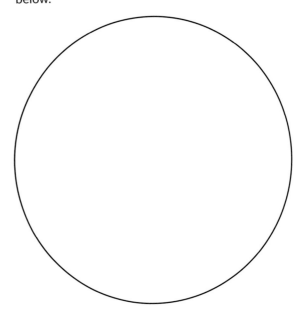

Figure 5.3 Preparing a wet mount slide.
(*Source: Gerdin, J. (2023). Health careers today. Elsevier.*)

8. Place the slide on the microscope stage and focus on the newspaper letter with the ×4 objective.

9. Compare the orientation of the letter 'e' on the slide with that of the image seen.

a. What term describes the orientation of the image in relation to the object?

_____

11. Move the slide sideways, upwards and downwards, while looking down the microscope.

a. How does the movement of the image compare with the movement of the object?

_____

Apply the Concepts

1. Describe and explain how a specimen that has been sectioned thickly would appear under the microscope.

_____

_____

_____

ACTIVITY 5.4: RESOLUTION

The most important feature of the light microscope is not its ability to magnify objects, but rather its **resolving power**. **Resolution** is a measure of the ability to recognise two individual but closely spaced points as separate. The human eye, on average, can only resolve points if they are more than 0.1 millimetre apart, whereas the light microscope can resolve points as little as 0.2 micrometres apart. Thus, the microscope enables the operator to see finer detail than is visible with the unaided eye.

This activity compares the resolving power of the eyes with that of the microscope and investigates the factors that affect resolution.

1. Cut out a small piece of coloured magazine paper and make a wet mount with it.

2. Examine the paper under the microscope at different magnifications.

   a. Describe any differences between the appearance of the paper to the naked eye and its appearance under the microscope.

   _____

   _____

3. With the ×10 objective in place, reduce the intensity of the light.

   a. What can be noted about the relationship between light intensity and resolution?

   _____

   _____

4. Set the light intensity to give optimal resolution. Now open and close the iris diaphragm.

   a. What effect does this have on resolution?

   _____

   _____

ACTIVITY 5.5: PREPARATION OF A STAINED WET MOUNT SLIDE

Many biological specimens are uncoloured and transparent when mounted on a glass **slide** with a glass **coverslip**, making it difficult to see any details clearly. Microscopists have devised a number of techniques for making objects more visible under the microscope. One popular way to do this is to stain the material so that its various components become coloured and visible.

This activity demonstrates the technique for making stained and unstained wet mounts of cheek cells.

1. Obtain two clean slides and label one slide 'U' (unstained) and the other 'S' (stained).

2. Place a small drop of saline solution in the centre of slide U.

3. Place a small drop of methylene blue/saline mixture in the centre of slide S.

4. Collect some cheek cells by gently scraping the inside of your cheek with the blunt end of a toothpick. Mix the material you have obtained with the fluid in the centre of slide U. Immediately dispose of your toothpick in the disinfectant container provided.

5. Repeat Step 4 with slide S.

6. Place a coverslip on each side.

7. Using the low power (×10) objective first, and then the high power (×40) objective, examine the stained slide and then the unstained slide and locate some cheek cells on both. Some cells will be separate and others may clump together.

8. Note that the cheek cells are very thin and may be difficult to see in the unstained specimen. You may need to increase contrast with the iris diaphragm to see them more clearly.

    a. Briefly describe the differences observed between the cells in the two slides.

    _____

    _____

    b. Approximately how many cells would fit across the diameter of the high power field of view?

    _____

9. Draw a diagram of two or three stained cells in the space below.

Magnification of diagram: × _____

10. Keep the stained preparation for use in the next activity.

Good Microscope Technique

When making sketches of objects under the microscope, pay attention to the following:
- Drawings should be as large as the space permits. Do not make them small simply because the object is small.
- Use a sharp pencil and draw clean, simple lines to show the shape and relative sizes of the structures observed. Avoid 'artistic' effects.
- Do not use shading to show darker areas; stippling or cross-hatching are better.
- Label as many structures in the diagram as possible by drawing a line from the structure to the label. Labels should be arranged such that lines never cross.
- Name each diagram and note whether the specimen is a transverse section (TS), longitudinal section (LS), or whole mount (wm).

Apply the Concepts

1. What is a Gram stain and what does it attempt to achieve?

    _____

    _____

2. Why is Gram staining important when antibiotics are prescribed for certain bacterial infections?

_____

_____

ACTIVITY 5.6: MEASURING SIZE WITH THE MICROSCOPE

The circle of light that can be seen when looking down the microscope is the **field of view**. Within the field of view, a magnified image of the specimen can be seen. At a higher power an enlarged image of a proportionately smaller part of the specimen can be seen. The diameter of the field of view at higher powers thus becomes progressively smaller, such that if the magnification is doubled, the diameter of the field of view is halved. If the diameter of the field of view is known, the size of objects being examined can be estimated. The field of view can be determined through the use of a **micrometer** scale (Fig. 5.4) and micrometer slide (Fig. 5.5).

This activity measures the diameters of the fields of view of a compound microscope and uses that information to estimate the actual size of an observed specimen.

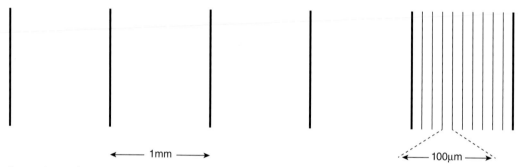

←——— 1mm ———→   ·←— 100µm —→·

Figure 5.4 A micrometer scale.

1. Take a micrometer (graticule) slide from its box and examine it. Notice that it has been marked in divisions of 1 mm and 100 micrometres (microns), as shown in Fig. 5.4.

2. Place the slide on the stage of the microscope and focus on it using the ×4 objective.

3. Adjust the position of the slide so that across the centre of the field a number of complete 1 mm divisions on the left-hand side and a number of smaller 100 micron divisions on the right-hand side can be observed, as shown in Fig. 5.5.

4. Measure the diameter of the field of view in mm and micrometres and record this in the table provided.

5. Repeat steps 2 and 3 for the ×10 and ×40 objectives. Note that with the ×40 objective, the field diameter will be less than 1 mm.

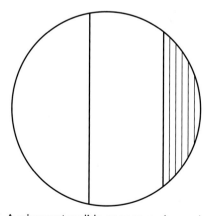

Figure 5.5 A micrometer slide as seen under a microscope.

6. The field diameter with the ×100 objective cannot be directly measured, but can be estimated from the diameter of the field with ×10 objective. Since the magnification is 10 times greater, the field will be one-tenth of the diameter.

7. Calculate the diameter of the field of view for the ×100 objective and record this in the table provided.

Objective lens	Ocular lens	Total magnification	Diameter of field of view	
			mm	μm
×4	×10			
×10	×10			
×40	×10			
×100	×10			

8. Re-examine the stained cheek cells from Activity 5.5 under high power (×40 objective).

   a. Approximately how many cells could fit across the field of view under the ×40 objective?

   _____

9. Estimate the diameter of a single cheek cell in micrometres, using the following formula:

$$\text{Diameter of one cell} = \frac{\text{Diameter of field of view (microns)}}{\text{No. of cells across field of view}}$$

$$= \text{_____ microns}$$

10. Now that the approximate actual diameter of a cheek cell is known, this information can be used to calculate the magnification of the drawing made in Activity 5.5.

11. Measure in millimetres the length of the drawing you made of a cheek cell. Convert this to micrometres.

12. Divide this number by the estimated diameter of an actual cheek cell, made in Step 9. The result is the magnification of the drawing.

13. Add the magnification of the drawing to the name of the diagram (e.g. human cheek cell wm ×2000). This means that the drawing is 2000 times larger than the cheek cell itself.

Good Microscope Technique

When making drawings of microscopic objects, always show the magnification of the drawing rather than the magnification of the lens combination used.

14. Estimate the diameter of red blood cells under high power using the prepared slides provided.

   a. Approximate diameter of a red blood cell
      = _____ microns

15. Does the estimated red blood cell diameter agree with published values? _____

Apply the Concepts

1. Determine the size (in microns) of the following cells using charts, books or microscope slides to assist:

   a. Smooth muscle cell _____

   b. Red blood cell _____

   c. White blood cell _____

   d. Platelet_____

   e. Sperm cell _____

   f. Ovum _____

   g. Bacterium_____

ACTIVITY 5.7: MICROSCOPY REVISION

An understanding of microscope components and their functions is essential to correct microscope technique, as is the preparation and documentation of specimens as part of general microscopy.

This activity provides an overview and revision of microscopy technique.

1. Complete the following sentences by filling in the blanks:

   a. The lenses closest to the observer's eyes are the
   _____, and those which are mounted on the revolving turret are the _____.

   b. The light source is focused by moving the _____, and the contrast of the image is adjusted by opening or closing the _____.

   c. When looking at a specimen for the first time, always use the _____ objective first.

   d. When using the high power objective, never use the _____ focus control knob.

   e. The image in a microscope is vertically and horizontally _____.

   f. When a specimen is moved to the left, its image moves to the _____.

   g. As magnification increases, the size of the image _____ and the diameter of the _____ decreases.

2. Explain what is meant by each of the following terms:

   a. Resolution_____

   b. Parfocal _____

   c. Field of view _____

   d. Working distance_____

   e. Coverslip _____

3. From the terms provided, choose one that matches each of the functions listed.

Coarse focus	Objective
Condenser	Resolution
Coverslip	Slide holder
Ocular	Stage
Fine focus	Voltage control
Iris diaphragm	Nosepiece

   a. Increases as magnification increases _____

   b. Used to change magnification _____

   c. Is located inside the condenser _____

   d. Adjusts light intensity_____

   e. Moves up and down during focusing_____

   f. Protects the specimen on the slide_____

   g. Positions the slide on the stage_____

Apply the Concepts

1. You are observing some cells through the high power objective of the microscope (Fig. 5.6). At this magnification, you have determined that the field of view is 400 microns across.

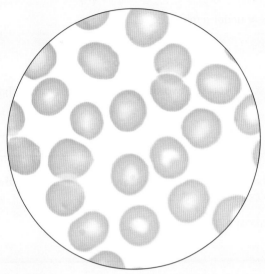

Figure 5.6 Cells observed under high power.
(Source: Turgeon, M. L. (2018). Linne & Ringsrud's clinical laboratory science: concepts, procedures, and clinical applications. Elsevier.)

a. What is the approximate diameter of a single cell?

_____

_____

b. You now make a sketch of one of these cells and measure the diameter of the cell in your drawing as 7.0 cm. What is the magnification of your diagram?

_____

2. A student examines a prepared slide of cheek epithelium cells under the low power of a microscope and has no trouble finding and focusing the cells. When she changes to high power, however, she is unable to bring the cells to clear focus.

a. Give three possible reasons why she could focus under low power but not high power.

_____

_____

_____

3. You are observing an object under low power and switch to high power for a closer view but the object is no longer there.

   a. What did you fail to do before switching to high power?

   _____

4. Draw the letter 'F' as it would appear under a microscope.

5. When you look through the microscope you see two overlapping images rather than a single image.

   a. What do you need to do to correct this?

   _____

6. You are observing white blood cells under high power. You are comfortable with the brightness of the field and the cells are correctly focused but you can see little detail of the cells.

   a. How could you increase the contrast of the image to see more detail?

   _____

   _____

Additional Resources

Histology Guide Virtual Microscopy Laboratory: The Cell
Histology Guide is an online resource providing a virtual microscopy laboratory experience by allowing users to view microscope slides from professional collections for the purpose of interpreting cellular and tissue structures as seen through a microscope.

histologyguide.com/slidebox/01-introduction.html

LabXchange: Microscopes
LabXchange provides a series of learning modules on a variety of topics. The microscopes module investigates different types of microscopes and how an image is formed in a compound microscope.

www.labxchange.org/library/items/lb:LabXchange:5d472313-e99e-3695-b777-5f27ffa4dc99:html:1

LabXchange: Staining Microscopic Specimens
LabXchange provides a series of learning modules on a variety of topics. The staining microscopic specimens module investigates different staining techniques, distinguishing cellular features, and the clinical applications of Gram staining.

www.labxchange.org/library/items/lb:LabXchange:261550f8-a1e1-3628-9324-a5ca34a97d49:html:1

Microscope Master
Microscope Master is an online repository providing information and resources on microscopy, with 'how to' guides, brand information, and background on specific fields of study.

www.microscopemaster.com/

The Virtual Microscope
The Virtual Microscope is a NASA-funded project that aims to provide an online method for exploring pre-captured image data through the ability to load and navigate specimens, change magnification and adjust image parameters.

virtual.itg.uiuc.edu/

Virtual 3D Microscope
An online 3D microscope offered by Oregon State University and created by mounting a camera on top of a microscope to provide a virtual simulation with 3D modelling software.

courses.ecampus.oregonstate.edu/bi206/virtual_scope/build.html

Virtual Labs: Using the Microscope
Virtual Labs provides a series of online simulated lab modules to help students learn basic laboratory techniques and practise methods used by lab technicians and researchers.

virtuallabs.nmsu.edu/micro.php

Virtual Microscope
Virtual Microscope is an online activity provided through BioNetwork which allows learners to interact with a virtual microscope to learn the components of a microscope, determine lens powers and magnification, and discuss care of the microscope.

www.ncbionetwork.org/educational-resources/elearning/interactive-elearning-tools/virtual-microscope

CHAPTER 6
Cells and Metabolism

Cells are the structural units of all living organisms, much as atoms are the fundamental building blocks of matter. The cells comprising an organism may be prokaryotic, where the genetic material exists freely within the cell, or eukaryotic, where the genetic material is enclosed within a membrane-bound nucleus. In addition, eukaryotic cells contain organelles, which are specialised membrane-bound compartments that perform specific tasks to maintain cell function. The study of cells is referred to as cytology. (Refer to Chapter 5: Microscopy, for further information on using microscopes.)

The cellular contents are bounded by the cell membrane, which acts as a barrier between internal and external fluids, regulates what substances enter and exit the cell, and protects the delicate internal cellular organelles. The semi-permeable, fluid nature of the cell membrane constitutes the cell's transport system. Substances such as nutrients are moved across the membrane into the cell based on solubility and size, usually in response to the cell's metabolic requirements.

Cells require nutrients to fuel biochemical reactions such as cell respiration, where cellular energy is synthesised in the form of adenosine triphosphate (ATP). ATP is the primary energy-transferring molecule that allows cells to divide, replicate, and undertake their programmed functions, thereby maintaining the life of the organism. (Refer to Chapter 22: Reproductive System and Heredity, for further information on cell division.)

LEARNING OUTCOMES

On completion of these activities, the student should be able to:

1. outline the theories associated with cell structure and function
2. identify and describe internal and external cell structures
3. describe the structures and functions of cell organelles using micrographs to identify structures
4. describe the composition and properties of the cell membrane
5. explain how surface-to-volume ratio affects transport of substances into cells and determines cell viability
6. identify and discuss the factors affecting transport across the cell membrane
7. differentiate between diffusion, osmosis and active transport, and explain the processes associated with each

LEARNING OUTCOMES—cont'd

8. outline the function of the sodium–potassium pump

9. define tonicity and explain how the concentration of different solutions affects osmotic processes

10. discuss the types and processes of bulk transport

11. outline the role of mitochondria in cell respiration

12. list the stages of cell respiration and outline the pathways and substrates involved in the production of cellular energy

13. discuss the structure of ATP and its role in cell metabolism

14. differentiate between aerobic and anaerobic respiration.

KEY TERMS

Active transport	Endocytosis	Mitochondrion
Adenosine triphosphate (ATP)	Eukaryotic	Nucleus
Aerobic	Exocytosis	Organelle
Anaerobic	Extracellular fluid	Passive transport
Bulk transport	Facilitated diffusion	Phospholipid
Cell	Flagella	Prokaryotic
Cell membrane	Golgi apparatus	Ribosome
Cell respiration	Hydrophilic	Rough endoplasmic reticulum
Cell theory	Hydrophobic	Simple diffusion
Centriole	Hypertonic	Semi-permeable membrane
Chemical energy	Hypotonic	Smooth endoplasmic reticulum
Cilia	Intracellular fluid	Sodium–potassium pump
Compartmentalisation	Isotonic	Surface-volume ratio
Cytoplasm	Metabolism	Tonicity
Diffusion	Microvilli	Vesicle

ACTIVITY 6.1: CELLULAR STRUCTURES AND ORGANELLES

Cells possess specialised internal and external structures. Internal structures or compartments are referred to as **organelles** (little organs) and perform various functions to maintain the life of the cell. Cells are classified based on whether or not they contain a nucleus, a word derived from the Greek for kernel or seed. The **nucleus** is a specialised organelle that contains genetic material. Cells that do not have a nucleus are referred to as **prokaryotic** (before nucleus), and those that do are referred to as **eukaryotic** (good nucleus). Eukaryotic cells typically contain a number of membrane-bound organelles, such as the **rough endoplasmic reticulum**, **smooth endoplasmic reticulum**, **mitochondria**, **Golgi apparatus** and **vesicles**, in addition to organelles that are not membrane-bound, such as ribosomes and **centrioles** (Fig. 6.1). The entire cell and its components are bounded by the **cell membrane**, which can sometimes feature surface specialisations such as **cilia**, **microvilli** and **flagella**. Not all cells contain each of these structures; however, many components are common to all human cells.

This activity highlights the structure and function of cellular components and organelles.

1. Identify the structures of the eukaryotic cell shown in Fig. 6.1, by assigning a letter using the terms provided.

   a. Cell membrane: _____

   b. Centriole: _____

   c. Cilia: _____

   d. Cytoplasm: _____

   e. Desmosome: _____

   f. Free ribosome: _____

   g. Golgi apparatus: _____

   h. Microfilament: _____

   i. Microtubule: _____

   j. Microvilli: _____

   k. Mitochondria: _____

   l. Nuclear envelope: _____

   m. Nuclear pore: _____

   n. Nucleolus: _____

   o. Nucleus: _____

   p. Ribosome: _____

   q. Rough ER: _____

   r. Smooth ER: _____

   s. Tight junction: _____

   t. Vesicle: _____

2. For each cellular structure listed below, briefly state its function.

   a. Cell membrane: _____

   _____

   _____

   b. Centriole: _____

   _____

   _____

   c. Cilia: _____

   _____

   _____

   d. Cytoplasm: _____

   _____

   _____

   e. Cytoskeleton: _____

   _____

   _____

   f. Golgi apparatus: _____

   _____

   _____

   g. Microvilli: _____

   _____

   _____

   h. Mitochondria: _____

   _____

   _____

   i. Nuclear envelope: _____

   _____

   _____

   j. Nuclear pore: _____

   _____

   _____

   k. Nucleolus: _____

   _____

   _____

   l. Nucleus: _____

   _____

   _____

   m. Ribosome: _____

   _____

   _____

   n. Rough endoplasmic reticulum: _____

   _____

   _____

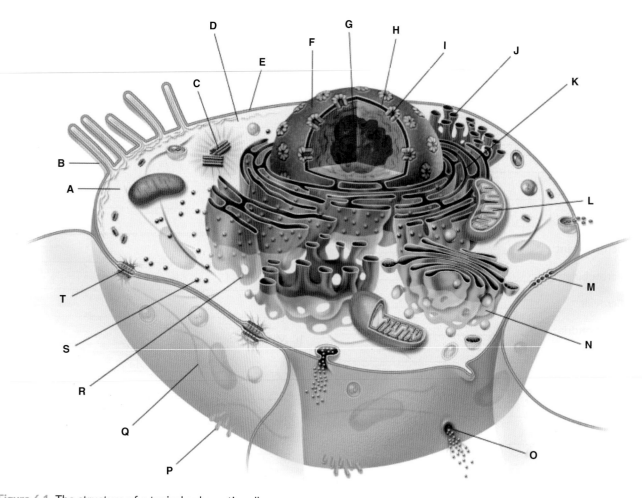

Figure 6.1 The structure of a typical eukaryotic cell.
(Source: Craft, J., Gordon, C., Huether, S. E., McCance, K. L., Brashers, V. L., & List, S. (2019). Understanding pathophysiology. Australia and New Zealand edition. Elsevier.)

o. Smooth endoplasmic reticulum: _____

_____

_____

p. Vesicle: _____

_____

_____

3. Consider the following questions:

a. Which structures form the endomembrane system of the cell and what is the function of this system?

_____

_____

_____

b. How are peroxisomes and lysosomes similar? How are they different?

_____

_____

_____

c. How are cilia and microvilli similar? How are they different?

_____

_____

_____

d. How are cilia and flagella similar? How are they different?

_____

_____

_____

Apply the Concepts

1. Explain why lysosomal disorders are often fatal.

_____

_____

_____

2. Explain why a disorder of the cilia may predispose an individual to respiratory infections.

_____

_____

_____

3. Explain why a disorder of the flagella may render a male infertile.

_____

_____

_____

Additional Activities

For additional activities visit Activity 6A: Cell Theories on Evolve®.

For additional activities visit Activity 6B: Identification of Cell Structures and Organelles on Evolve®.

ACTIVITY 6.2: PROPERTIES OF THE CELL MEMBRANE

The cell membrane is a fluid **phospholipid** bilayer that encloses the cellular contents and provides a physical barrier creating **compartmentation**. This physical barrier separates fluids such as the **cytoplasm** inside the cell, or **intracellular fluid**, and fluids outside the cell, or **extracellular fluid**, while regulating the transport of substances entering and exiting the cell (Fig. 6.2).

This activity highlights the composition and function of the cell membrane and its associated structures.

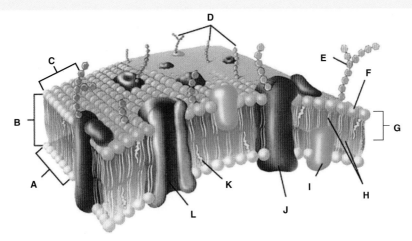

Figure 6.2 The cell (plasma) membrane composed of a phospholipid bilayer.

(Source: Craft, J., Gordon, C., Huether, S. E., McCance, K. L., Brashers, V. L., & List, S. (2019). Understanding pathophysiology. Australia and New Zealand edition. Elsevier.)

1. Identify the structures of the cell membrane shown in Fig. 6.2, using the terms provided.

   a. Carbohydrates: _____

   b. Cholesterol: _____

   c. External surface: _____

   d. Glycolipid: _____

   e. Glycoprotein: _____

   f. Hydrophilic head: _____

   g. Hydrophobic tail: _____

   h. Integral protein: _____

   i. Internal surface: _____

   j. Channel protein: _____

   k. Phospholipid: _____

   l. Phospholipid bilayer: _____

2. Consider the following questions:

   a. What are the three main components of the cell membrane?

   _____

   _____

   b. What is a phospholipid?

   _____

   _____

   c. How are phospholipids arranged in the cell membrane to form a phospholipid bilayer?

   _____

   _____

   _____

   d. Explain why the structure of the cell membrane is referred to as a fluid mosaic model.

   _____

   _____

   _____

   e. What are the functions of the glycolipids and glycoproteins in the cell membrane?

   _____

   _____

   f. List the six functions of the membrane-embedded proteins.

   _____

   _____

   _____

   _____

   g. Membrane proteins also have hydrophilic regions as well as hydrophobic regions. Which part of a membrane protein would you predict is hydrophilic and which is hydrophobic?

   _____

   _____

   _____

   h. List the three types of cell junctions and explain the characteristics of each.

   _____

   _____

   _____

3. Match the membrane properties listed below with the membrane structures responsible for that property. (Note: some membrane structures may be used more than once.)

   Membrane Properties

   1. Substances soluble in lipids move with relative ease between the cell and the surrounding medium.

   2. Many chemical reactions take place on the surface of cell membranes.

   3. Some substances that are capable of binding to proteins move into cells much faster than similar substances which cannot bind to proteins.

   4. Small particles, such as sodium ions, pass through membranes much more easily than large particles, such as polysaccharides.

   5. The size and nature of the charge on an ion affects the rate at which it moves across a membrane.

6. Membranes are good electrical insulators. The electrical charge outside a membrane is often different from the charge inside the membrane.

7. Uncharged particles cross membranes more rapidly than charged particles.

Membrane Structures

A. Cylindrical protein molecules form pores that penetrate the phospholipid bilayer.

B. A membrane is essentially a double layer of lipid molecules.

C. Some protein molecules can move from one side of a membrane to the other.

D. Many different protein molecules are embedded in the phospholipid bilayer.

E. Membrane pores are lined with groups which carry an electric charge.

Membrane property	Membrane structures
1.	_____
2.	_____
3.	_____
4.	_____
5.	_____
6.	_____
7.	_____

ACTIVITY 6.3: CELL MEMBRANE TRANSPORT MECHANISMS

The cell membrane is essential to the transport of substances into and out of the cell (Fig. 6.3). Diffusion refers to the movement of particles from an area of high concentration (where there are more particles) to an area of low concentration (where there are fewer particles). This process is dependent upon a concentration gradient. Only certain particles can cross the cell membrane directly (**simple diffusion**) without the aid of membrane-embedded transport proteins (**facilitated diffusion**). The simultaneous transport of a large quantity of particles or a single large particle, requires **bulk transport** methods. In addition, specialised membrane proteins driven by **active transport** and referred to as **sodium–potassium pumps** (Na^+–K^+ pumps), assist in transporting sodium and potassium ions against concentration gradients in order to stabilise ionic gradients across cell membranes (Fig. 6.4).

This activity outlines the mechanisms of trans-membrane cellular transport.

1. Identify each of the cellular transport mechanisms shown in Fig. 6.3:

   a. Mechanism 1:_____

   b. Mechanism 2:_____

   c. Mechanism 3:_____

   d. Mechanism 4:_____

   e. Mechanism 5:_____

2. Consider the following questions:

   a. Name three substances that are able to move directly across the cell membrane.

   _____

   _____

   _____

b. Simple diffusion and facilitated diffusion are also referred to by what other term?

   _____

c. How does water move across the cell membrane in the process of osmosis?

   _____

   _____

d. Glucose moves into many cells through facilitated diffusion. Why is this the case?

   _____

   _____

   _____

   _____

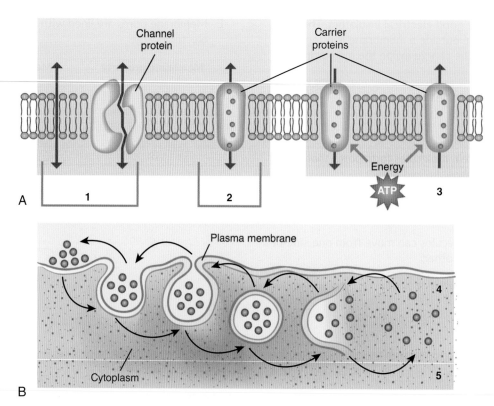

Figure 6.3 Cellular transport mechanisms. **A** Methods of diffusion. **B** Bulk transport.
(Source: Grodner, M., Escott-Stump, S., Dorner, S. (2020). Nutritional foundations and clinical applications: a nursing approach. Elsevier.)

e. What distinguishes passive transport from active transport?

_____

_____

_____

f. Explain why bulk transport is considered a form of active transport.

_____

_____

g. What are the two types of endocytosis?

_____

h. What is transported in phagocytosis?

_____

_____

i. What is transported in pinocytosis?

_____

_____

j. What is transported in exocytosis?

_____

_____

k. Why would a cell use endocytosis rather than a transport protein for transport?

_____

_____

3. Identify and explain the processes occurring in each of the stages shown in Fig. 6.4:

a. Stage A: _____

_____

b. Stage B: _____

_____

c. Stage C: _____

_____

d. Stage D: _____

_____

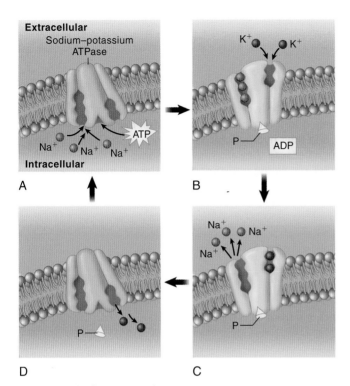

Figure 6.4 Sodium–potassium pump.
(Source: Patton, K. T., Thibodeau, G. A., & Hutton, A. (2019). Anatomy and physiology. Adapted international edition. Elsevier.)

4. Consider the following questions:

   a. What is the purpose of the Na$^+$-K$^+$ pump?

   _____

   _____

   b. Why is the Na$^+$-K$^+$ pump referred to as sodium–potassium ATPase?

   _____

   _____

   c. Why do sodium and potassium ions not enter the pump simultaneously?

   _____

   _____

   d. Why is the pump able to transport three sodium ions but only two potassium ions?

   _____

   _____

Apply the Concepts

1. What relationship do Na$^+$-K$^+$ pumps have with the nervous system?

   _____

   _____

2. What is digoxin and how does it affect Na$^+$-K$^+$ pumps?

   _____

   _____

3. Explain why H$^+$–K$^+$ ATPase is referred to as a proton pump.

   _____

   _____

4. What is a proton pump inhibitor?

   _____

   _____

ACTIVITY 6.4: POLARITY AND TRANSPORT ACROSS THE CELL MEMBRANE

The cell membrane is composed of phospholipids, which contain a **hydrophilic** (water-loving) head and two **hydrophobic** (water-fearing) tails. The phospholipids are arranged in a bilayer with their hydrophilic heads aligned towards the water-based internal and external environments, and their hydrophobic tails aligned to the inside of the membrane. This arrangement allows some items to pass through because they are small and non-polar (lipid-soluble) and excludes other items that are large and polar (water-soluble), regulating transport across the cell membrane.

This activity provides a visual model of diffusion across the cell membrane based on the polarity of substances.

 To conduct this activity, it is important to ensure the following safety precautions:

- *Methylene blue is a strong stain and can cause irritation.*
- *Scarlet R (Sudan IV) is a strong stain and can cause irritation.*
- *Ensure disposable gloves and safety glasses are worn at all times and the area is well-ventilated.*

1. This activity is best conducted in pairs.

2. Obtain two wide-mouthed test tubes, glass marker, deionised water, disposable pipettes, liquid paraffin, methylene blue, ethanol, scarlet R dye (Sudan IV), safety glasses and disposable gloves.

3. Ensure the test tubes are clean and dry. Label these 1 and 2.

4. Add 5 mL deionised water to test tube 1, using a pipette.

5. Add 5 mL liquid paraffin using a pipette. Note your observations.

   a. Does the paraffin mix with the water? Explain based on the polarity of both substances.

   _____

   _____

   _____

6. Add 2 drops methylene blue. Agitate the tube gently and note your observations.

   a. Which layer does the methylene blue dissolve in?

   _____

7. Add 6 drops scarlet R stain. Agitate the tube gently and note your observations.

   a. Which layer does the scarlet R dissolve in?

   _____

b. What do your observations indicate about the solubility of methylene blue and scarlet R?

   _____

   _____

   _____

8. Add 5 mL deionised water to test tube 2, using a pipette.

9. Add 2 drops methylene blue. Agitate the tube gently.

10. Add 5 mL paraffin using a pipette. Do not agitate the tube.

11. Add 5 mL ethanol using a pipette. Do not pour the ethanol into the tube, but gently trickle it down the side of the test tube. Do not agitate the tube.

12. Add 2 drops methylene blue. Do not agitate the tube. Note your observations.

13. Consider the following questions, assuming that test tube 2 represents a model cell membrane system:

   a. Which of the substances represents the internal cytoplasm of the cell, the cell membrane and the cell exterior?

   _____

   _____

b. If scarlet R represents a substance required by the cell, what does this indicate about the transport of non-polar substances across the cell membrane?

_____

_____

_____

c. If methylene blue represents a substance required by the cell, what does this indicate about the transport of polar substances across the cell membrane?

_____

_____

_____

d. In a cell, what would be required to allow polar substances to cross the cell membrane?

_____

_____

_____

ACTIVITY 6.5: DIFFUSION ACROSS MEMBRANES BASED ON PARTICLE SIZE

In order for a particle to cross a cell membrane via simple diffusion, the particle must be non-polar (lipid-soluble), such as cholesterol or steroids, or very small, such as oxygen or carbon dioxide. If the particles are not small enough, they will not be able to passively cross the membrane. Instead, they must be transported into the cell via facilitated diffusion, which requires membrane-embedded transport proteins. Both simple diffusion and facilitated diffusion require the presence of a concentration gradient to drive particle movement.

This activity investigates diffusion across cell membranes by comparing the diffusion of chemical compounds with different molar masses.

 To conduct this activity, it is important to ensure the following safety precautions:

- _Methylene blue is a strong stain and can cause irritation._
- _Wear safety glasses and disposable gloves when handling chemical compounds._
- _Dispose of chemical compounds as indicated by your demonstrator._

1. This activity is best conducted in pairs.

2. Determine the chemical formula and calculate the formula mass of the substances to be tested in the table provided.

3. Obtain a Petri dish (containing agar gel or edible gelatine), permanent marker, potassium permanganate, copper sulfate pentahydrate, methylene blue, Janus green, forceps, stopwatch, ruler, incubator, safety glasses and disposable gloves.

4. Score the underside of the Petri dish containing the gel into four quadrants with a black marker.

5. Place single, equal-sized granules of each substance to be tested in separate quadrants on the gel.

6. Gently press the granules into the gel with forceps to ensure good contact with the medium.

7. Leave the dish for 1 hour (placing the Petri dish in an incubator at 37°C will speed up the process).

8. After 1 hour, measure the diameter of the circle formed by the crystals in each quadrant with a ruler, recording your results in the table provided.

Substance tested	Chemical formula	Molar mass (g/mol)	Circle diameter (mm)
Potassium permanganate			
Copper sulfate pentahydrate			
Methylene blue			
Janus green			

9. Consider the following questions:

   a. What relationship exists between molar mass and particle size?

   _____

   _____

   _____

   b. What relationship seems to exist between molar mass and diffusion?

   _____

   _____

   _____

   c. How do the findings relate to simple diffusion into cells?

   _____

   _____

   _____

   d. Identify two substances that enter cells via simple diffusion.

   _____

   e. How are substances transported into cells when particle size increases to the point where diffusion is no longer possible?

   _____

   _____

   _____

   f. Identify two substances that cannot enter cells via simple diffusion.

   _____

   g. What other factors can affect diffusion into cells?

   _____

   _____

   h. How are simple diffusion and facilitated diffusion different? How are they similar?

   _____

   _____

   _____

   _____

ACTIVITY 6.6: DIFFUSION IN CELL MODELS (SURFACE–VOLUME RATIO)

Movement of materials into and out of cells must occur through the cell membrane. The size and surface area of the cell together determine the efficiency of **diffusion** into the cell. This relationship is referred to as the surface-area-to-volume ratio, or **surface–volume ratio**. In cells, a high surface-area-to-volume ratio greatly increases the efficiency of diffusion and absorption at the cell membrane, but can also lead to increased environmental exposure and water loss at the surface. Multicellular organisms are equipped with mechanisms to ensure survival despite the high surface-volume ratios of their cells.

In this activity, cubes of agar will act as cell models to determine the extent of diffusion. Agar is a gelatinous material which causes liquid media to gel into solids. The agar used in this activity has been impregnated with phenolphthalein, a colourless acid-base indicator that turns pink or red when it comes into contact with a base such as sodium hydroxide (NaOH). The extent of diffusion can be determined by how far the red colour penetrates into the cubes.

This activity demonstrates the effectiveness of diffusion based on the surface–volume ratio of an object.

 To conduct this activity, it is important to ensure the following safety precautions:

- *Sodium hydroxide (NaOH) is caustic and should not be handled with bare hands.*

- *Wear safety glasses and disposable gloves at all times during the activity.*

1. This activity is best conducted in pairs.

2. Obtain three cubes of prepared agar (1 × 1 cm, 3 × 3 cm, 5 × 5 cm), 500 mL glass beaker, 0.1 M NaOH, stopwatch, spoon, paper towels, knife, ruler, safety glasses and disposable gloves.

3. Place all three cubes into the empty beaker, so that the cubes do not touch each other or the sides of the beaker.

4. Calculate the surface area, volume, surface–volume ratio and surface-volume index of each cube, recording your calculations in the table provided. The surface-volume ratio can be expressed as a single number or index to compare the surface–volume ratio in the different cubes.

5. Pour the NaOH solution over the cubes to cover them completely.

6. Allow the cubes to remain submerged for a period of 12 minutes.

7. After 12 minutes, carefully remove the cubes from the solution with a spoon and place on a paper towel to drain.

8. Cut each cube in half with a knife to observe how far the NaOH has diffused into each cube. This can be determined by the red-coloured boundary inside each cube and measured with a ruler. The uncoloured area indicates where NaOH did not diffuse.

9. Calculate the volume of the uncoloured area within each cube, assuming that diffusion occurred evenly throughout the cube, recording your calculations in the table provided.

10. Calculate the volume of the coloured area within each cube, recording your calculations in the table provided.

11. Calculate the percentage of NaOH diffusion for each cube, recording your calculations in the table provided.

Cube size (cm)	Surface area[1] (cm^2)	Total volume[2] (cm^3)	Surface-volume ratio[3]	Surface-volume index[4]	Volume of uncoloured area[5] (cm^3)	Volume of coloured area[6] (cm^3)	Percentage of diffusion[7] (%)
1 × 1							
3 × 3							
5 × 5							

Notes:
1. Surface area = cube length (cm) × cube length (cm) × 6
2. Total volume = length × width × height
3. Surface-volume ratio = answer to (1) : answer to (2)
4. Surface-volume index = answer to (1) ÷ answer to (2)
5. Volume of uncoloured area = length × width × height of uncoloured area
6. Volume of coloured area = total volume − volume of uncoloured area
7. Percentage of diffusion = coloured area volume ÷ total cube volume × 100

12. Consider the following:

a. Why did the NaOH diffuse into the cube? Did any of the phenolphthalein diffuse out of the cube? Explain.

_____

_____

_____

b. Consider the surface-volume index for each cube and explain how this relates to differences in diffusion between the cubes.

_____

_____

_____

c. Into which cube was the largest percentage of volume reached by diffusion? Why?

_____

_____

_____

_____

d. Compare the surface-volume index with the percentage of diffusion for each cube. Explain whether there is a pattern between these two factors.

_____

_____

_____

e. Based on the information collected, explain whether it is biologically more practical for cells to be small or large.

_____

_____

_____

_____

ACTIVITY 6.7: CELLULAR OSMOSIS MODELS

Cell membranes are **semi-permeable** or selectively permeable. Water can only enter and exit cells via protein channels called aquaporins that span the thickness of the cell membrane. The water surrounding cells usually contains particles in solution. The water in this solution will move from an area of low particle concentration to an area of high particle concentration, down the osmotic gradient across the cell membrane. This will cause the water volume in the area of high particle concentration to increase, resulting in visible changes to the cell.

This activity demonstrates the process of osmosis in cells utilising a raw chicken egg as a model cell.

 To conduct this activity, it is important to ensure the following safety precautions:

• *Wear safety glasses and disposable gloves during the activity as hydrochloric acid may cause skin irritation.*

1. This activity is best conducted in pairs.

2. Obtain a raw chicken egg, 1000 mL measuring cylinder, 3.0 M HCl, stopwatch, paper towels, electronic scale, deionised water, 500 mL glass beaker, spoon, 0.9% NaCl solution, 20% NaCl solution, safety glasses and disposable gloves.

3. Place the egg carefully in the measuring cylinder.

4. Pour over enough HCl to completely cover the egg. The acid will dissolve the shell exposing the underlying membrane. This process should take about 3 minutes.

    a. Did a reaction occur? Explain the reaction chemically.

    _____

    _____

    _____

    b. Why is it necessary to remove the eggshell?

    _____

    _____

    _____

5. Leave any shell that remains on the surface of the egg intact as removing it may affect the integrity of the exposed membrane. It is important to handle the egg carefully as the exposed membrane is delicate and the egg is raw.

6. Place the egg on a paper towel to drain and gently pat dry.

7. Measure the mass of the egg using an electronic scale, recording the mass in the table provided.

8. Place the egg in the beaker and pour over enough deionised water to completely cover the egg.

9. Leave the egg in the solution for 8 minutes, then remove the egg to a paper towel with a spoon and gently pat dry.

10. Measure the mass of the egg as before, recording the mass in the table provided.

11. Place the egg on a spoon and gently rinse with cool tap water.

12. Place the egg in the beaker and pour over enough 0.9% NaCl solution to completely cover the egg.

13. Leave the egg in the solution for 8 minutes, then remove the egg to a paper towel with a spoon and gently pat dry.

14. Measure the mass of the egg as before, recording the mass in the table provided.

15. Place the egg on a spoon and gently rinse with cool tap water.

16. Place the egg in the beaker and pour over enough 20% NaCl solution to completely cover the egg.

17. Leave the egg in the water for 8 minutes, then remove the egg to a paper towel with a spoon and gently pat dry.

18. Measure the mass of the egg as before, recording the mass in the table provided.

19. Dispose of the egg as indicated by your instructor.

20. Calculate the changes in mass for the egg and record your findings in the table provided.

Solution	Initial mass (g)	Final mass (g)	Change in mass (g)	Tonicity of solution
Deionised water				
0.9% NaCl				
20% NaCl				

21. Consider the following:

a. Explain the principle of osmosis.

_____

_____

_____

_____

b. Explain the changes in the mass of the egg in each solution, based on the principle of osmosis.

_____

_____

_____

_____

c. What would happen if the egg was left in deionised water overnight?

_____

_____

_____

d. Explain what would happen if the egg were placed in 20% NaCl solution for 8 minutes and then placed in deionised water for 8 minutes.

_____

_____

_____

e. Explain whether anything other than water passed between the egg and the solutions.

_____

_____

_____

f. The 0.9% NaCl solution represents what type of fluid?

_____

Apply the Concepts

1. Normal saline is the only intravenous solution that can be infused at the same time as blood products. Explain why, based on tonicity.

_____

_____

_____

2. Why might deionised water followed by 5% glucose be administered to increase blood volume?

_____

_____

_____

ACTIVITY 6.8: OSMOSIS IN RED BLOOD CELLS (HAEMOLYSIS)

Red blood cells (RBCs) provide a perfect model for testing the effects of extracellular concentration (**tonicity**) on osmosis across cell membranes. Since they exist as single cells, the integrity of their cell membranes is not dependent on other cells. They also contain haemoglobin and, due to its red colour, this can be used to determine whether the cell is intact or not. When viable RBCs are placed in a solution similar to their internal concentration (an isotonic solution) very little nett movement of water occurs across the cell membrane and the cells maintain their characteristic biconcave shape. When RBCs are placed in a solution that is less concentrated than their internal concentration (a hypotonic solution), water moves into the cells via osmosis, causing the cells to swell and lose their biconcave shape. As water continues to enter the cell, the cell membrane will stretch and the cell will burst (lyse) allowing the haemoglobin to leak out and leave behind the empty cell. Alternatively, when RBCs are placed in a solution that is more concentrated than their internal concentration (a hypertonic solution), water moves out of the cells causing the cells to shrivel and crenate.

A suspension of viable RBCs is opaque. It is not possible to see through the suspension because the intact cells and their contained haemoglobin block the light. When the cells burst (haemolyse), the blood mixture will become a transparent red colour because the membranes no longer block the light and the released haemoglobin goes into solution, tinting the liquid red. Once the cells are dead, the suspension clears. The time taken for the RBCs to lyse can be measured based on the rate of clarification of the resulting suspension.

This activity demonstrates the effect of a series of salt (NaCl) solutions at different concentrations on RBC integrity due to osmosis.

 To conduct this activity, it is important to ensure the following safety precautions:

- *Body fluids will be used in this laboratory; exercise caution at all times.*

- *Wear disposable gloves, a disposable apron and safety glasses at all times during the activity as blood may harbour biological hazards.*

- *Additional precautions, including safe disposal of blood materials, may be required by your demonstrator.*

1. This activity is best conducted in groups of three.

2. Obtain 4 test tubes, glass marker, 0.145 M NaCl solution, 0.000 M deionised water, 0.065 M NaCl solution, 0.350 M NaCl solution, heparinised blood, Parafilm, stopwatch, desk lamp, white paper with black print, disposable pipettes, safety glasses and disposable gloves.

3. Label the test tubes 1 to 4 and half-fill each test tube with the solutions as indicated in the table provided.

4. Transfer 5 drops of heparinised blood into test tube 1.

5. Immediately seal the test tube with Parafilm and gently agitate the suspension by tilting the tube upside down once.

6. Start timing the reaction. This is time zero.

7. Immediately hold the test tube up to a bright light source, such as a desk lamp, with a test frame held between the tube and the light source (a square of white paper with black print on it will work as a test frame).

8. Continue to observe the print on the test frame through the test tube.

9. Stop the time when the print on the test frame can first be clearly seen through the suspension. This is the time taken for the suspension to haemolyse (become clear).

10. Record the time taken for the suspension to haemolyse in the table provided.

11. Repeat the procedure with the remaining test tubes.

12. Dispose of any blood and return any items having come in contact with blood as indicated by your demonstrator.

Test tube	Solution	NaCl concentration (M)	Time taken to haemolyse (s)	Relative rate of penetration[1] (s^{-1})
1	Isotonic	0.145		
2	Deionised water	0.000		
3	Hypotonic	0.065		
4	Hypertonic	0.350		

1. Relative rate of penetration (rrp) = 1 ÷ time (seconds)
If the time is greater than 10 minutes, record time as > 600 seconds and rrp as < 0.002 s^{-1}

13. Consider the following questions:

a. Why was deionised water used as a test solution? Is deionised water isotonic or hypotonic compared to the tonicity of the red blood cells?

_____

_____

b. Explain whether haemolysis occurred readily in the deionised water compared to the hypotonic solution.

_____

_____

c. Explain whether haemolysis readily occurred in the hypertonic solution.

_____

_____

_____

Apply the Concepts

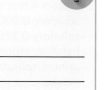

1. Relate the administration of physiological saline to the hydration of human body cells and tissues.

_____

_____

_____

Additional Activities

For additional activities visit Activity 6C: Yeast as an Active Transport Model on Evolve*.

For additional activities visit Activity 6D: *Amoeba* as a Vesicular Transport Model (Endocytosis) on Evolve*.

ACTIVITY 6.9: ORGANELLES ASSOCIATED WITH PROTEIN PROCESSING

The Golgi apparatus is a membranous organelle that processes and packages protein molecules received from the rough endoplasmic reticulum via small vesicles (Fig. 6.5). After entering the Golgi apparatus, proteins undergo a series of chemical modifications as they move through the cisternae and are packaged within a membranous vesicle when the process is complete. The vesicle migrates to, and merges with, the external cell membrane, releasing its contents outside the cell. Some vesicles remain inside the cell serving as storage vessels for the substance to be secreted.

This activity highlights the functional relationship between the rough endoplasmic reticulum and the Golgi apparatus in the production and packaging of proteins.

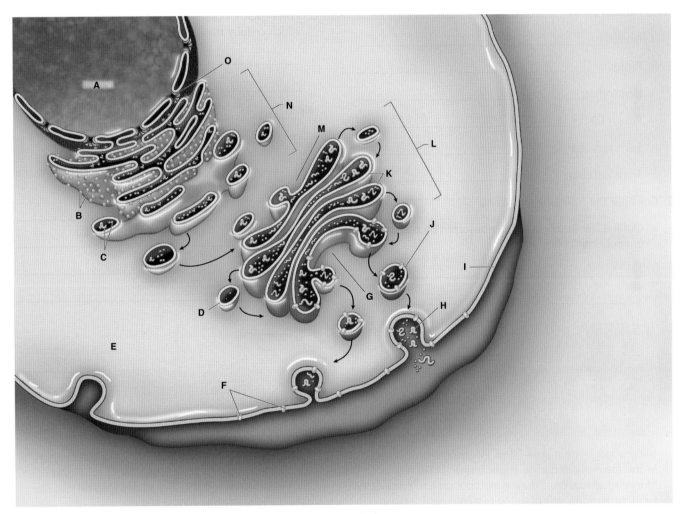

Figure 6.5 Rough endoplasmic reticulum and Golgi apparatus associations.
(Source: Patton, K. T., Thibodeau, G. A., & Hutton, A. (2016). Anatomy and physiology. Elsevier.)

1. Identify the structures of the trans-Golgi network shown in Fig. 6.5, using the terms provided.

   a. Cell membrane:_____

   b. Cis cisterna: _____

   c. Cisternae: _____

   d. Cytoplasm:_____

   e. Exocytosis:_____

   f. Golgi apparatus: _____

   g. Golgi vesicle: _____

   h. Membrane proteins: _____

   i. Nuclear pore: _____

   j. Nucleus:_____

   k. Proteins:_____

   l. Ribosomes:_____

   m. Rough ER: _____

   n. Secretory vesicle:_____

   o. Trans cisterna: _____

2. Consider the following questions:

   a. Outline the function of the ribosomes on the rough endoplasmic reticulum.

   _____

   _____

   b. How are items transported between the rough endoplasmic reticulum and the Golgi apparatus?

   _____

   _____

   _____

   c. The proximity of the nucleus to the rough endoplasmic reticulum and the Golgi apparatus has what functional significance?

   _____

   _____

   _____

   d. The vesicle exiting the cell in the diagram represents which cellular transport process?

   _____

   _____

   _____

   e. Disregarding the black arrows provided in the diagram, how can you tell that the vesicle at the bottom of the diagram is exiting and not entering the cell?

   _____

   _____

   _____

ACTIVITY 6.10: MITOCHONDRIA, CELL RESPIRATION AND ATP PRODUCTION

Mitochondria are matrix-filled, membrane-bound organelles that play a vital role in the production of cellular energy in the form of **adenosine triphosphate (ATP)** (Fig. 6.6). Cells utilise substances from the nutrient pool to undertake biochemical reactions during **metabolism** and produce ATP in a series of processes referred to as **cell respiration**. The term 'respiration' refers to the requirement for oxygen in human cells. Cells producing ATP in the presence of oxygen are termed **aerobic**, while those producing ATP in the absence of oxygen are termed **anaerobic**. Aerobic respiration is utilised by human cells as it produces ATP more efficiently than does anaerobic respiration, although some cells, such as skeletal muscle cells and red blood cells, are capable of anaerobic respiration. Anaerobic respiration pathways lead to fermentation and lactic acid production.

This activity highlights the structure of mitochondria and outlines the process of cell metabolism in the production of ATP.

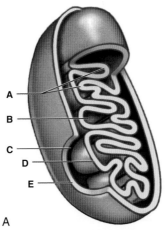

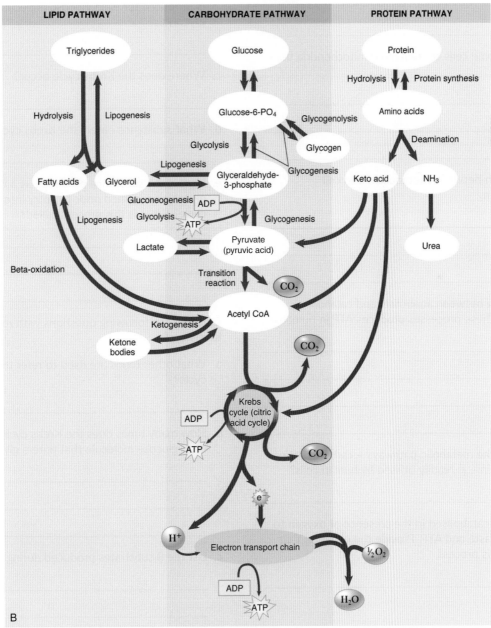

Figure 6.6 Cell respiration and ATP production. **A** Mitochondrion showing internal structures. **B** Metabolic pathways that produce ATP showing relationships between pathways.
*(Source: **A** Herlihy, B. (2022). The human body in health and illness. Elsevier. **B** Patton, K. T., Thibodeau, G. A., & Hutton, A. (2019). Anatomy and physiology. Elsevier.)*

1. Identify the structures of the mitochondrion shown in Fig. 6.6A, using the terms provided.

   a. Cristae: _____

   b. Inner membrane: _____

   c. Intermembranous space: _____

   d. Matrix:_____

   e. Outer membrane: _____

2. Consider the following, with reference to metabolism:

   a. Where are the enzymes responsible for producing ATP located within the mitochondrion?

   _____

   b. Why do some cells contain more mitochondria than others?

   _____

   _____

   _____

   c. Distinguish between metabolism and cell metabolism.

   _____

   _____

   _____

   d. Distinguish between anabolism and catabolism. Which of these processes produces ATP in humans?

   _____

   _____

   _____

   _____

   e. Which of the metabolic pathways – carbohydrate, lipid, protein – is readily utilised by human cells?

   _____

   f. Glucose is catabolised in the presence of oxygen to produce waste and ATP. Provide the equation that outlines this process.

   _____

   g. List the three stages of glucose catabolism (cell respiration).

   _____

   _____

3. Consider the following questions with reference to glycolysis:

   a. Where does glycolysis occur and is it an aerobic or anaerobic process?

   _____

   b. What is the final product of glycolysis and how much is produced for each glucose molecule entering glycolysis?

   _____

   c. Where does the Krebs cycle occur?

   _____

   d. What substance enters the Krebs cycle?

   _____

   e. How is the substance produced as a result of glycolysis modified prior to entry into the Krebs cycle? What is this process called?

   _____

   _____

   _____

4. Consider the following questions with reference to the Krebs cycle:

   a. What other terms are used to refer to the Krebs cycle?

   _____

   b. How many times does the Krebs cycle operate for each glucose molecule that enters glycolysis?

   _____

   _____

   _____

   c. List the 8 substrates produced during the Krebs cycle.

   _____

   _____

   _____

5. Consider the following questions with reference to the electron transport chain:

   a. What do NAD$^+$ and FAD$^+$ carry? How many does each carry? What is the destination of their cargo?

   _____

   _____

   _____

   b. Distinguish between substrate-level phosphorylation and oxidative phosphorylation. Where do each occur?

   _____

   _____

   _____

   _____

   c. Describe the process of chemiosmosis. Where does this occur?

   _____

   _____

   _____

   _____

   d. What is the name of the enzyme responsible for oxidative phosphorylation? Where are these enzymes located? What powers this enzyme to function?

   _____

   _____

   _____

   e. What purpose does oxygen serve in cell respiration and when is it needed?

   _____

   _____

   _____

6. How many net ATP molecules are produced as a result of:

   a. Glycolysis _____

   b. The Krebs cycle _____

   c. The electron transport chain _____

7. Consider the following questions with reference to metabolic pathways:

   a. What waste products are produced as a result of glucose catabolism?

   _____

   _____

   b. What product do the carbohydrate, lipid and protein catabolism pathways have in common?

   _____

   c. What useful and waste products are specific to the lipid catabolism pathway?

   _____

   _____

   d. What useful and waste products are specific to the protein catabolism pathway?

   _____

   _____

8. Consider the following questions with reference to ATP:

   a. Where is the energy required for cellular processes stored in ATP?

   _____

   _____

   b. How is this energy released?

   _____

   _____

   _____

   c. What is the origin of the energy stored in ATP bonds?

   _____

   _____

   d. What does the term phosphorylation refer to? Is this a reversible reaction?

   _____

   _____

   _____

Apply the Concepts

1. Muscle cells contain many mitochondria. Explain how this relates to their function.

_____

_____

_____

2. Identify two physiological effects that may result from a mitochondrial disorder.

_____

_____

_____

Additional Activities

For additional activities visit Activity 6E: Glucose and Sucrose Oxidation on Evolve°.

For additional activities visit Activity 6F: Aerobic Respiration and Carbon Dioxide Waste on Evolve°.

For additional activities visit Activity 6G: Yeast as an Aerobic and Anaerobic Cell Respiration Model on Evolve°.

Additional Resources

BBC Bitesize: Cellular Respiration
BBC Bitesize provides lessons, revision material and tests on a number of human biology-related topics, including cellular respiration and the production of ATP.
www.bbc.co.uk/bitesize/guides/zdq9382/revision/1

BioVisions
BioVisions provides a series of video animations with transcripts documenting cellular structures and processes. It is produced by Harvard University.
www.labxchange.org/org/BioVisions

Cell Image Library
The Cell Image Library is a repository for images and movies of cells from a variety of organisms and demonstrates cellular architecture and functions with high-quality images, videos and animations, with the goal of improving human health.
www.cellimagelibrary.org/home

CELLS alive!
CELLS alive! is an online resource capturing film and computer-enhanced images of living cells and organisms for education and medical research.
www.cellsalive.com/

Gizmos: Osmosis
An interactive simulation with lesson materials where users adjust the concentration of a solute on either side of a membrane in a cell and observe the system as it adjusts to the conditions through osmosis.
gizmos.explorelearning.com/index.cfm?method5cResource.dspDetail&ResourceID=418

Histology Guide Virtual Microscopy Laboratory: The Cell
Histology Guide is an online resource providing a virtual microscopy laboratory experience by allowing users to view microscope slides from professional collections for the purpose of interpreting cellular and tissue structures as seen through a microscope.
histologyguide.com/slidebox/01-introduction.html

Khan Academy: Metabolism and Thermoregulation
Video tutorials outlining the relationship between metabolism, temperature regulation and metabolic rate.
www.khanacademy.org/science/biology/principles-of-physiology#metabolism-and-thermoregulation

Osmosis – Cellular and Molecular Biology
The Cellular and Molecular Biology module of Osmosis provides videos, notes, quiz questions and links to further resources related to cells and cellular structures.
www.osmosis.org/library/md/foundational-sciences/cellular-and-molecular-biology

The Concord Consortium
The Concord Consortium provides a series of interactive simulations on a range of atomic, molecular and cellular topics in a number of languages.
www.labxchange.org/org/concordconsortium

The Histology Guide: The Cell
The Histology Guide is a virtual experience of using a microscope with zoom features. It is divided into topics and offers histological slides with labels and quizzes for each topic, such as cells. It is provided by the University of Leeds.
www.histology.leeds.ac.uk/cell/index.php

CHAPTER 7
Tissues and Organs

Humans are multicellular organisms. Their many different kinds of cells are organised into tissues. A tissue may be defined as a collection of cells, usually of similar origin, whose activities are coordinated to perform a common set of functions. There are four basic tissues in the human body: epithelial, connective, muscle and nervous tissue. The location of each tissue type within the body and individual organs is directly related to the individual structure and function of each tissue. (Refer to Chapter 12: Nervous System for further information on nervous tissue; Chapter 11: Muscular System for further information on skeletal muscle, and Chapter 16: Cardiovascular System for further information on cardiac muscle.) The study of tissues is referred to as histology. (Refer to Chapter 5: Microscopy, for further information on microscope use.)

Cells are arranged into tissues, and tissues are arranged into organs. An organ is a structurally distinct part of the body which performs a particular function. Typically, an organ is composed of several types of tissues that have a highly organised structural relationship with each other. Organs are then arranged into organ systems which are comprised of several different organs, each contributing a specific task to the overall role of the organ system.

LEARNING OUTCOMES

On completion of these activities, the student should be able to:

1. describe the classification, structure and function of epithelial tissue
2. compare and overview the characteristics of epithelial tissue
3. investigate diffusion and protection in epithelial tissue
4. describe the structure and function of epithelial exocrine glands
5. describe the classification, structure and function of connective tissue
6. compare and overview the characteristics of connective tissue
7. investigate the properties of fat and collagen within connective tissue
8. describe the classification, structure and function of muscle tissue
9. compare and overview the characteristics of muscle tissue

LEARNING OUTCOMES—cont'd

10. describe the classification, structure and function of nervous tissue

11. identify epithelial, connective, muscle and nervous tissues based on physical characteristics

12. conduct microscopic examinations of epithelial, connective, muscle and nervous tissues

13. identify epithelial, connective, muscle and nervous tissue associations within various organs.

KEY TERMS

Basement membrane
Blood
Bone
Cardiac muscle
Cartilage
Collagen
Connective tissue
Connective tissue proper
Dense connective tissue
Elastin
Endothelium

Epithelial tissue
Epithelium
Exocrine gland
Glandular epithelial tissue
Ground substance
Loose connective tissue
Matrix
Mesothelium
Muscle tissue
Nerve
Nervous tissue

Neuroglia
Neuron
Organ
Pseudostratified epithelium
Simple epithelium
Skeletal muscle
Smooth muscle
Stratified epithelium
Tissue

ACTIVITY 7.1: CLASSIFICATION OF EPITHELIAL TISSUE

Epithelial tissue, also referred to as epithelium, consists of sheets of cells that are held together in a brick-like arrangement. Classification is based on the shape and arrangement of the cells within the tissue (Fig. 7.1 and Fig. 7.2). Epithelial tissues exhibit polarity; that is, they consist of two surfaces – the apical surface which borders open spaces and the basal surface or basement membrane which faces underlying tissue. Epithelia that line internal body surfaces where the apical surface borders an internal cavity are referred to as endothelium, while epithelia that are found within serous membranes are referred to as mesothelium. Epithelial tissues cover body surfaces, line cavities and form glands. They are avascular, meaning they do not contain a blood supply; they also do not contain a nerve supply; however, cells at the apical surface may possess surface specialisations which assist in their overall function.

This activity investigates the classification of epithelial tissues based on cell shape and cell arrangement.

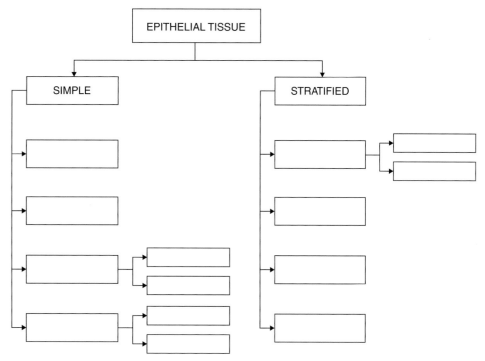

Figure 7.1 Classification scheme for epithelial tissue.

1. Complete the classification scheme for epithelial tissue in Fig. 7.1, using the terms provided below. (Note: Some terms are used more than once.)

Non-keratinised	Squamous	Keratinised
Columnar	Pseudostratified	Cuboidal
Transitional	Ciliated	Non-ciliated

a. Which epithelial tissues bear cilia on their apical surfaces?

_____

b. In transitional epithelium, what does the term 'transitional' refer to?

_____

_____

c. In pseudostratified epithelium, what does the term 'pseudostratified' refer to?

_____

_____

d. How does the term 'pseudostratified columnar ciliated epithelium' reflect the structure of this tissue?

_____

_____

_____

e. Stratified squamous tissue may be keratinised or non-keratinised. What is keratin and what does it contribute to the tissue?

_____

_____

2. Consider Fig. 7.2, which outlines the structural organisation of epithelial tissue in the body. Using the terms provided, answer the questions that follow. (Note: Some terms are used more than once.)

Simple	Squamous	Microvilli
Pseudostratified	Cuboidal	Goblet cells
Stratified	Columnar	Cilia
Transitional	Apical surface	Basement membrane

a. Identify the cell shape in:

   i. Diagram A: _____

   ii. Diagram B: _____

   iii. Diagram C: _____

b. Identify the cell arrangement in:

   i. Diagram H: _____

   ii. Diagram L: _____

   iii. Diagram J: _____

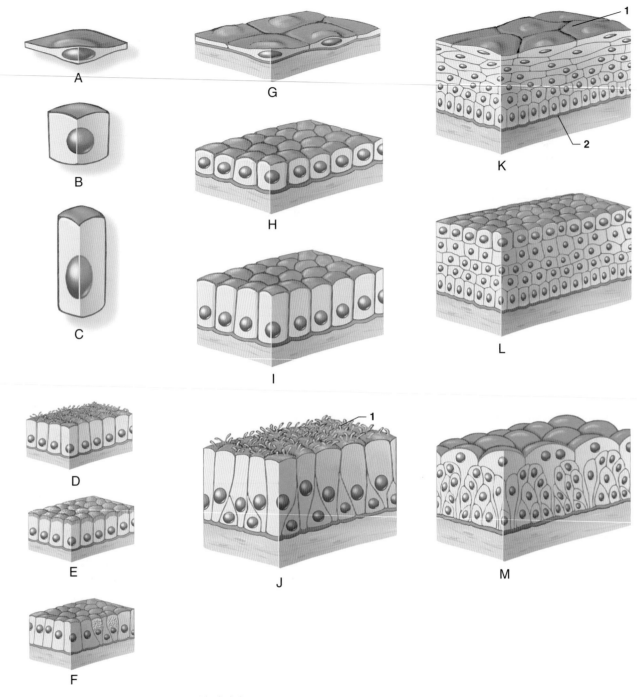

Figure 7.2 Structural organisation of epithelial tissue.
(Source: Patton, K. T., Thibodeau, G. A., & Hutton, A. (2016). Anatomy and physiology. Elsevier.)

c. Identify the tissue modifications in:

   i. Diagram D: _____

   ii. Diagram E: _____

   iii. Diagram F: _____

d. Identify the epithelial tissue in:

   i. Diagram G: _____

   ii. Diagram H: _____

iii. Diagram I: _____

iv. Diagram J: _____

v. Diagram K: _____

vi. Diagram L: _____

vii. Diagram M: _____

e. Identify the structures in diagram J:

   i. Structure 1: _____

f. Identify the structures in diagram K:

   i. Structure 1: _____

   ii. Structure 2: _____

3. In epithelial tissue, what is the purpose of:

  a. Cilia?

   _____

   _____

b. Microvilli?

  _____

  _____

c. Goblet cells?

  _____

  _____

Additional Activities

For additional activities visit Activity 7A: Identification of Epithelial Tissue on Evolve˚.

For additional activities visit Activity 7B: Microscopic Examination of Epithelial Tissue on Evolve˚.

ACTIVITY 7.2: OVERVIEW AND COMPARISON OF EPITHELIAL TISSUE

The arrangement of cells in epithelial tissue occurs in two ways: **simple epithelium** consists of a single layer of cells attached to the basement membrane, while **stratified epithelium** consists of multiple layers of cells attached to the basement membrane. **Pseudostratified epithelium** is technically a simple epithelium that consists of a single layer of cells of varying heights attached to the basement membrane, thereby giving the appearance of multiple cell layers. A comparison of epithelial tissue based on cell shape and arrangement reveals information about the function and, therefore, location of the tissue.

This activity provides an overview and comparison of the structure, location and functions of epithelial tissue.

1. Complete the table provided based on the structure, function and location of epithelial tissue.

Epithelial tissue	Structure	Function	Location
Simple squamous			
Simple cuboidal			
Simple columnar			
Stratified squamous			
Stratified cuboidal			
Stratified columnar			
Pseudostratified columnar			
Transitional			

2. Consider the following questions:

   a. What function do simple epithelial tissues have in common and why?

   _____

   _____

   b. What function do stratified epithelial tissues have in common and why?

   _____

   _____

   c. What function do cube-shaped and column-shaped cells have in common and why?

   _____

   _____

ACTIVITY 7.3: CELL ARRANGEMENT AND DIFFUSION IN EPITHELIAL TISSUE

Cell arrangement in epithelial tissue relates directly to its function. As a single cell layer, simple epithelia are suited to diffusion rather than protection, offering the least resistance to the transport of substances. Diffusion within tissues is crucial to delivering nutrients, exchanging gases and removing wastes, thereby supporting the function of vital organs. For this reason, simple epithelia are located within organs where these processes occur.

This activity examines diffusion in epithelial tissue based on cell arrangement.

 To conduct this activity, it is important to ensure the following safety precaution:

- *Wear disposable gloves at all times as methyl orange indicator is poisonous and may cause skin, eye and respiratory irritation.*

1. This activity is best conducted individually or in pairs.

2. Obtain an A4 sheet of graph paper (1 mm), scissors, forceps, methyl orange indicator, a ceramic tile or paper towel, pipettes, pencil, metric ruler (mm), stopwatch and disposable gloves.

3. From the sheet of graph paper, cut 12 individual squares approximately 3 cm × 3 cm in size (there should be 9 graph squares on each square of paper.)

4. On a ceramic tile or paper towel, place one paper square marking an 'X' on the paper in pencil and place another paper square on top. There should be two squares of paper forming a stack. This is tissue 1.

5. Next to this but not touching, place one paper square marking an 'X' on the paper in pencil and place another 3 paper squares on top. There should be 4 squares of paper forming a stack. This is tissue 2.

6. Next to this but not touching, place one paper square marking an 'X' on the paper in pencil and place another 5 paper squares on top. There should be 6 squares of paper forming a stack. This is tissue 3.

7. There should now be three stacks of paper squares, each containing a bottom square marked with an 'X'.

8. To each paper stack, gently add 3 drops of methyl orange indicator to the central grid of the uppermost paper square, holding the paper stack down at the edges.

9. If the indicator runs to the edge of the paper square, you will need to start again.

10. Wait for 2 minutes or until no methyl orange liquid remains on the top sheet.

11. Using forceps, gently lift and separate the paper layers starting from the top layer and count how many layers the methyl orange has penetrated in each stack.

12. Measure the area of penetration on the top layer and the lowest layer in each paper stack.

13. Record your results in the table provided.

Tissue	Number of layers	Number of layers penetrated	Area of penetration (top layer)	Area of penetration (lowest layer)	Layer with 'X' penetrated?
1	2 sheets				
2	4 sheets				
3	6 sheets				

14. Consider the following questions:

    a. Consider that the paper squares represent individual cells. Which epithelial cell shape is modelled by the square sheets of paper?

    _____

    b. Which layer present in epithelial tissue does the sheet with the 'X' represent?

    _____

    c. What type of epithelial cell arrangement does tissue 1 represent?

    _____

    d. What type of epithelial tissue does tissue 1 represent?

    _____

    e. Based on the number of layers penetrated and the areas of penetration, in tissue 1, which process would this tissue be suited to?

    _____

    f. What does this indicate about the function of this tissue?

    _____

    _____

    g. What type of epithelial arrangement do tissues 2 and 3 represent?

    _____

    h. What type of epithelial tissue do tissues 2 and 3 represent?

    _____

    i. Based on the number of layers penetrated, and the areas of penetration, in tissues 2 and 3, which process would these tissues be suited to?

    _____

    j. What does this indicate about the function of these tissues?

    _____

    _____

    _____

    _____

ACTIVITY 7.4: CELL ARRANGEMENT AND PROTECTION IN EPITHELIAL TISSUE

Stratified epithelia are suited more to protection than diffusion as multiple cell layers (stratification) offer the most resistance to forces and friction. External protection is crucial in maintaining the integrity and function of underlying tissues and associated structures. For this reason, stratified epithelia are located at the surface of structures where abrasion is likely to occur.

This activity examines protective function in epithelial tissue based on cell arrangement.

1. This activity is best conducted individually or in pairs.

2. Obtain 3 Kimwipes sheets, scissors, a ceramic tile or paper towel, a pipette and water.

3. Place the Kimwipes one on top of the other to form a stack.

4. Cut the Kimwipes stack down the middle to create two halves that are square and not rectangular.

5. Place one half on top of the other, then cut down the middle again to create two halves that are rectangular.

6. Place one half on top of the other, then cut down the middle again to create two halves that are square and not rectangular.

7. Each Kimwipes square represents one layer of squamous epithelial cells.

8. Remove one of the Kimwipes layers and place this on the ceramic tile or paper towel. This is tissue 1.

9. Place the remaining Kimwipes layers on the ceramic tile or paper towel next to, but without touching, tissue 1. This is tissue 2.

10. Fill the pipette with water and gently wet each of the tissues until they become damp but not saturated.

    a. Considering that these models are simulating human tissue, why is water added to each of the stacks?

    _____

    _____

11. Gently lift tissue 1 off the ceramic tile or paper towel, and holding the edges between both hands, gently pull the edges apart without using a tearing motion.

    a. How difficult was it to pull tissue 1 apart?

    _____

    _____

12. Gently lift tissue 2 off the ceramic tile or paper towel and repeat the process.

    a. How difficult was it to pull tissue 2 apart?

    _____

    _____

13. Consider the following questions:

    a. Which epithelial tissue is represented by tissue 1 and why?

    _____

    _____

    b. Which epithelial tissue is represented by tissue 2 and why?

    _____

    _____

    c. Which process would tissue 1 be better suited to and why?

    _____

    _____

    _____

    _____

    d. Which process would tissue 2 be better suited to and why?

    _____

    _____

    _____

    _____

Additional Activities

For additional activities visit Activity 7C: Structure, Function, and Secretion of Exocrine Glands on Evolve˙.

ACTIVITY 7.5: CLASSIFICATION OF CONNECTIVE TISSUE

Connective tissue acts to connect structures within the body (such as epithelial tissue to **muscle tissue**), and as such is widely distributed throughout the body. There are four main classes and several sub-classes of connective tissue. These are: **connective tissue proper** (which consists of **loose connective tissue** and **dense connective tissue**), **cartilage**, **bone** and **blood** (Fig. 7.3). Connective tissues are widely distributed throughout the body and their functions vary from binding, supporting, protecting, insulating, storing and transporting. This variety in function is based directly on the structure of the individual connective tissue (Fig. 7.4). Some organs, such as the brain, contain very little connective tissue, while others, such as bones, are composed primarily of connective tissue.

This activity investigates the classification of connective tissue based on tissue matrix.

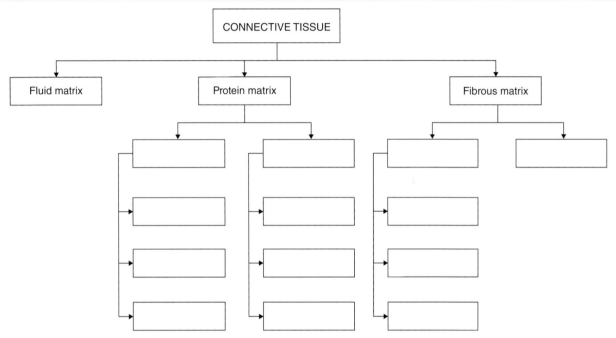

Figure 7.3 Classification scheme for connective tissue.

1. Complete the classification scheme for connective tissue in Fig. 7.3, using the terms provided below.

Regular	Dense	Hyaline	Bone
Fibro	Blood	Cartilage	Irregular
Elastic	Loose	Reticular	Areolar
	Adipose		

a. Which fibres are contained within a fluid matrix?

_____

b. Which fibres are contained within a protein matrix?

_____

c. Which fibres are contained within a fibrous matrix?

_____

d. Which connective tissue stores calcium?

_____

e. Which connective tissue stores fat?

_____

f. What is the function of -blast cells found in connective tissue?

_____

_____

g. What is the function of -cyte cells found in connective tissue?

_____

_____

h. Which connective tissues are vascular and which are avascular?

_____

_____

i. Explain why loose and dense connective tissues are often termed connective tissue proper.

_____

_____

2. Consider Fig. 7.4 which outlines the structural organisation of connective tissue in the body and using the terms provided, answer the questions that follow. (Note: Some terms are used more than once.)

Regular	Dense	Cartilage	Adipose
Fibrous	Blood	Areolar	Irregular
Elastic	Loose	Hyaline	Bone
Protein	Reticular		

a. Identify the connective tissue category represented in:

i. Diagram A: _____

ii. Diagram B: _____

iii. Diagram C: _____

iv. Diagram D: _____

v. Diagram E: _____

vi. Diagram F: _____

vii. Diagram G: _____

viii. Diagram H: _____

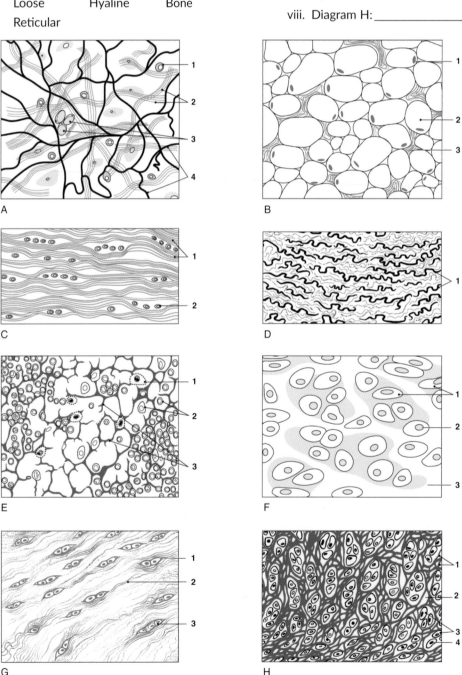

Figure 7.4 Structural organisation of connective tissue.

(Source: Waugh, A., & Grant, A. (2014). Ross & Wilson Anatomy and physiology in health and illness. Elsevier.)

b. Identify the type of matrix (protein or fibrous) in each of the connective tissues:

   i. Diagram A: _____

   ii. Diagram B: _____

   iii. Diagram C: _____

   iv. Diagram D: _____

   v. Diagram E: _____

   vi. Diagram F: _____

   vii. Diagram G: _____

   viii. Diagram H: _____

3. Identify each of the connective tissue structures shown in Fig. 7.4:

a. Diagram A:

   i. Structure 1: _____

   ii. Structure 2: _____

   iii. Structure 3: _____

   iv. Structure 4: _____

b. Diagram B:

   i. Structure 1: _____

   ii. Structure 2: _____

   iii. Structure 3: _____

c. Diagram C:

   i. Structure 1: _____

   ii. Structure 2: _____

d. Diagram D:

   i. Structure 1: _____

e. Diagram E:

   i. Structure 1: _____

   ii. Structure 2: _____

   iii. Structure 3: _____

f. Diagram F:

   i. Structure 1: _____

   ii. Structure 2: _____

   iii. Structure 3: _____

g. Diagram G:

   i. Structure 1: _____

   ii. Structure 2: _____

   iii. Structure 3: _____

h. Diagram H:

   i. Structure 1: _____

   ii. Structure 2: _____

   iii. Structure 3: _____

   iv. Structure 4: _____

4. In connective tissue, what is the purpose of:

a. Collagen fibres?

   _____

   _____

b. Elastic fibres?

   _____

   _____

c. Reticular fibres?

   _____

   _____

Additional Activities

For additional activities visit Activity 7D: Identification of Connective Tissue on Evolve˙.

For additional activities visit Activity 7E: Microscopic Examination of Connective Tissue on Evolve˙.

ACTIVITY 7.6: OVERVIEW AND COMPARISON OF CONNECTIVE TISSUE

The components of connective tissue include the tissue cells, extracellular matrix or ground substance secreted by the cells, and protein-based fibres that are present within the matrix. A comparison of connective tissues based on these factors reveals information about the function and, therefore, location of the tissue. As such, it is often necessary to examine different organs and various body structures in order to locate and study connective tissues.

This activity provides an overview and comparison of the components, location and functions of connective tissue.

1. Complete the table provided based on the components, location and functions of connective tissue.

| Connective tissue classes | Components | | | Tissue location | Tissue function |
	Cells present	Matrix structure	Types of fibres		
Blood					
Blood					
Connective tissue proper					
Loose connective tissue					
Areolar					
Adipose					
Reticular					
Dense connective tissue					
Regular					
Irregular					
Elastic					
Cartilage					
Hyaline					
Elastic					
Fibrocartilage					
Bone tissue					
Bone					

2. Consider the following questions:

   a. What function do loose connective tissues have in common and how does this relate to their structure?

   _____

   _____

   _____

   b. What function do dense connective tissues have in common and how does this relate to their structure?

   _____

   _____

   _____

   c. What function do cartilage tissues have in common and how does this relate to their structure?

   _____

   _____

   _____

   d. Which cell types are present in cartilage tissue and what are their functions?

   _____

   _____

   _____

   e. Compare the matrix of each class of connective tissue.

   _____

   _____

   _____

3. Place your index finger at the top of your ear pinna, fold it down towards the floor, then release it, noting what happens.

   a. Explain the result with reference to the structure of elastic cartilage.

   _____

   _____

   _____

   b. Compare the function of collagen and elastic fibres and relate this to their structure.

   _____

   _____

   _____

Apply the Concepts

1. Explain what occurs in liposuction and whether the results are permanent or temporary.

   _____

   _____

2. What is Marfan's syndrome?

   _____

   _____

3. What is a sarcoma?

   _____

   _____

ACTIVITY 7.7: PROPERTIES OF FAT AND COLLAGEN

Connective tissues are characterised by the density and composition of their extracellular matrix. The matrix of loose connective tissues tends to be gel-like and contains some fibres. In adipose tissue, however, there is little extracellular matrix. Instead, the adipose cells accumulate fat stores, contributing to the volume of the tissue. The matrix of dense connective tissues tends to be firm and is reinforced by collagen and elastin fibres. Collagen provides tensile strength while elastin provides stretch and recoil. These fibres contribute to the strength and flexibility of the tissue.

This activity examines the properties of fat and collagen as related to their functions in connective tissue.

 To conduct this activity, it is important to ensure the following safety precautions:

- *Wear safety glasses at all times as heated liquids may superheat and splutter causing permanent eye damage.*

- *Take care when handling and working around hotplates as they heat quickly and retain heat causing skin burns.*

Part 1: Thermal Properties of Fat

Adipose tissue is classified under connective tissue proper as a loose connective tissue. It consists of very little extracellular matrix, yet contains accumulated cellular fat stores. Fats have a relatively low thermal conductivity, meaning that they do not transfer heat well to other tissues or structures such as muscle or skin. Instead they act as an internal thermal insulator and reduce uncontrolled heat loss from the body to the environment. Even so, the maximum length of time humans can survive in 5°C water is about 30 minutes.

1. This activity is best conducted in groups of three or four.

2. Obtain 5 wide-mouthed test tubes, permanent marker, electronic scale, paper towels, popsticks, disposable pipettes, 5 thermometers, hotplate (placed on a heat mat), deionised water, olive oil, margarine, lard (pork fat), suet (beef fat), shaved ice, 5 × 200 mL beakers, 5 test tube holders, test tube rack, stopwatches and safety glasses.

3. Place the hotplate on the heat mat and turn the heat setting on the hotplate to medium and the stirrer setting (if available) to high.

4. Place approximately 150 mL of shaved ice into each 200 mL beaker and set aside.

5. Label the test tubes 1 to 5 with the permanent marker and place in the test tube rack.

6. To test tube 1, add 5 mL deionised water with a disposable pipette.

7. To test tube 2, add 5 mL olive oil with a disposable pipette.

8. To test tube 3, add 5 g margarine, measured by placing a paper towel onto the electronic balance and using a popstick to dispense the fat. Ensure that the fat is at the bottom of the test tube. (Note: margarine, lard and suet may be easier to portion and weigh when they are frozen. Samples will soften quickly after being placed in test tubes.)

9. To test tube 4, add 5 g suet measured by placing a paper towel onto the electronic balance and using a pop stick to dispense the fat. Ensure that the fat is at the bottom of the test tube.

10. To test tube 5, add 5 g lard measured by placing a paper towel onto the electronic balance and using a popstick to dispense the fat. Ensure that the fat is at the bottom of the test tube.

11. Insert a thermometer into each test tube and place the test tubes into the test tube holder.

12. Place the base of each test tube onto the hotplate, holding the test tube by the test tube holder. (Ensure that the bulb of the thermometer is suspended within the fat and not touching the base of the test tube.)

13. Start the stopwatch. (Each group member should be responsible for one test tube and one stopwatch.)

14. Gently stir the contents of the test tubes with the bulb of the thermometer to ensure that the contents are heated evenly, and the bulb of the thermometer is not touching the base of the tube.

15. Note the time taken for each test tube to reach 37°C, recording your results in the table provided.

16. Once 37°C has been reached, immediately remove each test tube from the hotplate and plunge them separately into the beakers filled with ice.

17. Start the stopwatch again, noting the time taken for the contents of each test tube to reach 5°C, and recording your results in the table provided.

18. Complete the information in the table provided, based on your observations.

Test tube number	Substance tested	Source (animal or vegetable)	Heating time (minutes)	Cooling time (minutes)	Heat retention time (minutes)	Rank (highest to lowest retention time)
1	Deionised water					
2	Olive oil					
3	Margarine					
4	Suet					
5	Lard					

19. Consider the following questions:

   a. What does heating the fats to 37°C represent?

   _____

   b. What does cooling the fats to 5°C represent?

   _____

   c. Why was it necessary to test water?

   _____

   d. How does the heat-retaining capacity of water compare to those of the fats tested?

   _____

   e. What does this indicate about the thermal properties of fats compared to water?

   _____

   _____

   f. Which group of fats tended to retain heat longer?

   _____

   g. What does this indicate about the thermal properties of this particular group of fats?

   _____

   _____

   _____

   h. The animal fats tested are representative of which human connective tissue?

   _____

   i. Where is this connective tissue found in the human body?

   _____

   _____

   j. Explain why water would not be an ideal substance for thermal insulation within the body.

   _____

   _____

   _____

   k. Explain what would occur if water was a thermal insulator within the body.

   _____

   _____

   _____

Part 2: Water-Retaining Properties of Collagen

Collagen is a fibrous protein that provides strength and flexibility to the extracellular matrix of some connective tissues. It can be found in cartilage, tendons, ligaments, bones and skin, and while it can be difficult to extract from animal tissues, an alternative can be obtained in the form of gelatine. Gelatine is a hydrolysed form of collagen taken from the skin, bone and connective tissues of animals. Hydrolysis has reduced the protein fibres to smaller peptide chains, producing a translucent, colourless and flavourless substance that is useful as a gelling agent in food, as well as in medical and industrial applications. Gelatine can absorb five to ten times its dry weight in water.

1. This activity is best conducted in groups of three or four.

2. Obtain 6 × 100 mL beakers, permanent marker, 100 mL measuring cylinder, dry gelatine powder, deionised water, plastic spoon, popstick, electronic scale and stopwatch.

3. Label each beaker 1 to 6 with the permanent marker.

4. Place beaker 1 on the electronic scale and tare the scale to zero.

5. Add 5 g of dry gelatine powder to the beaker with the plastic spoon.

6. Repeat this process with each of the beakers.

7. To beaker 1, add 5 mL deionised water and stir quickly with a popstick. This is sample 1.

8. To beaker 2, add 15 mL deionised water and stir quickly with a popstick. This is sample 2.

9. To beaker 3, add 25 mL deionised water and stir quickly with a popstick. This is sample 3.

10. To beaker 4, add 35 mL deionised water and stir quickly with a popstick. This is sample 4.

11. To beaker 5, add 45 mL deionised water and stir quickly with a popstick. This is sample 5.

12. To beaker 6, add 55 mL deionised water and stir quickly with a popstick. This is sample 6.

13. Allow the beakers to stand for 30 minutes.

14. Calculate the ratio of gelatine to water in each of the beakers, recording your results in the table provided.

15. Calculate the percentage of water in each of the beakers, recording your results in the table provided.

16. Touch the surface of the contents in each beaker and describe the firmness, recording your observations in the table provided.

17. Tilt each beaker slightly to the side to test for the flow of the contents, recording your observations in the table provided.

18. Poke your finger into each of the beakers to test whether the contents support the shape of your finger, recording your observations in the table provided.

19. Remove some of the contents of each beaker with a popstick and press between your fingers to test for strength, recording your observations in the table provided.

	Sample 1	Sample 2	Sample 3	Sample 4	Sample 5	Sample 6
Gelatine-to-water ratio						
Percentage of water						
Test characteristics						
Gel firmness						
Gel flow						
Supports shape						
Gel strength						

20. Consider the following questions:

    a. Based on the test characteristics, which samples would be more suited to functions associated with flexibility? Explain.

    _____

    _____

    b. In which connective tissues might these functions be required?

    _____

    _____

    c. Based on the test characteristics, which samples would be more suited to functions associated with strength? Explain.

    _____

    _____

    d. In which connective tissues might these functions be required?

    _____

    _____

    e. Was the gelatine able to absorb five to ten times its dry weight in water and produce a gel? Explain.

    _____

    _____

    _____

    _____

    f. Cartilage matrix contains collagen and up to 80% water. Relate the water content of cartilage to the water retaining properties of gelatine (collagen).

    _____

    _____

    _____

    _____

Apply the Concepts

1. Explain why an understanding of the thermal properties and capacities of various substances is important in human physiology.

   _____

   _____

   _____

2. What is a fat embolism and how does it occur?

   _____

   _____

   _____

3. Why is a fat embolism potentially dangerous?

   _____

   _____

   _____

ACTIVITY 7.8: CLASSIFICATION OF MUSCLE TISSUE

Three types of **muscle tissue** occur in the human body. These are **skeletal muscle**, **cardiac muscle** and **smooth muscle** (Fig. 7.5). All are composed of elongated cells bound together in bundles or sheets. Each cell has the ability to contract or shorten, thus causing movement of body parts. Classification of muscle is based on either the structural characteristics of the muscle cells within the tissue or the location of the tissue.

This activity investigates the classification of muscle tissue based on structure and function.

1. Consider Fig. 7.5, which outlines the classification of muscle tissue in the body and using the terms provided, answer the questions that follow. (Note: Some terms are used more than once.)

Involuntary	Bundled	Skeletal
Cylindrical	Sheets	Voluntary
Spindle	Cardiac	Branching
Nucleus	Muscle cell	Striations
Smooth	Intercalated discs	

a. Identify the cell shape in:

   i. Diagram A: _____

   ii. Diagram B: _____

   iii. Diagram C: _____

b. Identify the cell arrangement in:

   i. Diagram A: _____

   ii. Diagram B: _____

   iii. Diagram C: _____

2. Identify each of the muscle tissues and associated structures shown in Fig. 7.5:

   a. Diagram A:

   i. Structure 1: _____

   ii. Structure 2: _____

   iii. Structure 3: _____

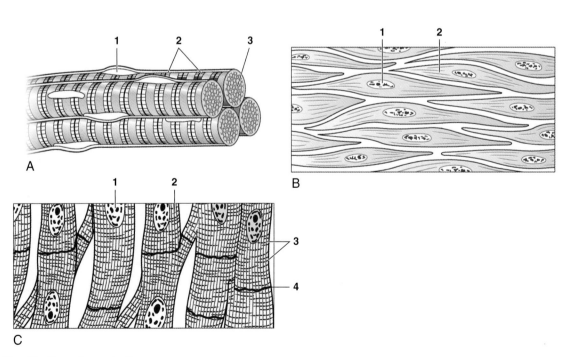

Figure 7.5 Classification of muscle tissue.
(Source: Waugh, A., & Grant, A. (2014). Ross & Wilson Anatomy and physiology in health and illness. Elsevier.)

b. Diagram B:

    i. Structure 1: _____

    ii. Structure 2: _____

c. Diagram C:

    i. Structure 1: _____

    ii. Structure 2: _____

    iii. Structure 3: _____

    iv. Structure 4: _____

d. Identify how the muscle tissue is controlled in:

    i. Diagram A: _____

    ii. Diagram B: _____

    iii. Diagram C: _____

3. Consider the following questions:

a. What is the purpose of bundling in skeletal muscle?

_____

_____

b. What is the purpose of sheet formation in smooth muscle?

_____

_____

c. What is the purpose of branching in cardiac muscle?

_____

_____

d. Where can skeletal muscle be found in the body?

_____

_____

e. Where can smooth muscle be found in the body?

_____

_____

f. Where can cardiac muscle be found in the body?

_____

_____

Additional Activities

For additional activities visit Activity 7F: Identification of Muscle Tissue on Evolve˚.

For additional activities visit Activity 7G: Microscopic Examination of Muscle Tissue on Evolve˚.

ACTIVITY 7.9: OVERVIEW AND COMPARISON OF MUSCLE TISSUE

Skeletal muscle is associated with the skeleton and during contraction exerts pulling forces on bone, enabling movements associated with locomotion, posture, body maintenance and object manipulation. Cardiac muscle is found within the walls of the heart, and as its cells spontaneously contract and relax, their rhythm is modified by the autonomic nervous system to regulate heartbeat. Smooth muscle is found within the walls of internal organs, and through spontaneous slow contraction, it allows for movements associated with the mixing, propulsion and expulsion of their contents.

This activity provides an overview and comparison of structure, location and functions of muscle tissue.

1. Complete the table provided based on the structure, function and location of muscle tissue.

Characteristic	Skeletal muscle	Cardiac muscle	Smooth muscle
Uninucleate or multi-nucleate cells			
Cylindrical or tapered cells			
Visible striations			
Parallel or branching cells			
Fibres in bundles or sheets			
Voluntary or involuntary			
Location			

2. Consider the following questions:

   a. What is the purpose of multiple nuclei per muscle cell in skeletal muscle?

   _____

   _____

   b. What is the purpose of sheet formation in cardiac and smooth muscle?

   _____

   _____

   c. Cardiac and smooth muscle are coordinated by which division of the nervous system?

   _____

   d. Skeletal muscle is coordinated by which division of the nervous system?

   _____

Additional Activities

For additional activities visit Activity 7H: Identification of Nervous Tissue on Evolve˙.

For additional activities visit Activity 7I: Microscopic Examination of Nervous Tissue on Evolve˙.

ACTIVITY 7.10: TISSUE IDENTIFICATION OF INTERNAL ORGANS

An organ is a discrete, specialised body structure responsible for a particular function or activity that no other organ can perform. Organs commonly consist of all four types of tissue whose activities are integrated in such a way as to produce the function of the organ (Fig. 7.6).

This activity identifies the location of various tissue types within selected internal organs.

1. Identify the tissues present in each of the organs shown in Fig. 7.6.

   a. Diagram A:

      i. Tissue 1:_____

     ii. Tissue 2:_____

    iii. Tissue 3:_____

    iv. Tissue 4:_____

     v. Tissue 5:_____

   b. Diagram B:

      i. Tissue 1:_____

     ii. Tissue 2:_____

    iii. Tissue 3:_____

    iv. Tissue 4:_____

     v. Tissue 5:_____

   c. Diagram C:

      i. Tissue 1:_____

     ii. Tissue 2:_____

    iii. Tissue 3:_____

    iv. Tissue 4:_____

     v. Tissue 5:_____

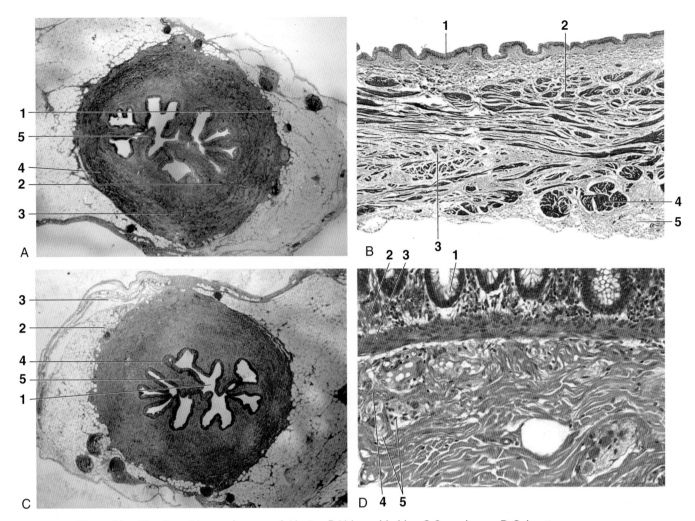

Figure 7.6 Tissue identification of internal organs. **A** Ureter. **B** Urinary bladder. **C** Oesophagus. **D** Colon.
*(Source: **A**, **C** Barros, A. A., Oliveira, C., Reis, R. L., Lima, E., & Duarte, A. R. C. (2017). In vitro and ex vivo permeability studies of paclitaxel and doxorubicin from drug-eluting biodegradable ureteral stents. Journal of Pharmaceutical Sciences, 106(6), 1466–1474. **B**, **D** Young, B., Woodford, P., & O'Dowd, G. (2014). Wheater's functional histology: A text and colour atlas. Elsevier.)*

d. Diagram D:

   i. Tissue 1:_____

   ii. Tissue 2:_____

   iii. Tissue 3:_____

   iv. Tissue 4:_____

   v. Tissue 5:_____

2. Consider the following questions:

  a. Where is the epithelial tissue located in each organ and why?

    _____

    _____

b. Where is the connective tissue located in each organ and why?

    _____

    _____

c. Where is the muscle tissue located in each organ and why?

    _____

    _____

d. Which type of muscle is present in each of these organs and why?

    _____

    _____

e. Where is the nervous tissue located in each organ and why?

_____

_____

f. Why is nervous tissue difficult to locate in each of these organs?

_____

_____

Apply the Concepts

1. What is a biopsy and what is its purpose?

_____

_____

_____

2. What is an autopsy and what is its purpose?

_____

_____

_____

3. What is necrosis and how does it occur?

_____

_____

_____

4. What is organ failure and how does it occur?

_____

_____

_____

Additional Resources

Anatomy Next
An anatomical directory of the organ systems and associated structures of the human body accompanied by detailed anatomical illustrations and 3D user interaction guides.

www.anatomy.net/

Anatomy TV
Anatomy TV provides interactive learning tools related to the study of anatomy and physiology in the form of 3D models, dissections, imaging, clinical conditions, physiology, functional anatomy, guided learning and assessments.

www.anatomy.tv/welcomer

AnatomyZone
AnatomyZone provides numerous video tutorials and interactive 3D models on various regions of the human body.

anatomyzone.com/

Atlas of Microscopic Anatomy – A Functional Approach
A digital library of labelled histological and micrographic images with structural and functional explanations from the University of Iowa.

www.anatomyatlases.org/MicroscopicAnatomy/MicroscopicAnatomy.shtml

Blue Histology
Laboratory and lecture notes with labelled histological images of tissues and major organ systems of the body, produced by the University of Western Australia.

lecannabiculteur.free.fr/SITES/UNIV%20W.AUSTRALIA/mb140/Lectures.htm

Clinical Anatomy
An interactive resource covering the anatomy and physiology of a number of body regions, including videos, a radiological atlas, anatomical illustrations and anatomy labs, affiliated with the University of British Columbia.

www.clinicalanatomy.ca/

Histology Guide Virtual Microscopy Laboratory: Tissues
An online resource providing a virtual microscopy laboratory experience, by allowing users to view microscope slides from professional collections for the purpose of interpreting cellular and tissue structures as seen through a microscope.

histologyguide.com/slidebox/02-epithelium.html
histologyguide.com/slidebox/03-connective-tissue.html
histologyguide.com/slidebox/05-cartilage-and-bone.html
histologyguide.com/slidebox/06-nervous-tissue.html
histologyguide.com/slidebox/04-muscle-tissue.html

Histology Lab Videos
A series of histology laboratory lessons presented as a series of videos produced by the University of Wisconsin.

videos.med.wisc.edu/events/140

KenHub
An integrated platform that brings together multiple learning tools, such as video tutorials, adaptable quizzes, detailed articles and high-quality atlas images.

www.kenhub.com/

MedPics Histology
Selectable histology lessons with interactive histological images of tissues and major organ systems of the body, produced by the University of California.

medpics.ucsd.edu/index.cfm?curpage=main&course=hist

Osmosis – Introduction to Histology
The Introduction to Histology module of Osmosis provides videos, notes, quiz questions and links to further resources related to histology and microscopy.

www.osmosis.org/library/md/foundational-sciences/histology

The Histology Guide: Tissue Types
The Histology Guide is a virtual experience of using a microscope with zoom features divided into topics and offering histological slides with labels and quizzes for each topic such as tissues. It is provided by the University of Leeds.

www.histology.leeds.ac.uk/tissue_types/index.php

Virtual Histology
Annotated interactive histological cell and body system images and lessons from Loyola University Chicago.

zoomify.lumc.edu/

Zygote Body
Zygote Body is a free 3D platform allowing user interaction with a model human body and providing visualisation of the various organ systems and structures of the body.

www.zygotebody.com/

CHAPTER 8
Body Orientation and Homeostasis

The human body is a complex system with a multi-level structural hierarchy ranging from atoms at the chemical level to the entire organism. The study of the structures of the body forms the basis of anatomy and the study of their function is the science of physiology. Structure and function are inseparable: form and function are complementary. The chief structures responsible for vital functions are the organs, which are assembled into organ systems based on their common role in the body; however, the organ systems also display functional integration in that they work together to maintain overall body function. Most organs are located in body cavities lined with specialised membranes that offer support and protection. As it is important for health professionals to accurately reference and communicate the locations of specific organs within these cavities, the use of body planes and directional terms based on the anatomical position is employed.

The functions of the organs and organ systems of the body require continuous monitoring and adjustment against internal changes. This is achieved through homeostasis, where the body's internal environment is kept within optimal functioning limits, and deviations are stabilised by negative feedback mechanisms.

LEARNING OUTCOMES

On completion of these activities, the student should be able to:

1. describe the structural levels of organisation in the human body
2. identify the major organ systems in the human body and explain their functional integration
3. state the anatomical position
4. apply body planes and directional terms to communicate the location of anatomical structures
5. identify the body cavities, abdominopelvic quadrants and regions, and apply these to communicate the location of internal structures
6. apply dissection techniques to demonstrate body planes and directional terms, noting differences in the resulting sections
7. discuss the structural and functional importance of the serous membranes
8. define homeostasis and the describe the components and processes of homeostatic control systems

LEARNING OUTCOMES—cont'd

9. explain and apply the principles of homeostatic feedback mechanisms to physiological processes

10. explain how positive and negative feedback processes stabilise homeostatic fluctuations

11. explain the mechanisms associated with temperature regulation (thermoregulation) and the processes of heat exchange

12. explain the homeostatic mechanisms associated with exercise.

KEY TERMS

Abdominopelvic quadrant	Frontal	Positive feedback
Abdominopelvic region	Homeostasis	Receptor
Anatomical position	Inferior	Sagittal
Anatomy	Median	Serous cavity
Anterior	Negative feedback	Serous fluid
Body cavity	Organ	Serous membrane
Body plane	Organ system	Superior
Cavity	Organism	Thermoregulation
Control centre	Parietal serosa	Transverse
Control system	Physiology	Visceral serosa
Effector	Posterior	

ACTIVITY 8.1: STRUCTURAL ORGANISATION AND ORGAN SYSTEMS

In the study of **anatomy** and **physiology**, the human body is found to have a number of structural levels of organisation, beginning at the simplest chemical level and progressing to the entire organism (Fig. 8.1). This is the structural hierarchy within the human body. The body also contains many individually functioning **organs**, which are organised into **organ systems**. These organ systems function independently, but are also integrated so that they work together to maintain optimal functioning of the **organism**.

This activity provides an overview of the structural organisation in the human body with emphasis on organ systems and interactions.

1. What is anatomy and what is physiology? How are they related?

_____

_____

_____

_____

2. What does the principle of complementarity of structure and function refer to?

_____

_____

_____

_____

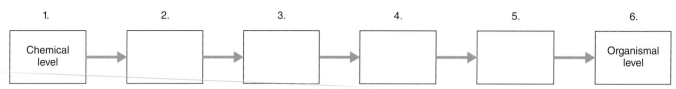

Figure 8.1 Levels of structural organisation.

3. Consider the flow diagram in Fig. 8.1, which outlines the levels of structural organisation in the human body. Complete each box by providing the structural level of organisation. (The first and final boxes have been completed to provide perspective.)

4. For each level of organisation, provide an overview of structural arrangement (including the first and final boxes.)

   a. Box 1: _____
   _____

   b. Box 2: _____
   _____

   c. Box 3: _____
   _____

   d. Box 4: _____
   _____

   e. Box 5: _____
   _____

   f. Box 6: _____
   _____

5. Consider each of the organ systems of the body outlined in Fig. 8.2 (opposite). In the table provided, identify each of the organ systems indicated in the diagram, list two organs belonging to the organ system, and the main function of the organ system.

Organ system	Two organs identified	Main function
1.		
2.		
3.		
4.		
5.		
6.		

Organ system	Two organs identified	Main function
7.		
8.		
9.		

6. Consider the following questions:

   a. Two organ systems have been incorporated into the organ system at number 2. Explain why these two organ systems are often considered together.

   _____
   _____
   _____

   b. Two organ systems have been incorporated into the organ system at number 6. Explain why these two organ systems are often considered together.

   _____
   _____
   _____

7. Fill in the following table, based on the organ groups listed:

   a. In column 1, circle the organ that does not belong in the list.

   b. In column 2, identify the organ system to which the circled organ belongs.

   c. In column 3, identify the organ system formed by the remaining organs.

Organ that does not belong (circle)	Organ system that circled organ belongs to	Organ system formed by the remaining organs
Brain Nerves Pancreas Spinal cord		

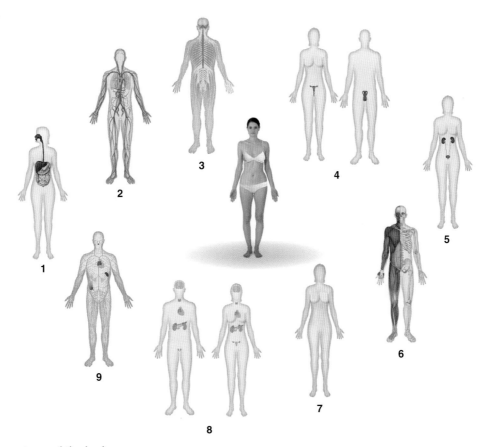

Figure 8.2 Organ systems of the body.
(Source: Hombach-Klonisch, S., Klonisch, T., & Peeler, J. (Eds.). (2019). Sobotta clinical atlas of human anatomy. Elsevier.)

Organ that does not belong (circle)	Organ system that circled organ belongs to	Organ system formed by the remaining organs
Stomach Large intestine Oesophagus Lungs		
Bladder Ureter Urethra Brain		
Uterus Spleen Ovaries Prostate		

8. Consider the interactions between some of the organs and organ systems within the human body in Fig. 8.3.

   a. Identify each of the body systems indicated in the diagram.

      i. System A: _____

      ii. System B: _____

      iii. System C: _____

      iv. System D: _____

      v. System E: _____

      vi. System F: _____

   b. If system A was removed, what effect would this have on system F?

      _____

      _____

      _____

      _____

   c. If system B was removed, what effect would this have on system F?

      _____

      _____

      _____

      _____

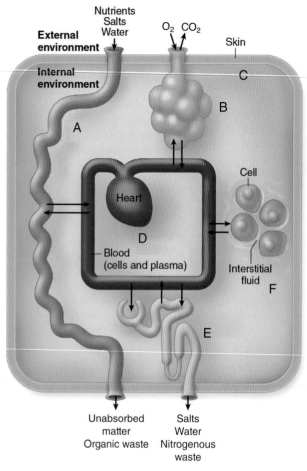

Figure 8.3 A model of organ system integration.
Source: Patton, K. T., Thibodeau, G. A., & Hutton, A. (2019). Anatomy and physiology. Adapted international edition. Elsevier.)

d. If system E was removed, what effect would this have on system D?

_____

_____

_____

_____

e. If system D was removed, what effect would this have on systems A and F?

_____

_____

_____

_____

f. If system D was removed, what effect would this have on systems E and F?

_____

_____

_____

_____

g. Which common processes integrate these systems functionally?

_____

_____

_____

_____

Apply the Concepts

1. Identify three essential physiological survival needs of the human organism.

_____

_____

_____

ACTIVITY 8.2: BODY PLANES AND DIRECTIONAL TERMS

In the study of anatomy and physiology, the ability to convey the location of an organ, limb, or structure is crucial in order to communicate the correct information. The use of everyday words and phrases to achieve this can often be cumbersome and ambiguous. To eliminate confusion and provide accurate information, specific terms are used to describe location according to **body planes (frontal, sagittal, transverse)** and directions (**anterior, posterior, superior, inferior**), based on the **anatomical position** (Fig. 8.4). These terms are also used in many health professions.

This activity outlines the relationships between body planes and directional terms and utilises specific terms to determine locations of body structures.

1. This activity is best conducted in pairs.

2. Obtain a human subject and have them assume the anatomical position.

   a. What is the anatomical position?

   _____

   b. Why is the anatomical position important in the study of the human body?

   _____

   _____

   c. Which parts of the subject are considered axial?

   _____

   _____

   d. Which parts of the subject are considered appendicular?

   _____

   _____

   _____

3. Consider the terms in Fig. 8.4, where directional terms have been included in addition to the body planes.

   a. Identify each of the planes indicated.

      i. Plane 1: _____

      ii. Plane 2: _____

      iii. Plane 3: _____

   b. The frontal plane divides the body into which portions?

   _____

   _____

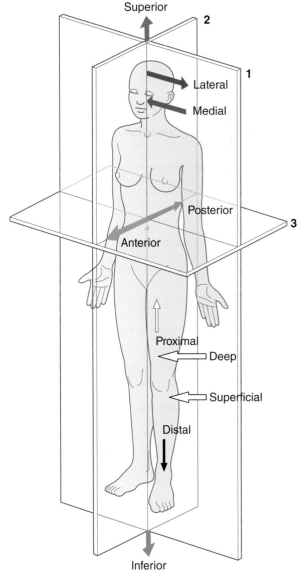

Figure 8.4 Body planes and directional terms.
(Source: Soames, R. W. (2019). Anatomy and human movement: Structure and function. Elsevier.)

c. The sagittal plane divides the body into which portions?

_____

_____

_____

d. Where is the midsagittal plane located?

_____

_____

_____

e. The transverse plane divides the body into which portions?

_____

_____

_____

f. Where is the transverse plane located?

_____

_____

_____

g. How are the frontal and sagittal planes similar?

_____

_____

_____

4. In the following three boxes, and using charts and models to assist, draw a lung according to the section outlined within each box.

Frontal section

Sagittal section
Transverse section

a. Compare the advantages and disadvantages of frontal and sagittal sections over a transverse section.

_____

_____

_____

_____

5. Complete each directional statement by selecting the correct term from the list provided, and using Fig. 8.4 to assist.

Anterior	Distal
Posterior	Superficial
Lateral	Deep
Medial	Superior
Proximal	Inferior

a. The head is _____ to the thorax.

b. The elbow is _____ to the wrist.

c. The stomach is _____ to the spine.

d. The skin is _____ to the skeleton.

e. The ankles are _____ to the waist.

f. The lungs are _____ to the breastbone.

g. The liver is _____ to the skin.

h. The heart is _____ to the arm.

i. The knee is _____ to the waist.

j. The hips are _____ to the navel.

6. How do superior and inferior differ from proximal and distal?

_____

_____

_____

7. Identify the area of the body indicated by each of the anatomical regions provided.

a. Axillary: _____

b. Cephalic: _____

c. Cervical: _____

d. Digital: _____

e. Gluteal: _____

f. Inguinal: _____

g. Lumbar: _____

h. Patellar: _____

i. Pedal: _____

j. Plantar: _____

ACTIVITY 8.3: PLANES AND SECTIONS (DISSECTION)

To fully appreciate the positions of the various planes and the information that can be gained from them, it is useful to use the process of dissection. The resulting sections can then provide perspective as to the anatomical arrangement of the structures found within the object. This arrangement varies with the section, providing anatomical information about concealed structures.

This activity demonstrates the application of sectioning processes and compares the characteristics of the resulting sections.

1. This activity is best conducted in pairs.

2. Obtain two bananas (stems removed), an apple, field mushroom, cucumber (varieties with large seeds are ideal), a chef's knife, chopping board and magnifying glass.

3. Place one banana on the chopping board and, using the knife, make a sagittal cut directly through the median plane of the banana.

a. Are the resulting sections identical?

_____

b. Would it have been easier to determine the median plane on the apple? Explain.

_____

_____

_____

_____

4. Place the second banana on the chopping board and, using the knife, make a frontal cut through the banana.

a. Are the resulting sections identical?

_____

b. What are the correct terms for the resulting sections?

_____

c. Would it have been easier to make a frontal cut through the apple?

_____

_____

5. Place the apple on the chopping board and using the knife, make a transverse cut through the apple.

a. Are the resulting sections identical?

_____

b. A transverse section is also known by what other term?

_____

c. When might a transverse section be useful?

_____

_____

6. Take the superior portion of the apple and make a transverse cut through the portion.

7. Repeat this process with the inferior portion of the apple. You should now have four sections.

a. Are the resulting sections identical?

_____

b. How do the sections differ?

_____

_____

8. Place the mushroom on the chopping board and using the knife, make two intermediate cuts on either side of the median line.

a. How many sections are formed as a result of these cuts?

_____

_____

b. Are the resulting sections identical?

_____

_____

c. If two intermediate cuts had been performed on the apple, would the resulting sections be identical? Explain.

_____

_____

_____

9. Place the cucumber on the chopping board and using the knife, make a transverse cut through the cucumber.

a. Are the resulting sections identical?

_____

10. Take the superior portion of the cucumber only and make a sagittal cut directly through the median plane.

11. Compare the features visible in the cut surfaces of the transverse and sagittal sections with the magnifying glass.

a. Are the visible features identical?

_____

_____

b. How do the visible features differ?

_____

_____

_____

Apply the Concepts

1. Why are sections used in the study of anatomy?

_____

_____

_____

2. Identify three ways that body planes are applied in healthcare.

_____

_____

_____

ACTIVITY 8.4: BODY CAVITIES, QUADRANTS AND REGIONS

Many of the body's internal organs are situated in **body cavities** because of the internal protection provided (Fig. 8.5). Within these cavities, the organs often overlap each other, making it difficult to describe their exact locations for the purpose of anatomical referencing. To address this issue, and because the majority of these organs are located in the abdominopelvic cavity, this cavity can be divided into **abdominopelvic quadrants** and regions (Fig. 8.6). The abdominopelvic quadrants are formed when a transverse and **median** plane pass through the umbilicus (belly button) at right angles, resulting in four quadrants. The **abdominopelvic regions** are formed when two transverse and two parasagittal planes are positioned on the abdomen in a grid, resulting in nine regions.

This activity outlines the locations, divisions, and structures associated with the body cavities, quadrants and regions for the purpose of anatomical description.

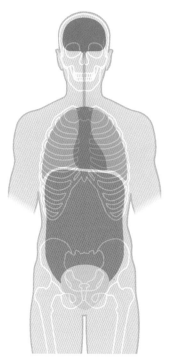
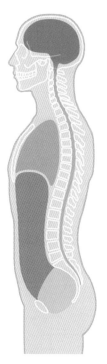

Figure 8.5 The body cavities.
(Source: Waugh, A., & Grant, A. (2018). Ross & Wilson anatomy and physiology in health and illness. Elsevier.)

1. Consider the body cavities and their locations in Fig. 8.5.

   a. Where is the mediastinum located and what is found in this location?

   _____

   _____

   b. Which cavity is shaded purple?

   _____

   c. Identify one organ that is found within this cavity.

   _____

   d. Which cavity is shaded blue?

   _____

   e. Identify one organ that is found within this cavity.

   _____

   f. The cavity shaded blue can be further divided into two smaller cavities. Identify these cavities and the organs they contain.

   _____

   _____

   g. Which cavity is shaded pink?

   _____

   h. Identify one organ that is found within this cavity.

   _____

   i. Which cavity is shaded yellow?

   _____

   j. Identify one organ that is found within this cavity.

   _____

   k. Which structure separates the cavities shaded blue and pink?

   _____

   l. Which structures protect the organs contained within the cavity shaded purple?

   _____

m. Which structure protects the organs contained within the cavity shaded blue?

_____

n. Which structure protects the organs contained within the cavity shaded yellow?

_____

o. Which structures partly protect the organs contained within the cavity shaded pink?

_____

2. For each of the smaller body cavities listed below, identify its location and what is contained within it.

a. Oral: _____

_____

b. Nasal: _____

_____

c. Orbital: _____

_____

d. Middle ear: _____

_____

e. Synovial: _____

_____

3. Consider the quadrants and regions of the abdominopelvic cavity in Fig. 8.6.

a. Identify each of the quadrants in Fig. 8.6A.

i. Quadrant 1: _____

ii. Quadrant 2: _____

iii. Quadrant 3: _____

iv. Quadrant 4: _____

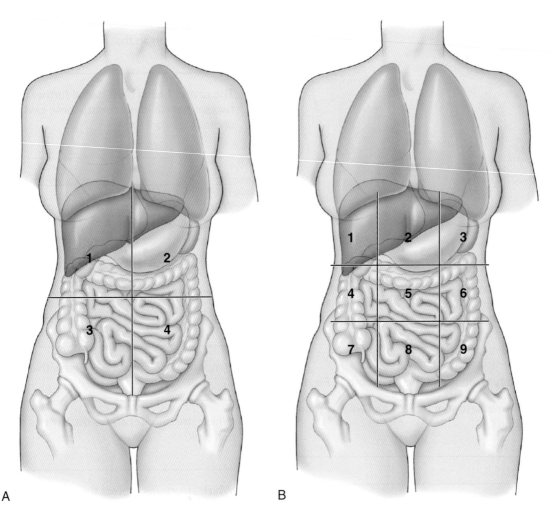

A   B

Figure 8.6 The abdominopelvic cavity. **A** Four quadrants. **B** Nine regions.
(Source: Herlihy, B. (2018). The human body in health and illness. Elsevier.)

b. Identify an organ located in each of the quadrants in Fig. 8.6A.

i. Quadrant 1: _____

ii. Quadrant 2: _____

iii. Quadrant 3: _____

iv. Quadrant 4: _____

c. Identify each of the regions in Fig. 8.6B.

i. Region 1: _____

ii. Region 2: _____

iii. Region 3: _____

iv. Region 4: _____

v. Region 5: _____

vi. Region 6: _____

vii. Region 7: _____

viii. Region 8: _____

ix. Region 9: _____

d. Identify an organ located in each of the regions in Fig. 8.6B.

i. Region 1: _____

ii. Region 2: _____

iii. Region 3: _____

iv. Region 4: _____

v. Region 5: _____

vi. Region 6: _____

vii. Region 7: _____

viii. Region 8: _____

ix. Region 9: _____

4. What information do quadrants and regions provide?

_____

_____

5. Which health issue may be indicated if an individual is experiencing pain in:

a. Region 1? _____

_____

b. Region 2? _____

_____

c. Region 4? _____

_____

d. Region 7? _____

_____

e. Region 9? _____

_____

ACTIVITY 8.5: SEROUS MEMBRANE MODELS

The walls of the body cavities are lined with a thin, double-layered **serous membrane**, or serosa, which folds in on itself much like a pocket. The outer portion of the membrane which lines the cavity walls is the **parietal serosa**, while the inner portion of the membrane which lines the internal organs is the **visceral serosa**. The space between these layers is the **serous cavity** and is filled with **serous fluid**. The purpose of this fluid is to reduce friction between the cavity wall and the cavity organs as they slide against each other during their normal activities.

This activity demonstrates the efficiency of serous membranes and the fluids they secrete.

1. This activity is best conducted in pairs.

2. Obtain a small funnel, 2 party balloons, tap water and a 100 mL measuring cylinder.

3. Measure 40 mL tap water in the measuring cylinder.

4. Place the funnel in the neck of one of the balloons and fill with the water in the measuring cylinder.

5. Tie the end of the balloon so that no water can escape.

6. Inflate the second balloon with air so that it is the same size as the balloon filled with water.

7. Tie the end of the balloon so that no air can escape.

8. Hold the balloon filled with the water in the palm of your hand, and gently press into the balloon with your finger, aiming to touch the palm of your hand.

9. Repeat the process with the balloon filled with air.

   a. Which balloon offered more resistance? Suggest a reason for this observation.

   _____

   _____

   _____

   _____

10. Relating this model to the structure of serous membranes, what is being represented by:

   a. Your finger?

   _____

   b. The inner balloon wall?

   _____

   c. The cavity between the balloon walls containing water?

   _____

   d. The water between the balloon walls?

   _____

   e. The outer balloon wall?

   _____

11. How does this arrangement relate to the function of the serous membranes and serous fluid?

   _____

   _____

   _____

   _____

   _____

   _____

   _____

Apply the Concepts

1. What is ascites and how does it occur?

   _____

   _____

   _____

2. What is effusion and how does it occur?

   _____

   _____

   _____

Additional Activities

For additional activities visit Activity 8A: Body Cavities and Internal Structures (Rat Dissection) on Evolve®.

ACTIVITY 8.6: HOMEOSTATIC CONTROL SYSTEMS

The body's internal environment requires continual monitoring and adjustment against changes. This is achieved through homeostasis. **Homeostasis** occurs through the coordinated efforts of the body's cells, tissues, organs and organ systems, so that the body's internal environment is kept within optimal functioning limits. This homeostatic **control system** involves detection of the change via a **receptor**, coordination of a response to the change via a **control centre**, and finally, distribution of the response to the change via an **effector** (Fig. 8.7).

This activity outlines the principles and processes of homeostatic control systems within the body.

1. Define homeostasis.

   _____

   _____

   _____

   a. What does it mean to maintain homeostasis within the body?

      _____

      _____

      _____

2. Considering the term 'homeostasis':

   a. What does the prefix *homeo-* refer to?

      _____

   b. What does the suffix *-stasis* refer to?

      _____

3. Compare the terms 'homeostasis' and 'homeodynamics'. How might the term 'homeodynamics' better represent the mechanism known as homeostasis?

   _____

   _____

   _____

4. Consider the homeostatic feedback system in Fig. 8.7, which shows how deviations or imbalances in function are brought into balance.

   a. Identify the three main components of the homeostatic control system, indicated by the boxes in the diagram.

      _____

      _____

      _____

   b. Identify the four processes of the homeostatic control system, indicated by the numbered arrows in the diagram.

      _____

      _____

      _____

   c. Explain the process indicated by arrow 1.

      _____

      _____

      _____

   d. What is the function of the component in box A?

      _____

      _____

      _____

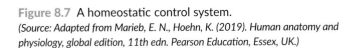

Figure 8.7 A homeostatic control system.
(Source: Adapted from Marieb, E. N., Hoehn, K. (2019). Human anatomy and physiology, global edition, 11th edn. Pearson Education, Essex, UK.)

e. Explain the process indicated by arrow 2.

_____

_____

_____

f. What is the function of the component in box B?

_____

_____

_____

g. Explain the process indicated by arrow 3.

_____

_____

_____

h. What is the function of the component in box C?

_____

_____

_____

i. Explain the process indicated by arrow 4.

_____

_____

_____

j. What effect will the process at arrow 4 have on the process at arrow 1?

_____

_____

_____

5. Consider the process at arrow 4 and the effect it has on the process at arrow 1.

a. What is represented by the process at arrow 4 if it has an enhancing effect on arrow 1?

_____

_____

_____

b. What is represented by the process at arrow 4 if it has an inhibiting effect on arrow 1?

_____

_____

_____

ACTIVITY 8.7: HOMEOSTATIC FEEDBACK MECHANISMS (POSITIVE AND NEGATIVE FEEDBACK)

Homeostatic control systems rely on information feedback processes in order to monitor and respond to deviations in the body's internal environment. This is achieved through positive and negative feedback mechanisms, where **positive feedback** amplifies the deviation and **negative feedback** reduces the deviation (Fig. 8.8). The combination of positive and negative feedback mechanisms working together to counteract internal changes, is essential in maintaining the body's internal environment within optimal functioning limits.

This activity outlines the roles of positive and negative feedback as homeostatic mechanisms.

1. Define negative feedback.

_____

_____

a. Provide one example of a negative feedback pathway.

_____

2. Define positive feedback.

_____

_____

a. Provide one example of a positive feedback pathway.

_____

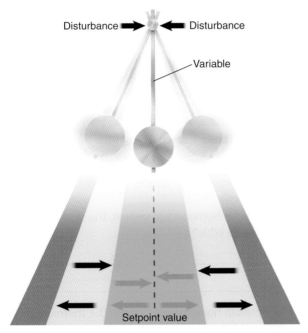

Figure 8.8 Fluctuation and balance of homeostatic variables.
(Source: Patton, K. T., Thibodeau, G. A., (2016). Anatomy and physiology, 9th edn. Mosby Elsevier, St Louis.)

3. Consider the model representing homeostatic balance and fluctuations in Fig. 8.8.

   a. On the diagram, which set of arrows indicates positive feedback?

   _____

   b. On the diagram, which set of arrows indicates negative feedback?

   _____

   c. If the setpoint value for a given variable is indicated by the dashed line, what does the green area represent?

   _____

   d. If the setpoint value for a given variable is indicated by the dashed line, what do the yellow areas represent?

   _____

   e. If the setpoint value for a given variable is indicated by the dashed line, what do the red areas represent?

   _____

4. Explain why most homeostatic mechanisms involve negative feedback rather than positive feedback.

   _____

   _____

   _____

   a. Why is positive feedback necessary?

   _____

   _____

   b. Is positive feedback practical over extended periods of time? Explain.

   _____

   _____

5. How will a receptor that is not functioning affect the negative feedback loop?

   _____

   _____

   _____

6. In humans, fluctuations around a setpoint value, but within a reference range for a particular variable, indicate that homeostatic mechanisms are functioning at optimal levels.

   a. Predict what will happen if a variable strays outside the optimal reference range.

   _____

   _____

   b. Predict what will happen if a variable continues to stray outside the optimal reference range for extended periods of time.

   _____

   _____

ACTIVITY 8.8: A MODEL TEMPERATURE REGULATION SYSTEM

The homeostatic regulation of temperature (**thermoregulation**) involves the coordination of a number of different structures located throughout the body. The negative feedback mechanism of thermoregulation involves the typical components of a homeostatic control system – a receptor, control centre and effector. These components work together to maintain a stable internal body temperature during periods of heat and cold (Fig. 8.9).

This activity utilises a home heating system to model the concept of temperature homeostasis in the human body.

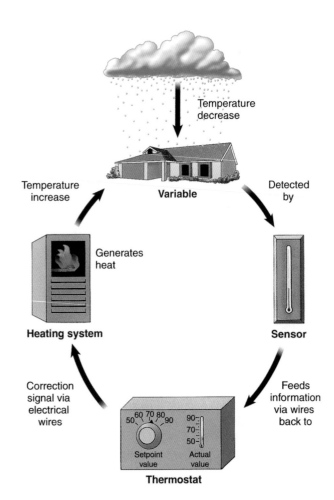

Figure 8.9 A thermoregulatory homeostatic control system.
Source: Patton, K. T., Thibodeau, G. A., & Hutton, A. (2019). Anatomy and physiology. Adapted international edition. Elsevier.)

1. Consider the homeostatic feedback system in Fig. 8.9, which applies the example of a house thermostat to represent thermoregulation within the human body.

   a. In a human homeostatic system, the external temperature decrease represents which component?

   _____

   b. In a human homeostatic system, the sensor represents which component?

   _____

   _____

   c. In a human homeostatic system, the thermostat represents which component?

   _____

   _____

   d. In a human homeostatic system, the heating system represent which component?

   _____

   _____

   e. Explain how this system operates to maintain a consistent temperature within the house (place the homeostatic components in brackets).

   _____

   _____

   _____

   _____

   _____

   _____

2. Assume that the thermostat of the house in Fig. 8.9 is set to 25°C and detects the external temperature by means of a sensor. The outside temperature is 15°C. The thermostat functions by turning the heating system on and off based on the external temperature. The temperature inside the house is measured every hour over 5 hours, and the result is represented on a graph (Fig. 8.10).

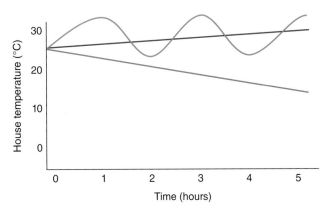

Figure 8.10 Internal house temperature (°C) based on changes in external temperature over time (hours).

3. Considering each of the components discussed in the scenario, which parts of a human homeostatic control system would be represented by the:

a. Internal temperature? _____

b. External temperature? _____

c. Thermometer? _____

d. Thermostat? _____

e. Heating system? _____

4. Consider the following questions with reference to Fig. 8.10:

a. Which line best represents the temperature inside the house over the 5-hour period?

_____

b. Explain why the other two lines do not represent the scenario described.

_____

_____

_____

_____

c. Is it possible to determine when the heating system turns on and off based on the graph? Explain by marking these events on the graph.

_____

_____

_____

_____

d. Based on the graph, explain why the house temperature does not remain constant at 25°C.

_____

_____

_____

e. Describe how this scenario is similar to and different from changes in body temperature.

_____

_____

_____

_____

ACTIVITY 8.9: THERMOREGULATORY MECHANISMS

Core body temperature can be affected by exercise, heat stress, fever and inflammation, hot environments and cold exposure. Normal physiological functioning generally occurs between 35–40°C; however, some function is also possible between 30–35°C and 40–45°C, the boundaries at which thermoregulation ceases. A sustained core body temperature below 35°C increases the risk of cardiac dysrhythmias, cessation of respiratory movements and cardiac arrest, while a sustained core body temperature above 40°C increases the risk of heat stroke and irreversible cell damage. The purpose of thermoregulation is to increase or decrease core body temperature through the process of negative feedback, thereby maintaining core body temperature within stable, functional limits (Fig. 8.11).

This activity provides an overview of the structures and processes associated with temperature regulation (thermoregulation) in the human body.

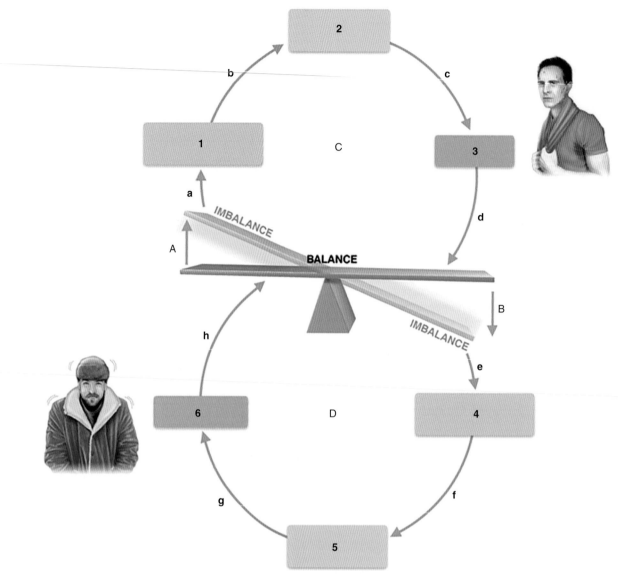

Figure 8.11 Thermoregulatory feedback loops.
(Source: Adapted from Marieb, E. N., Hoehn, K. (2019). Human anatomy and physiology, global edition, 11th edn. Pearson Education, Essex, UK.)

1. Consider the thermoregulatory feedback loops in Fig. 8.11.

   a. Identify the stimulus at A:

   _____

   b. Identify the stimulus at B:

   _____

2. Identify each component of the homeostatic feedback system indicated by the boxes and provide a brief description of its location.

   a. Box 1: _____

   _____

   b. Box 2: _____

   _____

   c. Box 3: _____

   _____

   d. Box 4: _____

   _____

   e. Box 5: _____

   _____

   f. Box 6: _____

   _____

3. Which thermoregulatory process does the feedback loop at C outline?

_____

_____

4. Outline the homeostatic processes indicated by the arrows in feedback loop C and include the boxed components in the feedback loop.

a. Arrow a: _____

_____

b. Box 1: _____

_____

c. Arrow b: _____

_____

d. Box 2: _____

_____

e. Arrow c: _____

_____

f. Box 3: _____

_____

g. Arrow d: _____

_____

5. Is feedback loop C an example of negative or positive feedback? Explain.

_____

_____

_____

_____

6. Which thermoregulatory process does the feedback loop at D outline?

_____

_____

_____

7. Outline the homeostatic processes indicated by the arrows in feedback loop D and include the boxed components in the feedback loop.

a. Arrow e: _____

_____

b. Box 4: _____

_____

c. Arrow f: _____

_____

d. Box 5: _____

_____

e. Arrow g: _____

_____

f. Box 6: _____

_____

g. Arrow h: _____

_____

8. Is feedback loop D an example of negative or positive feedback? Explain.

_____

_____

_____

ACTIVITY 8.10: TEMPERATURE AND HEAT EXCHANGE MECHANISMS

One aspect of the thermoregulatory feedback mechanism involves heat exchange, which occurs at the body's surface. There are four mechanisms by which heat is exchanged at the skin during thermoregulation: conduction, convection, radiation and evaporation. Heat is lost or gained by the transfer of energy. Heat always flows down a thermal gradient from a region of higher temperature to one of lower temperature. Depending on the conditions, some or all of the four mechanisms of heat exchange may act to maintain core body temperature within functional limits.

This activity demonstrates the ways in which heat is lost from the body in the regulation of body temperature.

1. This activity is best conducted in pairs.

2. Obtain 4 laboratory thermometers, 2 × 250 mL beakers or cups, boiling water, tap water, cotton wool or tissue, a piece of card and a stopwatch.

3. Pour 100 mL of boiling water into one of the beakers and put the 4 thermometers into the liquid.

4. Keep the thermometers in the hot water until their readings become steady.

5. Into the other beaker, introduce 100 mL room temperature tap water.

6. When the temperature readings become steady, complete the activities that follow, recording your results in the table provided.

Thermometer 1

a. Note the temperature on the thermometer and record this in the table.

b. Place the thermometer quickly into the beaker with room temperature water and start the timer.

c. Once the timer reaches 1 minute, note and record the temperature on the thermometer.

Thermometer 2

a. Note the temperature on the thermometer and record this in the table.

b. Wipe the bulb of the thermometer dry quickly with a piece of cotton wool and start the timer.

c. Hold the thermometer in the air by the end opposite to the bulb without moving it.

d. Once the timer reaches 1 minute, note and record the temperature on the thermometer.

Thermometer 3

a. Note the temperature on the thermometer and record this in the table.

b. Wipe the bulb of the thermometer dry quickly with a piece of cotton wool and start the timer.

c. Hold the thermometer by the end opposite to the bulb, and fan the bulb in the air with the piece of card.

d. Once the timer reaches 1 minute, note and record the temperature on the thermometer.

Thermometer 4

a. Note the temperature on the thermometer and record this in the table.

b. Take the thermometer out of the water (do not dry it) and start the timer.

c. Hold the thermometer in the air by the end opposite to the bulb without moving it.

d. Once the timer reaches 1 minute, note and record the temperature on the thermometer.

7. Calculate the temperature change in each condition.

Thermometer number	Initial temperature (°C)	Final temperature (°C)	Temperature change (°C)	Rank (most to least heat lost)	Heat loss mechanism
1					
2					
3					
4					

8. Consider the following questions:

   a. To which medium, air or water, does a hot body lose more heat in a given time?

   _____

   _____

   b. Which thermometer and process represents heat loss via sweating? How is the heat transferred?

   _____

   _____

   c. Which thermometer and process represents heat loss via fever? How is the heat transferred?

   _____

   _____

   d. Which thermometer and process represents heat loss via breathing and respiration? How is the heat transferred?

   _____

   _____

   e. Which thermometer and process represents heat loss via application of a cold pack? How is the heat transferred?

   _____

   _____

   f. If the heat loss mechanism that was indicated by thermometer 2 increased in the body, how could the body compensate to avoid excessive heat loss?

   _____

   _____

   g. If the heat loss mechanism that was indicated by thermometer 4 was not able to occur in the body, explain the effect this would have on thermoregulation.

   _____

   _____

Additional Activities

For additional activities visit Activity 8B: Thermoregulation During Exercise on Evolve˙.

For additional activities visit Activity 8C: Exercise Homeostasis on Evolve˙.

Additional Resources

Clinical Anatomy

An interactive resource focusing on the anatomy of major body systems, including videos, a radiological atlas, anatomical illustrations and anatomy labs from the University of British Columbia.

www.clinicalanatomy.ca/

eduMedia: Homeostasis

An online platform providing innovative resources and interactive animations on a variety of human body topics, including homeostasis relating to a number of body systems.

www.edumedia-sciences.com/en/curriculum/1914-homeostasis

Gizmos: Human Homeostasis

An interactive simulation with lesson materials where users adjust the levels of clothing, perspiration and exercise to maintain a stable internal temperature as the external temperature changes.

gizmos.explorelearning.com/index.cfm?method=cResource. dspDetail&resourceID=519

Guided Tour of the Visible Human

The Visible Human Project has generated over 18000 digitised sections of the human body, providing 2D and 3D tours to teach key concepts in human anatomy.

www.madsci.org/,lynn/VH/

Khan Academy: Body Structure and Homeostasis

Video tutorials outlining the relationship between various organs and systems of the body and their contribution to homeostasis.

www.khanacademy.org/science/biology/principles-of-physiology/ body-structure-and-homeostasis/e/body-structure-and- homeostasis

Osmosis – Introduction to Anatomy

The Introduction to Anatomy module of Osmosis provides videos, notes, quiz questions and links to further resources related to the anatomical regions of the human body.

www.osmosis.org/library/md/foundational-sciences/anatomy

Teach Me Anatomy

A comprehensive anatomy encyclopedia resource containing over 700 images and lessons on a variety of body regions, with registration options.

teachmeanatomy.info/

Visible Body

An interactive modelling platform providing 3D visualisation of the human body, including an overview of anatomical planes and cavities.

www.visiblebody.com/blog/anatomy-and-physiology-anatomical- planes-and-cavities

Visible Human Browsers

Fully interactive human body scans of various body sections created by the Leiden University Medical Centre, the Netherlands.

www.caskanatomy.info/browser/index.html

CHAPTER 9
The Integumentary System

An organ is a structurally distinct part of the body and performs a specific function. Typically, an organ is composed of several types of tissue which have a highly organised structural relationship with each other. A typical example of an organ that contains all four tissue types – epithelial, connective, muscle and nervous tissue – is the skin. The skin and its associated structures, such as the cutaneous glands (sudoriferous and sebaceous), hair and nails, share common functions. The functions of the skin, while mostly protective, also include cutaneous sensation, vitamin D production, excretion, thermoregulation, and as a blood reservoir. The skin and its associated structures form the integumentary system. The integumentary system contains self-repairing components that are able to withstand varying degrees of mechanical and chemical trauma, thereby protecting underlying structures.

LEARNING OUTCOMES

On completion of these activities, the student should be able to:

1. describe the structure and function of the skin
2. explain the layers of skin and the structures located within each layer
3. describe the structure and function of the epidermis
4. explain the protective characteristics of the epidermis
5. describe the structure and function of the dermis
6. outline the structural and functional relationship between the dermis and epidermis
7. explain the structure and function of cutaneous glands and receptors
8. explain the structure and function of nails
9. explain the structure and function of hair and hair follicles
10. conduct microscopic and physical examinations of integumentary structures.

KEY TERMS

Apocrine sweat gland	Hypodermis	Reticular dermis
Cerumen	Keratin	Sebaceous gland
Ceruminous gland	Keratinocytes	Sebum
Cutaneous sensory receptor	Meissner's (tactile) corpuscles	Skin
Dermis	Melanin	Sudoriferous gland
Eccrine sweat gland	Melanocytes	Sweat
Epidermis	Nails	Thick skin
Hair	Pacinian (lamellar) corpuscles	Thin skin
Hair follicle	Papillary dermis	

ACTIVITY 9.1: STRUCTURE AND FUNCTION OF THE SKIN

Human skin is a large organ composed of multiple tissue types. It is waterproof, stretchable, washable, and capable of self-repair. It also has a major role in thermoregulation. The **skin** consists of two layers, the epidermis and dermis (Figure 9.1). The **epidermis** is the outermost avascular layer providing protection, while the **dermis** is the underlying vascular layer, providing strength and flexibility. The **hypodermis** underlies the dermis and forms the subcutaneous tissue. It is not considered part of the skin but shares some of the skin's protective functions.

This activity provides an overview of the structure and function of human skin.

1. Identify and briefly describe the four main functions of skin.

   _____

   _____

   _____

   _____

2. Identify the structures of the skin shown in Fig. 9.1, by assigning a letter to each of the terms provided.

   a. Adipose tissue: _____

   b. Arrector pili muscle: _____

   c. Artery: _____

   d. Dermis: _____

   e. Eccrine sweat gland: _____

   f. Epidermis: _____

   g. Free nerve ending: _____

   h. Hair follicle: _____

   i. Hair root: _____

   j. Hair shaft: _____

   k. Meissner's corpuscle: _____

   l. Pacinian corpuscle: _____

   m. Papillary layer: _____

   n. Pore: _____

   o. Reticular layer: _____

   p. Root hair plexus: _____

   q. Sebaceous gland: _____

   r. Sensory nerve fibre: _____

   s. Stratum basale: _____

   t. Stratum corneum: _____

   u. Stratum granulosum: _____

   v. Stratum lucidum: _____

   w. Stratum spinosum: _____

   x. Subcutaneous tissue: _____

   y. Vein: _____

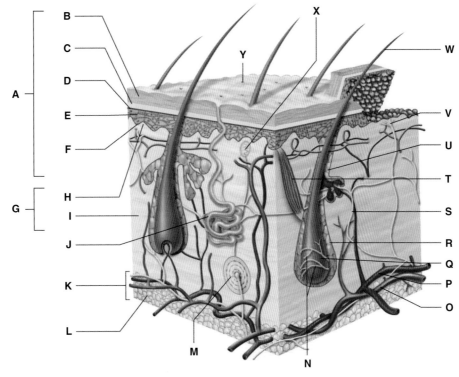

Figure 9.1 Structural organisation of the skin.
(Source: Crisp, J., Douglas, C., Rebeiro, G., & Waters, D. (2021). Potter & Perry's fundamentals of nursing, ANZ edition. Elsevier, Sydney.)

3. Group the skin structures in Fig. 9.1, according to the classifications that follow.

Epithelial tissue	
Glandular tissue	
Connective tissue	
Muscle tissue	
Nervous tissue	

4. Select one structure from each of the groups above, identify the layer of skin in which it is found, and briefly describe its function within the skin.

   a. Epithelial tissue

      i. Example: _____

      ii. Skin layer: _____

      iii. Function: _____

          _____

   b. Glandular tissue

      i. Example: _____

      ii. Skin layer: _____

      iii. Function: _____

          _____

   c. Connective tissue

      i. Example: _____

      ii. Skin layer: _____

      iii. Function: _____

          _____

d. Muscle tissue

    i. Example: _____

    ii. Skin layer: _____

    iii. Function: _____

    _____

e. Nervous tissue

    i. Example: _____

    ii. Skin layer: _____

    iii. Function: _____

    _____

Apply the Concepts

1. What are freckles and how do they occur?

    _____

    _____

    _____

2. What is a nevus and how does it occur?

    _____

    _____

    _____

3. What are liver spots and how do they occur?

    _____

    _____

    _____

4. What is a basal cell carcinoma and in which layer of the skin does it occur?

    _____

    _____

    _____

5. What is a malignant melanoma and in which layer of the skin does it occur?

    _____

    _____

    _____

ACTIVITY 9.2: IDENTIFICATION AND FUNCTION OF EPIDERMAL LAYERS

The characteristics of skin are related to the functions of the underlying structures that it covers. **Thick skin** consists of five layers and is located on areas of the body subject to abrasion, such as the palms of the hands, fingertips and soles of the feet (Fig. 9.2), while **thin skin** consists of four layers and is located over the rest of the body. The layers identified in thick and thin skin refer to the epidermis only and do not include the dermis.

This activity examines the arrangement of skin layers using a histological micrograph.

1. Identify each of the layers found in the thick skin shown in Fig. 9.2, using Fig. 9.1 to assist.

   a. Layer A: _____

   b. Layer B: _____

   c. Layer C: _____

   d. Layer D: _____

   e. Layer E: _____

   f. Layer F: _____

   g. Layer G: _____

   h. Layer H: _____

   i. Layer I: _____

2. Consider the following questions:

   a. Which tissue type comprises the epidermis?

   _____

   b. What is the function of the epidermis?

   _____

   _____

   c. Which tissue type comprises the dermis?

   _____

   d. What is the function of the dermis?

   _____

   _____

   e. Which tissue type comprises the hypodermis?

   _____

   f. What is the function of the hypodermis?

   _____

   _____

   g. How is the structure of layer A suited to its function?

   _____

   _____

   _____

   h. What is found in layer A?

   _____

   i. What is found in layer C?

   _____

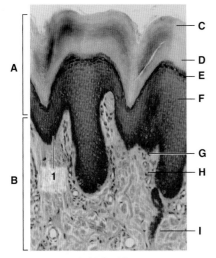

Figure 9.2 Structure of thick skin.
(Source: Patton, K. T., Bell, F. B., Matusiak, D. J., & Wood, S. R. (2021). Anatomy and physiology laboratory manual. Elsevier.)

j. What is found in layer D?

_____

k. What is found in layer E?

_____

l. What is found in layer F?

_____

m. What is found in layer G?

_____

n. Which of these layers is not found in thin skin and why?

_____

_____

o. What is found at structure 1 and what is its function?

_____

_____

p. Why does the appearance of layer A change from layer G to layer C?

_____

_____

3. Identify the function of the following cells in the epidermis:

a. Keratinocytes: _____

_____

b. Melanocytes: _____

c. Dendritic (Langerhans) cells:

_____

d. Merkel (tactile) cells:

_____

4. How is the structure of layer B suited to its function?

_____

_____

_____

a. What is found in layer B?

_____

b. What is found in layer H?

_____

c. What is found in layer I?

_____

5. Is the dermis or epidermis better nourished? Explain.

_____

_____

_____

_____

Apply the Concepts

1. How does the skin contribute to the body's first line of defence?

_____

_____

_____

2. Explain why wrinkles occur.

_____

_____

_____

3. In which layers of the skin are subcutaneous injections delivered and why?

_____

_____

_____

4. How is the skin involved in vitamin D synthesis?

_____

_____

_____

Additional Activities

For additional activities visit Activity 9A: Microscopic Examination of the Skin on _Evolve_.

For additional activities visit Activity 9B: Physical Examination of the Skin on _Evolve_.

ACTIVITY 9.3: EXAMINATION OF FRICTION RIDGES

The friction ridges of the fingertips overlay the ridges in the **papillary dermis** underneath, forming a pattern unique to each individual that does not alter over time. Fingerprints are typically formed from the aqueous-based secretions of the **eccrine glands** of the fingers and palms. The resulting latent fingerprints usually consist of water, small traces of amino acids, chlorides and sebaceous fatty acids and triglycerides. The patterns of the friction ridges of the fingertips are readily transferred as fingerprints when they contact a surface. Fingerprints can be visualised through simple fingerprinting methods and the resulting configurations examined. There are three basic fingerprint configurations according to the Henry Classification System: arch patterns have no deltas, loop patterns have one delta, and whorl patterns have two deltas (Fig. 9.3).

This activity uses the processes of latent fingerprinting and iodine fuming to observe the pattern of friction ridges on fingerprints.

Part 1: Latent Fingerprinting

Latent or invisible fingerprints are commonly made visible through the use of powders but can also be made visible when the fingers are covered with an opaque substance such as soot, grease, blood or ink. This is then transferred onto a surface when contact occurs between the fingertip and the surface.

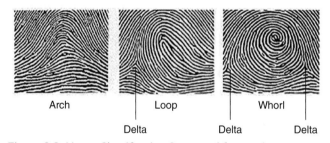

Figure 9.3 Henry Classification System of fingerprints.
(Source: Science Source)

1. This activity is best completed individually.

2. Obtain two pieces of 5 cm × 5 cm white paper, a 2B graphite pencil, 20 mm wide clear adhesive tape, scissors and a magnifying glass.

3. Colour one of the pieces of paper solidly with the 2B pencil until the white paper can no longer be seen.

4. Place your right thumb firmly in the middle of the pencil-coloured paper without moving it around so that your thumb becomes coated with graphite.

5. Cut 6 cm of adhesive tape and, avoiding touching the tape as much as possible, place your coated thumb in the middle of the tape on the adhesive side pressing firmly into the tape.

6. Remove your thumb and tape the adhesive side of the tape onto the second clean piece of paper.

7. The fingerprint should now be visible.

8. Classify the fingerprint using the Henry Classification System provided (Fig. 9.3).

   a. Do friction ridges in fingerprints represent the crests or the troughs of the epidermal tissue?

   _____

   b. Where are the sweat pores associated with the friction ridges located?

   _____

   c. To what structures did the graphite adhere to create the fingerprint?

   _____

Part 2: Iodine Fuming

Iodine fuming is a process whereby an aqueous-based secretion such as **sweat** or **sebum**, which contains organic molecules such as amino acids, chlorides and fatty acids, is exposed to iodine fumes. The iodine fumes react with the organic molecules present in the secretion, forming a brown-coloured change-transfer complex. This allows the pattern of organic residue left behind by the fingerprint to be observed.

⚠ To conduct this activity, it is important to ensure the following safety precautions:

- *Iodine may cause an allergic reaction in some individuals, especially those with shellfish allergies. Avoid contact with iodine where allergies are indicated.*

- *Iodine crystals should be used and dispensed in a fume hood, as inhalation may cause respiratory tract irritation.*

1. This activity is best completed individually.

2. Obtain a pair of forceps, 5 cm × 5 cm white paper, iodine crystals, spatula, weigh boat, electronic scale, 200 mL glass jar with lid, stopwatch, magnifying glass and a fume hood.

3. Place 2 g iodine crystals into the glass jar and close the lid tightly. This is the iodine developing jar. Place the jar in the fume hood.

4. Using the forceps, grasp the square of paper by the corner in order to avoid touching the sides of the paper with your fingers.

5. Place your right thumb firmly in the middle of the paper without moving it around, to make a fingerprint. This process will work effectively if the thumb is sweaty.

6. If your thumb is dry, you should rub it along your neck, temple or hairline.

7. Place the piece of paper into the iodine developing jar in the fume hood, ensuring that the lid is tightly secured.

8. Wait 20 minutes for the fingerprint to develop.

9. Remove the paper from the developing jar and examine the fingerprint with a magnifying glass.

10. Classify the fingerprint using the Henry Classification System provided (Fig. 9.3).

11. The fingerprint will slowly fade over time, so you may wish to take a photograph of the print.

    a. How did the fingerprint become visible?

    _____

    _____

    b. What does this indicate about the composition of eccrine sweat produced at the friction ridges?

    _____

    _____

    _____

    c. Which method produced the best fingerprint? Suggest a reason for this.

    _____

    _____

    _____

Apply the Concepts

1. Explain the functional significance of friction ridge swelling with prolonged exposure to water.

   _____

   _____

   _____

2. How do transdermal patches deliver medication to underlying tissues?

   _____

   _____

   _____

3. Why are transdermal patches not applied to the palms of the hands and soles of the feet?

   _____

   _____

   _____

ACTIVITY 9.4: EXAMINATION OF EPIDERMAL CELLS

The epidermis is composed of stratified squamous epithelial tissue that is infiltrated with keratin. **Keratin** acts as an epithelial cell-binding agent which then hardens to protect the skin against abrasion and penetration. **Melanin**, a dark pigment produced by melanocytes, acts to protect the nuclei of maturing keratinocytes from ultraviolet (UV) damage. Both keratinocytes and **melanocytes** arise from the stratum basale, or basal layer. The stratum corneum, also called the horny layer due to its cornification with keratin, is the outermost epidermal layer that is visible. It consists of 20 to 30 cell layers and comprises three-quarters of the epidermal thickness. Cells of the stratum corneum are regularly shed in the form of flakes as cells from underlying layers move upwards. Collection and examination of epidermal skin cells and debris is valuable clinically and diagnostically.

This activity studies epidermal cells via microscopic examination.

 To conduct this activity, it is important to ensure the following safety precautions:

- *Methylene blue is a strong stain and can cause irritation.*

- *Ensure disposable gloves are worn at all times and the area is well ventilated.*

Part 1: Skin Scraping

Skin scraping is a technique often employed in dermatology for obtaining skin samples to test for parasitic, fungal and yeast infestations. Skin scraping may be conducted dry or wet, with application of mineral oil (to mobilise any parasites) or with potassium hydroxide (to dissolve skin cells, rendering microorganisms visible).

1. This activity is best conducted individually.

2. Obtain a microscope, clean microscope slide, coverslip, plastic scraper, deionised water, methylene blue, disposable pipettes and disposable gloves.

3. Add 1 drop of deionised water to the microscope slide.

4. Add 1 drop of methylene blue to the water on the microscope slide.

5. Add 1 drop of water to the back of your forearm, and with the plastic scraper, gently but firmly scrape the skin to remove surface material without drawing blood.

6. Transfer the collected material to the water drop on the slide by gently mixing the material into the water droplet.

7. Place the coverslip on top.

8. View the slide under low power then move to high power but do not use oil immersion.

9. Draw a diagram of what you can see in the space below and label any structures you identify.

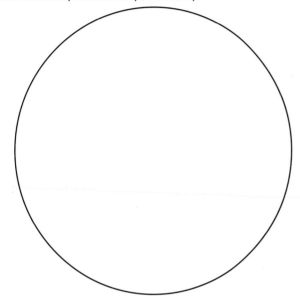

Magnification of diagram: × _____

a. Were epithelial cells of the epidermis visible?

_____

b. Suggest a possible reason for this.

_____

_____

_____

Part 2: Tape Stripping

Tape stripping is a technique often employed in dermatology research to investigate skin barrier function and the penetration of topically applied drugs. It has an advantage over skin biopsies as it allows for collection of epidermal cells without scarring and discomfort, and collects only epidermal cells without dermal and subcutaneous tissue. In addition, tape stripping yields cell layers that originate from various depths of the epidermis because of furrows in the skin.

1. This activity is best conducted individually.

2. Obtain a microscope, a clean microscope slide, methylene blue, clear adhesive tape, scissors, forceps, disposable pipettes, liquid soap, paper towels and disposable gloves.

3. Wash your hands with liquid soap and water and gently pat dry with paper towels.

4. Allow any remaining water to air dry until your hands are completely dry.

5. Cut 4 cm of clear adhesive tape, handling it carefully to avoid placing your fingerprints on the tape.

6. Press the tape firmly onto the back of your hand, adhesive side down.

7. Pull the tape off with the forceps to avoid fingerprints and mount the tape onto the microscope slide with the adhesive side down.

8. Don a pair of disposable gloves.

9. Lift one corner of the tape with the forceps and place 1 drop of methylene blue onto the microscope slide just under the tape.

10. The methylene blue will move under the tape across the slide.

11. View the slide under low power then move to high power, but do not use oil immersion.

12. Draw a diagram of what you can see in the space below and label any structures you identify.

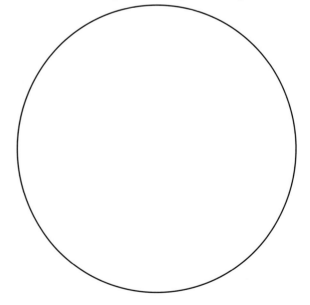

Magnification of diagram: × _____

a. Were epithelial cells of the epidermis visible?

_____

b. What type of arrangements did the cells form?

_____

_____

c. Did the methylene blue assist with visualising cell structures?

_____

_____

d. Which cell structures were visible under the microscope and at what magnification were they visible?

_____

_____

13. Compare the slide from Part 1 with the slide from Part 2.

a. In which slide were epithelial cells clearly visible?

_____

b. Suggest a possible reason for this.

_____

_____

_____

Apply the Concepts

1. What is dermatitis and how does it occur?

_____

_____

_____

2. What is eczema and how does it occur?

_____

_____

_____

3. What is psoriasis and how does it occur?

_____

_____

_____

4. What is pompholyx and how does it occur?

_____

_____

_____

ACTIVITY 9.5: ACTIVITY, LOCATION, AND DISTRIBUTION OF ECCRINE SWEAT GLANDS

Sudoriferous glands, or sweat glands, are distributed across most of the skin surface. **Eccrine sweat glands** are abundant on the palms of the hands, soles of the feet and forehead, and produce sweat which is primarily water with traces of salts, metabolic wastes and microbial peptides. **Apocrine sweat glands** are located within the axillary and anogenital regions and produce sweat which is viscous and contains an oily compound and proteins.

The starch-iodine test, also known as Minor's test, is a qualitative medical test that is used to evaluate sudoriferous gland function and was first described by Victor Minor in 1928. Minor's test can be used as a diagnostic tool to evaluate underactive sweating (hypohidrosis) and overactive sweating (hyperhidrosis), and can be used to confirm Horner's Syndrome, where decreased sweating is a symptom of damage to sympathetic nerves of the autonomic nervous system.

This activity highlights the function, location and distribution of eccrine sweat glands.

 To conduct this activity, it is important to ensure the following safety precautions:

- *Iodine may cause an allergic reaction in individuals with shellfish allergies. Avoid contact with iodine where allergies are indicated.*

1. This activity is best conducted in pairs.

2. Obtain tincture of iodine, an eyedropper, cotton swabs, cotton balls, corn starch, millimetre ruler, an exercise bike, a water-erasable ink marker and a stopwatch.

3. For subject number 1, place a drop of iodine tincture at the base of the left palm of the hand (near the heel of the hand).

4. Spread it around with a cotton swab until an area of about 2.5 cm is covered.

5. Repeat this process placing the iodine tincture on the inside of the left wrist where a watchband would be.

6. Repeat this process placing the iodine tincture inside the left axilla.

7. Allow the tinctures to air-dry.

8. Gently dust the tinctured areas with a thin layer of corn starch using a cotton ball.

9. Encourage sweating by increasing the room temperature or exercising using the exercise bike for 5 minutes.

10. Note any changes to the areas of skin where the iodine and corn starch were added.

    a. What do you observe?

    _____

b. What is the physiological significance of the colour change?

_____

_____

_____

c. Were some dots larger than others? Explain based on sweat gland function.

_____

_____

_____

11. Count the number of purple dots that appear on the surface of the skin, recording your results in the table provided. (If a large number of dots is present, provide an estimate.)

12. Measure the distance between 4 dots using the millimetre ruler, recording the mean distance between the dots in the table provided.

Location	Number of dots	Mean distance between dots
Palm of left hand		
Inside left wrist		
Left axilla		

13. Consider the following questions:

    a. In which location were the sweat glands more numerous?

    _____

    _____

    b. In which location did the sweat glands indicate a higher density?

    _____

    _____

    c. What does the density of sweat glands indicate about the function of the skin in that location?

    _____

    _____

    _____

14. For subject number 2, mark a 2.5 cm spiral with the water-erasable ink marker in the same locations as for subject number 1.

15. Repeat this process for the same locations on the right side of the body.

16. Note the time taken for the ink spirals to disappear in each location, recording your results in the table provided.

Location	Time taken to disappear (left side)	Time taken to disappear (right side)
Palm of hand		
Inside wrist		
Axilla		

17. Consider the following questions:

    a. Explain why the ink does not rub off easily after it dries but disappears on contact with sweat.

    _____

    _____

    _____

    b. Suggest a reason for the disappearance of the water-soluble ink due to contact with the water in sweat.

    _____

    _____

    _____

    c. Did the time taken for the ink to disappear vary according to the part of the body?

    _____

    d. How long did it take for the ink in the axillae to begin to fade?

    _____

    e. How long did it take for the ink in the axillae to disappear?

    _____

    f. Was there a difference in the time taken for the ink to disappear on both sides of the body?

    _____

    _____

    g. If a time difference was observed between both sides of the body, what does this indicate about the function of sweat glands across the body?

    _____

    _____

    _____

Apply the Concepts

1. What is bromhidrosis and how does it occur?

_____

_____

_____

2. What is hyperhidrosis and how does it occur?

_____

_____

_____

Additional Activities

For additional activities visit Activity 9C: Characteristics of Cutaneous Glands on Evolve˙.

For additional activities visit Activity 9D: Microscopic Examination of Cutaneous Glands on Evolve˙.

For additional activities visit Activity 9E: Distribution of Cutaneous Sensory Receptors (Thermoreceptors) on Evolve˙.

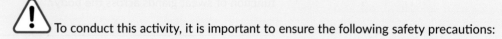

ACTIVITY 9.6: FLUID PENETRATION IN THE EPIDERMIS

The epidermis consists of four distinct cell types, found in four distinct layers in thin skin and five distinct layers in thick skin. The stratum corneum of the epidermis provides a thick, nearly waterproof barrier that prevents fluid loss to the environment, but also prevents excess fluid absorption and pathogen penetration into underlying layers of the skin. **Keratinocytes**, located in the epidermis, produce the fibrous protein keratin, while sebum, produced by the sebaceous glands located in the dermis, is an oily, lipid-based secretion. Together, keratin and sebum act to protect and waterproof the epidermis.

This activity demonstrates the structure of the skin epidermis and its effects on fluid penetration.

⚠ To conduct this activity, it is important to ensure the following safety precautions:

- *Methyl orange indicator is poisonous and may cause skin, eye and respiratory irritation.*
- *Scarlet R (Sudan IV) is a strong stain and can cause irritation.*
- *Methylene blue is a strong stain and can cause irritation.*
- *Ensure disposable gloves are worn at all times and the area is well ventilated.*

Part 1: Epidermal Diffusion and Protection

The epidermis consists of keratinised cells which are further waterproofed by sebum produced by embedded sebaceous glands, producing a unique biological barrier to the external environment.

1. This activity is best conducted individually or in pairs.

2. Obtain an A4 sheet of graph paper (1 mm), scissors, forceps, stopwatch, methyl orange indicator, a ceramic tile or paper towel, deionised water, paraffin oil, disposable gloves, 2.5 cm wide dialysis tubing (moistened and cut open), and disposable pipettes.

3. From the sheet of graph paper, cut 14 individual squares approximately 3 cm × 3 cm in size (there should be 9 graph squares on each square of paper).

4. On a ceramic tile or paper towel, place 5 paper squares on top of each other forming a stack. This is tissue 1.

5. Next to this but not touching, place 4 paper squares on top of each other forming a stack.

6. Obtain another paper square and to this add 2 drops of water.

7. Using gloved hands, gently work the water into the paper square until it becomes damp.

8. Place the damp paper square on top of the four paper squares in the previously created stack. This is tissue 2.

9. Next to this but not touching, place 4 paper squares on top of each other forming a stack.

10. Obtain another paper square and to this add 2 drops paraffin oil.

11. Using gloved hands, gently work the oil into the paper square until it becomes translucent. Blot away any excess oil with a tissue.

12. Place the oiled paper square on top of the 4 paper squares in the previously created stack. This is tissue 3.

13. Next to this but not touching, place 4 paper squares on top of each other forming a stack.

14. Obtain a piece of dialysis tubing that has been moistened with water and cut open to form a flat ribbon.

15. Trim the dialysis tubing to a 3 cm × 3 cm square and place this on top of the 4 paper squares in the previously created stack, ensuring that the dialysis tubing remains flat and does not contain folds. This is tissue 4.

16. There should now be four stacks of paper squares each containing five layers.

17. To each paper stack, gently add 3 drops of methyl orange indicator to the central grid of the uppermost paper square, holding the paper stack down at the edges.

18. If the indicator runs to the edge of the paper square, you will need to start again.

19. Wait for 2 minutes.

20. Using forceps, gently lift and separate the paper layers starting from the top layer and count how many layers the methyl orange has penetrated in each stack.

21. Record your results in the table provided.

Tissue number	Tissue composition	Number of layers penetrated
Tissue 1	5 sheets of paper	
Tissue 2	4 sheets of paper + 1 damp sheet	
Tissue 3	4 sheets of paper + 1 oiled sheet	
Tissue 4	4 sheets of paper + 1 dialysis tubing sheet	

22. Consider the following questions:

a. Which tissue layer in skin do tissues 1 to 4 represent?

_____

b. What tissue type comprises this skin layer?

_____

c. Why was it necessary to construct tissue 1?

_____

_____

d. Noting the area of spread on the bottom sheet of the graph paper, was penetration greater in tissue 1 or tissue 2?

_____

e. What can be concluded about fluid penetration in tissues 1 and 2 and why?

_____

_____

_____

f. Is vegetable oil water-soluble or water-insoluble?

_____

g. What effect does the paraffin oil have on fluid penetration in tissue 3?

_____

_____

h. What does the paraffin oil in the top layer of tissue 3 represent?

_____

_____

i. Relate the results to the function of sebum in the skin.

_____

_____

_____

j. Dialysis tubing is composed of what material?

_____

_____

k. What effect does the dialysis tubing have on fluid penetration in tissue 4?

_____

_____

_____

l. What does the dialysis tubing in the top layer of tissue 4 represent?

_____

_____

m. Relate the results to the function of keratin in the skin.

_____

_____

_____

_____

n. Based on the number of layers penetrated by the methyl orange in tissues 3 and 4, what does this indicate about the function of this tissue?

_____

_____

_____

Part 2: Epidermal Barrier Penetration

The epidermis of the skin is protected by keratin and sebum, which provide a barrier to microorganisms attempting to penetrate the skin.

1. This activity is best conducted individually or in pairs.

2. Obtain an A4 sheet of graph paper (1 mm), scissors, forceps, Sudan IV stain, 2 paper towels, olive oil, stopwatch, disposable pipettes and disposable gloves.

3. From the sheet of graph paper, cut 2 individual squares approximately 3 cm × 3 cm in size.

4. Place the paper towels one on top of the other to create an absorptive base.

5. Place one of the paper squares on the paper towels. This is tissue 1.

6. To the other paper square, add 2 drops of olive oil.

7. Using gloved hands, gently work the oil into the paper square until it becomes translucent. Blot away any excess oil with a tissue.

8. Place the oiled paper square next to the dry paper square on the paper towel without touching. This is tissue 2.

9. To each paper square, gently add 3 drops of Sudan IV stain to the central grid of the paper square, holding the paper down at the edges.

10. If the stain runs to the edge of the paper square, you will need to start again.

11. Wait for 20 minutes.

12. Using forceps, gently lift each paper square to determine if the Sudan IV stain has penetrated through to the paper towels.

13. Record your results in the table provided.

Paper type	Paper penetrated? (yes/no)
Dry paper	
Oiled paper	

14. Consider the following questions:

a. What does the olive oil in tissue 2 represent?

_____

_____

b. Why did the Sudan IV stain penetrate tissue 1 more readily than tissue 2?

_____

_____

_____

Apply the Concepts

1. Can skin that is moisturised be moisturised further? Explain.

   _____

   _____

   _____

2. How do skin creams act to moisturise the skin?

   _____

   _____

   _____

3. How does sunburn occur?

   _____

   _____

   _____

4. What causes the symptoms associated with sunburn?

   _____

   _____

   _____

5. How do sunscreens work to prevent sunburn?

   _____

   _____

   _____

ACTIVITY 9.7: STRUCTURE AND FUNCTION OF NAILS

Nails are modifications of the epidermis, which forms scale-like structures on the dorsal surfaces and distal portions of the fingertips and toes (Fig. 9.4). Nails provide a clear, protective covering as can be seen from their free edges, which assist with picking up small objects and scratching surfaces. Nails are composed of keratin; however, in contrast to the soft keratin found in the epidermis, nails are composed of hard keratin which is more resilient. The underlying dermis in the nail bed contains a rich capillary network which causes nails to appear pink, a feature which can also be used diagnostically.

This activity provides an overview of the structure and function of nails.

1. Identify the structures of the nail shown in Fig. 9.4, using the terms provided. (Note: some terms are used more than once.)

   a. Bone: _____

   b. Cuticle: _____

   c. Free edge: _____

   d. Lunula: _____

   e. Nail bed: _____

   f. Nail body: _____

   g. Nail matrix: _____

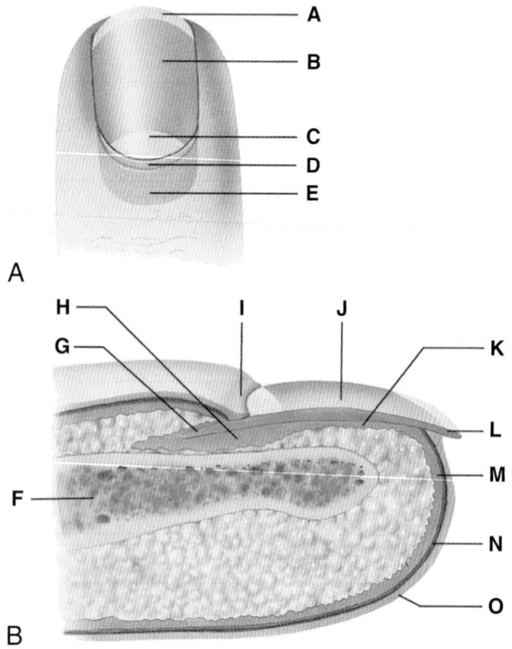

   h. Nail root: _____

   i. Stratum corneum: _____

   j. Stratum germinativum: _____

   k. Stratum granulosum: _____

2. Briefly state the function of each of the following nail structures:

   a. Cuticle: _____
   _____

   b. Free edge: _____
   _____

   c. Lunula: _____
   _____

   d. Nail bed: _____
   _____

   e. Nail body: _____
   _____

   f. Nail matrix: _____
   _____

   g. Nail root: _____
   _____

3. What is the relationship between the nail root and the lunula?

   _____
   _____
   _____

Figure 9.4 Nail structure. **A** Surface view. **B** Sagittal section. (*Source: Patton, K.T., Thibodeau, G.A., & Douglas, M. (2011). Essentials of anatomy and physiology. Mosby, St Louis.*)

ACTIVITY 9.8: PHYSICAL EXAMINATION OF THE NAILS

A physical examination of the nails can provide an insight into any structural changes, which often reflect alterations to underlying physiology (Fig. 9.5). This information can be applied clinically to determine the presence of a number of conditions; however, further clinical testing is always recommended to assess for causative pathology.

This activity examines the appearance, characteristics and surface structures of the nails.

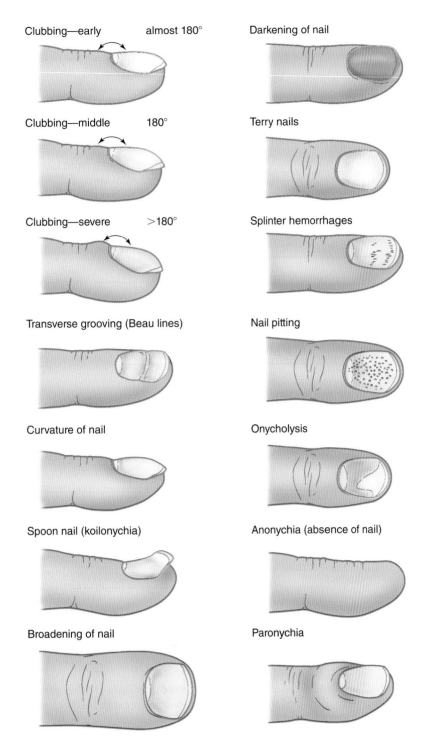

Figure 9.5 Nail conditions.
(Source: Ball, J. W., Dains, J. E., Flynn, J. A., Solomon, B. S., & Stewart, R. W. (2019). Seidel's guide to physical examination: An interprofessional approach. Elsevier.)

1. This activity is best conducted in pairs.

2. Obtain a magnifying glass or hand lens and a desk lamp.

3. Examine the surface of the nails on the subject's right hand noting the colour, length and shape.

4. Note the lunula, cuticle and nail body on each nail of the right hand, referring to Fig. 9.4 to assist with identification.

   a. Is the lunula visible on each nail of the right hand? Explain.

   _____

   _____

   _____

5. Note the colour of the nail body.

   a. What colour are the nail bodies and why?

   _____

   _____

   _____

6. Turn the subject's hand laterally and examine the nails from a sagittal view.

7. Refer to Fig. 9.5 to assist with your examination.

   a. Do any of the nails being examined display any of the characteristics indicated?

   _____

Apply the Concepts

1. In a physical assessment, what do the following nail conditions indicate physiologically?

   a. Clubbing: _____

   b. Transverse grooving: _____

   c. Spooning (koilonychia): _____

   d. Pitting: _____

   e. Onycholysis: _____

   f. Paronychia: _____

ACTIVITY 9.9: NAIL STRUCTURE

Nails are claw-like extensions of the fingers and toes that correspond to the nails of other primates and the claws found in other animals. Indeed, nails are composed of the same type of keratin found in the hooves, hair, claws and horns of other vertebrates. Nails consist of a number of functional structures; however, it is the nail matrix that produces cells that eventually become the nail plate (Fig. 9.6). The size, length and thickness of the nail matrix will determine the width and thickness of the nail plate, while the shape of the fingertip bone determines whether the nail plate is flat, arched or hooked.

This activity examines the structure of nails using a histological micrograph.

1. Identify each of the structures found in the fingernail shown in Fig. 9.6, referring to Fig. 9.4 to assist with identification.

   a. Structure 1: _____

   b. Structure 2: _____

   c. Structure 3: _____

   d. Structure 4: _____

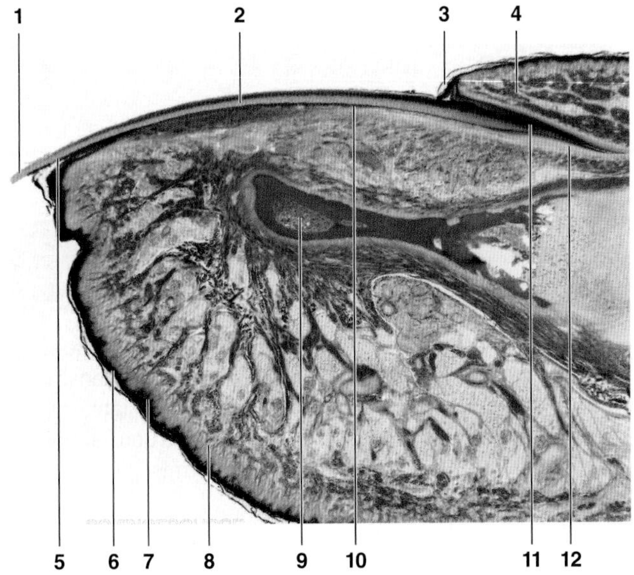

Figure 9.6 Fingernail structure.
(Source: Alvin Telser/Science Source)

h. Structure 8: _____

i. Structure 9: _____

j. Structure 10: _____

k. Structure 11: _____

l. Structure 12: _____

2. Consider the following questions:

a. How does the structure of the nail matrix differ from that of the nail plate?

_____

_____

b. How might damage to the nail matrix affect nail growth?

_____

_____

_____

_____

e. Structure 5: _____

f. Structure 6: _____

g. Structure 7: _____

Apply the Concepts

1. What diagnostic significance does the colour of the nail beds have?

_____

_____

_____

2. Why do some hospital admission forms ask patients to remove nail polish prior to admission for a surgical procedure?

_____

_____

_____

3. What is a hangnail and how does it occur?

_____

_____

_____

4. What is an ingrown nail and how does it occur?

_____

_____

_____

_____

Additional Activities

For additional activities visit Activity 9F: Microscopic Examination of Nails on Evolve.

ACTIVITY 9.10: STRUCTURE OF HAIR

Hair can be found over the entire surface of the body with the exception of the palms of the hands, soles of the feet, lips, nipples and parts of the external genitalia. Depending on the location of the hair, as well as its thickness and density, it can provide sensory information about the skin surface, guard against physical trauma, protect against sunlight, and assist in thermoregulation. Hair grows from **hair follicles** located within the dermis of the skin, forming a structural unit (Fig. 9.7). The hair follicles, although located within the dermis, are actually tubular pockets of the epidermis.

This activity provides an overview of the structure and function of human hair.

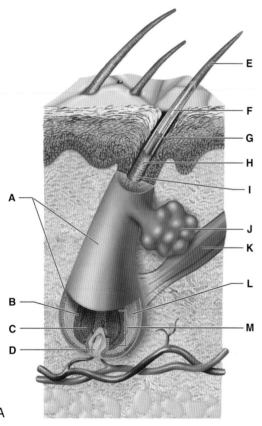

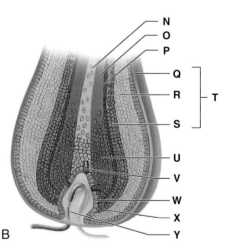

Figure 9.7. Hair follicle. **A** Hair follicle and related skin structures. **B** Hair follicle wall and hair bulb.
(Source: Patton, K. T., Bell, F.B., Thompson, T., & Williamson, P. (2018). Anatomy and physiology. Elsevier.)

1. Identify the structures of the hair shown in Fig. 9.7, by assigning a letter to each of the terms provided. (Note: some terms have more than one letter).

   a. Arrector pili muscle: _____

   b. Cortex: _____

   c. Cuticle: _____

   d. Dermal root sheath: _____

   e. External root sheath: _____

   f. Glassy membrane: _____

   g. Hair bulb: _____

   h. Hair follicle wall: _____

i. Hair matrix: _____

j. Hair root: _____

k. Hair shaft: _____

l. Internal root sheath: _____

m. Medulla: _____

n. Melanocyte: _____

o. Papilla: _____

p. Sebaceous gland: _____

q. Stratum basale: _____

2. Briefly state the function of each of the following hair structures:

a. Cortex: _____

_____

b. Cuticle: _____

_____

c. Hair bulb: _____

_____

d. Hair follicle: _____

_____

e. Hair matrix: _____

_____

f. Medulla: _____

_____

g. Melanocyte: _____

_____

h. Papilla: _____

_____

3. What is found in the:

a. Cortex? _____

_____

b. Cuticle? _____

_____

c. Medulla? _____

_____

4. Blood supplied to the hair bulb is drawn from which layer of the skin?

_____

_____

5. In which layer of the skin is the hair follicle located?

_____

6. Identify the location of the following segments of hair:

a. Bulb: _____

_____

b. Root: _____

_____

c. Shaft: _____

_____

7. Identify the characteristics and location of:

a. Terminal hair: _____

_____

_____

b. Vellus hair: _____

_____

_____

Apply the Concepts

1. How does the application of hair conditioner affect the hair shaft?

_____

_____

_____

2. How do hair bleaching and hair colourants affect the hair shaft?

_____

_____

_____

ACTIVITY 9.11: STRUCTURE AND FUNCTION OF THE HAIR FOLLICLE

Like the nails, hair is composed of hard keratin. This is deposited in the base of the hair follicle at the hair matrix by blood vessels located in the papilla. The hair matrix consists of dividing cells which are pushed upwards as they mature, fuse and become keratinised, while new cells replace them (Fig. 9.8). This causes the hair shaft to grow longer as the process is repeated. Hair follicles undergo growth cycles in which they are active or inactive; however, a variety of conditions can affect the health of the hair follicles and, subsequently, the texture of the hair and the rate at which it grows.

This activity examines the structure and function of a hair follicle using histological micrographs.

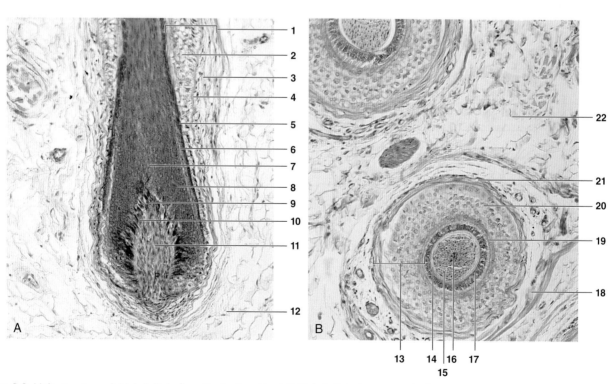

Figure 9.8 Hair structure. **A** Hair follicle (longitudinal section). **B** Hair follicle (cross-section).
(Source: Patton, K. T., Thibodeau, G. A., & Hutton, A. (2019). Anatomy and physiology. Adapted international edition. Elsevier.)

1. Identify each of the structures found in the hair follicle shown in Fig. 9.8A, referring to Fig. 9.7 to assist.

   a. Structure 1: _____

   b. Structure 2: _____

   c. Structure 3: _____

   d. Structure 4: _____

   e. Structure 5: _____

   f. Structure 6: _____

   g. Structure 7: _____

   h. Structure 8: _____

   i. Structure 9: _____

   j. Structure 10: _____

   k. Structure 11: _____

   l. Structure 12: _____

2. Identify each of the structures found in the hair follicle shown in Fig. 9.8B, referring to Fig. 9.7 to assist.

   a. Structure 13: _____

   b. Structure 14: _____

   c. Structure 15: _____

   d. Structure 16: _____

   e. Structure 17: _____

   f. Structure 18: _____

   g. Structure 19: _____

   h. Structure 20: _____

   i. Structure 21: _____

   j. Structure 22: _____

3. Consider the following questions:

   a. What is the peripheral connective tissue sheath?

   _____

   b. What is the glassy membrane?

   _____

   c. What is the epithelial root sheath?

   _____

   d. How are the texture and curliness of hair determined by the hair shaft?

   _____

   _____

   _____

Apply the Concepts

1. Which process is responsible for the production of white hairs?

   _____

   _____

   _____

2. Which process is responsible for hair loss (alopecia)?

   _____

   _____

   _____

Additional Activities

For additional activities visit Activity 9G: Microscopic Examination of Hair Structures on Evolve.

Additional Resources

Australian College of Dermatologists: A to Z of Skin

The A to Z of Skin database, provided by the Australian College of Dermatologists, offers information about common skin conditions, problems, symptoms, causes, and how they are diagnosed and treated.

www.dermcoll.edu.au/a-to-z-of-skin/

BBC Bitesize: Skincare

A short lesson providing information about UV light from the sun and the damage it can cause to skin and DNA through free-radical reactions, with associated test material.

www.bbc.co.uk/bitesize/guides/zbwtbdm/revision/1

DermIS Dermatology Information System

DermIS is a dermatology information service offering elaborate image atlases, complete with diagnoses and differential diagnoses, case reports and additional information on almost all skin diseases.

www.dermis.net/dermisroot/en/home/index.htm

Dermnet: Skin Disease Atlas

Dermnet is a dermatology source dedicated to online medical education though articles, photos and videos providing information on a wide variety of skin conditions through innovative media.

www.dermnet.com/

DermNet NZ

DermNet NZ is a resource about the skin providing more than 2500 topic pages and 25 000 clinical and dermatopathology images, supported by the New Zealand Dermatological Society Incorporated.

www.dermnetnz.org/

Histology Guide Virtual Microscopy Laboratory: Skin

Histology Guide is an online resource providing a virtual microscopy laboratory experience, by allowing users to view microscope slides from professional collections for the purpose of interpreting cellular and tissue structures as seen through a microscope.

histologyguide.com/slidebox/11-skin.html

Innerbody Research: Integumentary System

Innerbody Research provides objective, science-based advice to help readers make more informed choices about home health products and services with most up-to-date reviews, guides and research, including information about various body systems.

www.innerbody.com/anatomy/integumentary

Osmosis – Integumentary System

The Integumentary System module of Osmosis provides videos, notes, quiz questions and links to further resources related to the integumentary system.

www.osmosis.org/library/md/foundational-sciences/physiology#integumentary_system

The Histology Guide: The Skin

The Histology Guide is a virtual experience of using a microscope with zoom features divided into topics and offering histological slides with labels and quizzes for each topic such as skin. It is provided by the University of Leeds.

www.histology.leeds.ac.uk/skin/index.php

CHAPTER 10
The Skeletal System and Joints

The skeletal system comprises the bones of the skeleton, the joints or articulations formed where bone endings converge, and the tissues which comprise, maintain and integrate these structures. The human skeleton is composed of 206 bones of varying size and shape, which act to provide support for the limbs and trunk, protection for soft and vital organs, and attachment sites for muscles and tendons, facilitating movement.

Bones, while seemingly lifeless, contain living tissues that are remodelled throughout life and play a vital role in mineral storage and the maintenance of blood calcium levels. This is achieved through coordinated events involving endocrine organs which regulate the activities of resident bone cells. In addition, red bone marrow situated within the medullary cavities of certain bones, is active in the process of haematopoiesis – the production of blood cells, each with specialised functions. (Refer to Chapter 15: Blood, for further information on blood cells.) Due to its metabolic properties and abundant blood supply, bone is capable of self-repair when damaged or fractured.

LEARNING OUTCOMES

On completion of these activities, the student should be able to:

1. identify the functions and locations of bones in the skeleton
2. distinguish between the axial and appendicular skeleton, and associated structures
3. classify and identify bones based on their shape
4. identify the macroscopic structures of a long bone
5. identify the microscopic structure of skeletal tissues and bone
6. compare the structural differences between compact and spongy bone
7. explain the processes associated with calcium regulation
8. explain the composition of the bone matrix
9. compare the structure and function of the organic and inorganic components of bone
10. identify various types of bone fractures and explain the process of bone healing
11. classify joints according to structure and function
12. explain synovial joint structure, classification and function
13. describe synovial joint movement and range of motion (ROM).

KEY TERMS

Appendicular skeleton	Collagen	Osteoid
Articulation	Compact bone	Osteon
Axial skeleton	Fibrous joint	Parathyroid hormone (PTH)
Bone	Fracture	Range of motion (ROM)
Bone marrow	Joint	Skeletal system
Bone matrix	Ossification	Skeleton
Calcitonin	Osteoblast	Spongy bone
Cartilage	Osteoclast	Synovial joint
Cartilaginous joint	Osteocyte	Trabeculae

Additional Activities

For additional activities visit Activity 10A: Bones of the Skeleton on Evolve˙.

ACTIVITY 10.1: BONE CLASSIFICATION AND IDENTIFICATION

Human bones exhibit a variety of shapes and sizes related to their locations and functions. To simplify the wide variation in bone morphology, bones are classified according to their shape, which does not necessarily relate to their size. Classifying bones according to shape assists in understanding how the bone fits within the skeleton and how surrounding structures interact with the bone. In addition, bone shape also provides functional information when bone ends form **joints** or **articulations**.

This activity explores the classification, identification and morphology of various bone shapes.

1. This activity is best conducted in pairs.

2. Obtain an articulated skeleton or refer to Fig. 10A.1A.

3. Identify and list two bones classified according to the following bone shapes:

   a. Long bone: _____

   b. Short bone: _____

   c. Sesamoid bone: _____

   d. Flat bone: _____

   e. Irregular bone: _____

4. You have been provided with 10 sealed and numbered bags each containing one bone.

5. Without opening the bags, feel the shape of each bone through the bag.

6. Identify each of the bone shapes provided using the following terms and determine the location of each bone on an articulated skeleton or Fig. 10A.1A.

   Long   Short   Sesamoid   Flat   Irregular

   a. Bone 1: _____

      i. Location: _____

   b. Bone 2: _____

      i. Location: _____

   c. Bone 3: _____

      i. Location: _____

   d. Bone 4: _____

      i. Location: _____

e. Bone 5: _____

   i. Location: _____

f. Bone 6: _____

   i. Location: _____

g. Bone 7: _____

   i. Location: _____

h. Bone 8: _____

   i. Location: _____

i. Bone 9: _____

   i. Location: _____

j. Bone 10: _____

   i. Location: _____

7. Consider the following questions:

a. Where are most long bones located in the human skeleton?

_____

b. What is the general function of long bones?

_____

_____

c. Where are most short bones located in the human skeleton?

_____

d. What is the general function of short bones?

_____

_____

e. Where are most irregular bones located in the human skeleton?

_____

f. What is the general function of irregular bones?

_____

_____

g. Where are most flat bones located in the human skeleton?

_____

h. What is the general function of flat bones?

_____

_____

i. Where are most sesamoid bones located in the human skeleton?

_____

j. What is the general function of sesamoid bones?

_____

_____

k. Sesamoid bones are a sub-type of which bone shape?

_____

l. Sesamoid bones are so named because of their resemblance to what?

_____

ACTIVITY 10.2: MACROSCOPIC AND MICROSCOPIC BONE STRUCTURE

The bones of the body can be examined for macroscopic and microscopic structures (Fig. 10.1). Macroscopic structures relate to bone morphology and give clues about bone associations with surrounding structures, while microscopic structures relate to bone composition are involved in the maintenance of the body's calcium balance. Microscopic structures can be identified in most bones as belonging to two distinct tissues – **compact bone** (or cortical bone), which is dense and provides protection and strength, and **spongy bone** (or cancellous bone), which is less dense and allows for slight compression in bone ends or where stresses arrive from many directions.

This activity outlines the macroscopic and microscopic structure of bones.

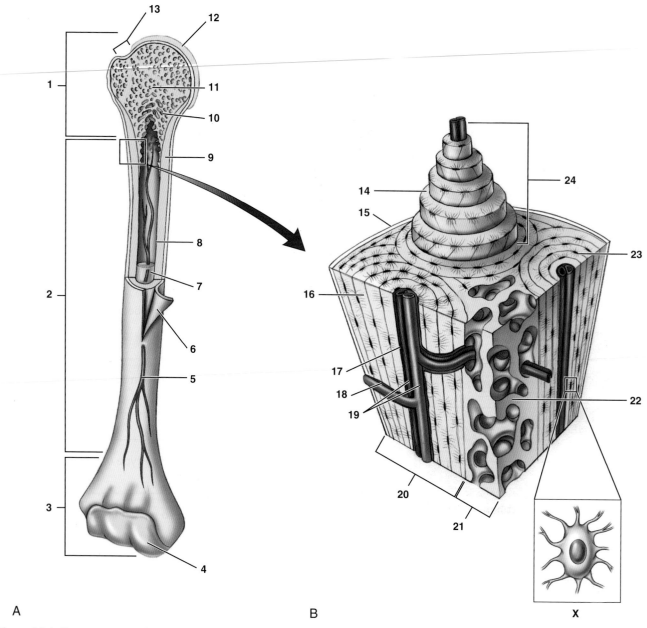

Figure 10.1 Bone structure. **A** Macroscopic (gross) structure. **B** Microscopic structure.
(Source: Herlihy, B. (2018). The human body in health and illness. Elsevier.)

1. Identify each of the numbered structures shown in Fig. 10.1:

   a. Structure 1: _____

   b. Structure 2: _____

   c. Structure 3: _____

   d. Structure 4: _____

   e. Structure 5: _____

   f. Structure 6: _____

   g. Structure 7: _____

   h. Structure 8: _____

   i. Structure 9: _____

   j. Structure 10: _____

   k. Structure 11: _____

   l. Structure 12: _____

   m. Structure 13: _____

   n. Structure 14: _____

o. Structure 15: _____

p. Structure 16: _____

q. Structure 17: _____

r. Structure 18: _____

s. Structure 19: _____

t. Structure 20: _____

u. Structure 21: _____

v. Structure 22: _____

w. Structure 23: _____

x. Structure 24: _____

2. Consider the following questions:

a. What is the function of structure 6?

_____

_____

b. What is contained in structure 7?

_____

_____

c. What is the function of structure 8?

_____

_____

d. What is contained in structure 10?

_____

_____

e. What is the function of structure 12?

_____

_____

f. What is the function of structure 13?

_____

_____

g. What is the function of structure 14?

_____

_____

h. What is the function of structure 16?

_____

_____

i. What is the function of structure 17?

_____

_____

j. What is the function of structure 18?

_____

_____

k. What is the function of structure 22?

_____

_____

l. What is structure X?

_____

m. What is the function of structure X?

_____

_____

n. Structure X is located within which of the structures shown?

_____

o. What is the metaphysis?

_____

_____

p. Compact bone is composed of which structural units?

_____

q. Spongy bone is composed of which structural units?

_____

r. The structural units of spongy bone form in response to what?

_____

_____

Apply the Concepts

1. What is ostealgia and how does it occur?

_____

_____

_____

_____

ACTIVITY 10.3: EXAMINATION OF A LONG BONE

The overall examination of bones provides information about their composition, their relationship to surrounding structures, and how they work in unison with those structures to achieve functions such as movement and protection.

This activity examines the macroscopic (gross) structure of a beef bone and the composition of bone marrow.

⚠ To conduct this activity, it is important to ensure the following safety precautions:

- *Wear disposable gloves and safety glasses at all times during the activity as fresh specimens may harbour pathogenic microorganisms.*

- *Exercise care when handling dissection tools.*

- *Additional precautions, including safe disposal of animal material, may be required by your demonstrator.*

Part 1: Examination of a Long Bone

Macroscopic bone structures are more easily distinguished in long bones due to the overall elongated shape of the bone, and this information can be related to microscopic structures observed under the microscope.

1. This activity is best conducted in groups of two or three.

2. Obtain a beef bone, a metal spatula, 25 mL beaker, hotplate (placed on a heat mat), disposable pipettes, scarlet R dye (Sudan IV), microscope slides, coverslips and a compound microscope.

3. Don the disposable gloves and place the beef bone on the dissecting tray or bench covering.

4. Using the magnifying glass and blunt probe, carefully identify and examine the following structures:

a. Periosteum

i. Where is the periosteum located?

_____

ii. Does the periosteum separate from the bone easily? Explain.

_____

_____

iii. What is the function of the periosteum?

_____

_____

b. Bone markings

i. Where are the bone markings located?

_____

ii. How do the bone markings appear?

_____

_____

iii. What are bone markings?

_____

_____

iv. What are the functions of bone markings?

_____

_____

c. Diaphysis

i. Where is the diaphysis located?

_____

ii. How does the surface of the diaphysis appear?

_____

_____

iii. What is the diaphysis composed of?

_____

d. Medullary cavity

i. Where is the medullary cavity located?

_____

ii. What is found in the medullary cavity?

_____

_____

e. Epiphyses

i. Where are the epiphyses located?

_____

ii. What are the epiphyses composed of?

_____

iii. What is found in the cavities within the epiphyses?

_____

f. Epiphyseal plate

i. Where is the epiphyseal plate located?

_____

ii. What is the epiphyseal plate?

_____

_____

iii. What is an epiphyseal line?

_____

_____

g. Articular cartilage

i. Where is the articular cartilage located?

_____

ii. What is articular cartilage composed of?

_____

iii. What is the function of articular cartilage?

_____

_____

h. Endosteum

i. Where is the endosteum located?

_____

ii. How does the endosteum appear?

_____

_____

iii. What is the function of the endosteum?

_____

_____

5. Retain the beef bone for Part 2 of this activity.

Part 2: Examination of Bone Marrow Composition

Many long bones contain an observable medullary cavity containing red bone marrow, the site of haematopoiesis. Examination of **bone marrow** provides an insight into its nature as a connective tissue and its role in the manufacture of the formed elements of blood.

1. This activity is best conducted in pairs.

2. Obtain a metal spatula, 25 mL beaker, hotplate, disposable pipettes, scarlet R dye, microscope slides, coverslips and a compound microscope.

3. Using the metal spatula, scrape samples from the bone marrow, placing them directly into the beaker (you will need to collect enough to fit into a 1 cm × 1 cm cube).

4. Place the beaker on the hotplate; turn up the heat setting and the stirrer setting (if available) to high and heat until just melted (ensure that you watch this carefully as the marrow will melt quickly).

5. Working quickly, place a drop of the marrow onto a microscope slide with a disposable pipette.

6. Add 1 drop of scarlet R dye with a disposable pipette, mixing together well with the tip of the pipette and apply a coverslip.

7. View the slide with the microscope starting with the ×4 objective and progressing to the ×40 objective.

8. For best results, direct your viewing towards the periphery of the specimen.

9. Draw a diagram of what you can see in the space below.

Magnification of diagram: × _____

10. Consider the following questions:

a. Scarlet R dye detects the presence of which macromolecule and why?

_____

_____

b. How did the marrow sample appear under the ×40 objective?

_____

_____

c. What does this indicate about the chemical composition of bone marrow?

_____

_____

Additional Activities

For additional activities visit Activity 10B: Identification of Skeletal Tissues on Evolve°.

For additional activities visit Activity 10C: Microscopic Examination of Skeletal Tissues on Evolve°.

ACTIVITY 10.4: COMPONENTS AND MODELS OF BONE

Cartilage, in the form of hyaline cartilage or fibrocartilage, is the foundation of developing and healing bone. Cartilage is comprised of approximately 80% water, the remainder including organic collagen, a fibrous protein. This provides a flexible matrix within which inorganic calcium salts, mainly calcium phosphate, can be deposited, acting to strengthen the bone tissue over time. This characteristic is common to both compact bone and spongy bone, yet these bone types are found in different locations within the skeleton.

This activity demonstrates the organic and inorganic components of bone and examines the structural differences between compact and spongy bone.

Part 1: Organic and Inorganic Bone Components

The bone matrix consists of an organic component, the **osteoid**, composed primarily of collagen and water from the foundational cartilage tissue, and the inorganic salt component, primarily calcium phosphate. The characteristics that these components impart to bone can be compared to provide structural information about bone.

1. This activity is best completed in groups of two or three.

2. Obtain one 250 mL beaker, two 100 mL beakers, a permanent marker, 100 mL measuring cylinder, gelatine powder, deionised water, 5 calcium tablets, mortar, pestle, electronic scale, hotplate (placed on a heat mat), popsticks, three 20 mL syringes, masking tape, a test tube rack (or 250 mL beaker), weigh boat, 2 test tubes, 1.0 M HCl and a stopwatch.

3. Label the syringes 1 to 3, and the 100 mL beakers 1 and 2, with the permanent marker.

4. Remove the syringe plungers and place a piece of masking tape over the narrow tip of each syringe to seal the opening, but allow for easy removal.

5. Place the syringes in the test tube holder with the narrow tip facing downwards.

6. Place the 250 mL beaker on the electronic scale and tare the scale to zero.

7. Carefully add 20 g gelatine to the beaker and remove from the scale.

8. Measure 100 mL of deionised water with the measuring cylinder and add to the beaker, mixing well with a popstick.

9. Place the beaker on the hotplate; turn up the heat setting and the stirrer setting (if available) to high and heat until the mixture is melted and no solids remain, stirring with a popstick occasionally.

10. Pour 20 mL of the gelatine mixture into syringe 1 and allow to set.

11. Pour 20 mL of the gelatine mixture into beakers 1 and 2.

12. Using the mortar and pestle, crush one calcium tablet into a powder and add to beaker 1 with the gelatine mixture, stirring well with a popstick.

13. Pour this mixture into syringe 2 and allow to set.

14. Using the mortar and pestle, crush four calcium tablets into a powder and add to beaker 2 with the gelatine mixture, stirring well with a popstick.

15. Pour this mixture into syringe 3 and allow to set.

16. The syringes may be placed in the refrigerator for 15–30 minutes to reduce the setting time.

17. Once set, place a plunger into each syringe and press to expel the contents onto the laboratory bench, ensuring that the contents are expelled in parallel rows rather than in a pile.

18. Note the force required to expel the contents from each syringe.

    a. Which syringe required greater force to expel the contents?

    _____

19. Examine the expelled contents from each syringe noting the texture and consistency.

    a. What percentage of water did the initial gelatine mixture contain and what does this represent physiologically?

    _____

    _____

    b. The contents of which syringe showed the greatest flexibility when the strands were pulled and why?

    _____

c. The contents of which syringe showed the least flexibility when the strands were pulled and why?

_____

_____

d. Suggest a possible reason for the differences in flexibility and density between the strands when force is applied.

_____

_____

_____

_____

20. Label test tubes 1 and 2 with the permanent marker.

21. Measure 1 g of the contents from syringe 1 into a weigh boat with an electronic scale and place in test tube 1.

22. Measure 1 g of the contents from syringe 2 into a weigh boat with an electronic scale and place in test tube 2.

23. Add 5 mL HCl with a disposable pipette to each test tube and start timing each reaction with a stopwatch, agitating the tubes gently during the process.

24. Note the time taken for the contents in each test tube to completely dissolve below:

   a. Test tube 1: _____

   b. Test tube 2: _____

   c. Which gas was produced? _____

   d. Which component of the syringe mixtures did the HCl dissolve?

   _____

   _____

   e. Which physiological action in bone does the additional of HCl replicate and why?

   _____

   _____

   f. Suggest a possible reason for the different times taken for the contents of test tubes 1 and 2 to dissolve based on the composition of the mixtures in each of the test tubes.

   _____

   _____

   _____

25. Reserve the remaining gelatine mixture for Part 2 of this activity.

26. If time permits, allow the expelled syringe contents to air dry for 1 hour or overnight and examine the degree of flexibility in each.

27. Consider the following questions:

   a. Which part of bone tissue is considered non-living?

   _____

   _____

   b. Which part of bone tissue is considered living?

   _____

   _____

   c. What is the bone matrix and what is its composition?

   _____

   _____

   d. Which part of the bone matrix is organic and what is its composition?

   _____

   _____

   _____

   e. What is the origin of the organic component of bone?

   _____

   _____

   f. Which component of the bone matrix is composed of collagen?

   _____

   _____

   g. How is the collagen matrix of bone strengthened to withstand tension?

   _____

   _____

   h. Which part of the bone matrix is inorganic and what is its composition?

   _____

   _____

   i. What is the origin of the inorganic component of bone?

   _____

   _____

Part 2: Compact and Spongy Bone Models

There are two types of bone tissue – compact or cortical bone, and spongy or cancellous bone. Although both are composed of organic and inorganic components, the internal microscopic structure of each differs. Compact bone is dense, hard and consists of concentric **osteons** or Haversian systems, while spongy bone is light, porous and consists of **trabeculae** interspersed with intertrabecular spaces. The internal structure of bone tissue determines its location within bones and the skeleton.

1. This activity is best completed in groups of two or three.

2. Obtain the gelatine mixture from Part 1, two 100 mL beakers, a permanent marker, 8 calcium tablets, mortar, pestle, electronic scale, hotplate (placed on a heat mat), popsticks, weight boat (or watch glass), dry yeast, sugar, cling film, stopwatch, paper towels, knife and a magnifying glass.

3. Label the beakers 1 and 2 with the permanent marker.

4. Place the gelatine mixture from Part 1 on the hotplate to ensure a liquid consistency if the mixture has begun to solidify.

5. Using the mortar and pestle, crush 8 calcium tablets into a powder and add to the gelatine mixture from Part 1, stirring well with a popstick.

6. Measure 1 g dried yeast and 1 g sugar into the weigh boat with the electronic scale and add these to beaker 2.

7. Pour 20 mL of the gelatine mixture into beakers 1 and 2, stirring the contents of beaker 2 well with a popstick.

8. Cover beaker 2 with cling film and allow the mixtures in both beakers to set for 30 minutes.

9. Once the time has elapsed, examine the side of each beaker noting the appearance of each of the mixtures.

    a. Which mixture represents the structure of compact bone and why?

    _____

    b. Which mixture represents the structure of spongy bone and why?

    _____

10. Gently remove the mixtures carefully from each beaker onto a paper towel, by running a popstick around the inside rim of each beaker, so that two discs are extracted.

11. Gently press each disc between your fingers to determine its flexibility.

    a. Which disc allowed for greater absorption of force and why?

    _____

    _____

12. Gently cut each disc in half with a knife, so that the interior can be seen and examine the cross-section of each disc with the magnifying glass.

    a. Which disc indicated greater density and why?

    _____

    _____

13. If time permits, allow the discs to air dry for 1 hour or overnight and examine the degree of flexibility in each.

14. Consider the following questions:

    a. Disc 1 simulated which type of bone?

    _____

    b. Where is compact bone located within a long bone and how does its location relate to its function?

    _____

    _____

    c. Disc 2 simulated which type of bone?

    _____

    d. The air pockets in disc 2 represent which bone structures?

    _____

    e. The material in between the air pockets in disc 2 represent which bone structures?

    _____

    f. The air pockets in disc 2 were created by which component?

    _____

    g. In spongy bone, the air pockets simulated in disc 2 are created by which component?

    _____

    h. Where is spongy bone located within a long bone and how does its location relate to its function?

    _____

    _____

Apply the Concepts

1. Explain why hydroxyapatite is widely used in dentistry.

_____

_____

_____

ACTIVITY 10.5: CALCIUM REGULATION

The density of the inorganic salt portion (calcium phosphate) of the bone matrix is maintained through a series of biochemical processes (Fig. 10.2). This involves endocrine control via hormones and a number of organ systems, such as the urinary and digestive systems, which affect the retention, absorption and excretion of calcium. These processes contribute to calcium homeostasis in the body, which is directly related to blood calcium concentration.

This activity outlines the structures and processes involved in calcium regulation.

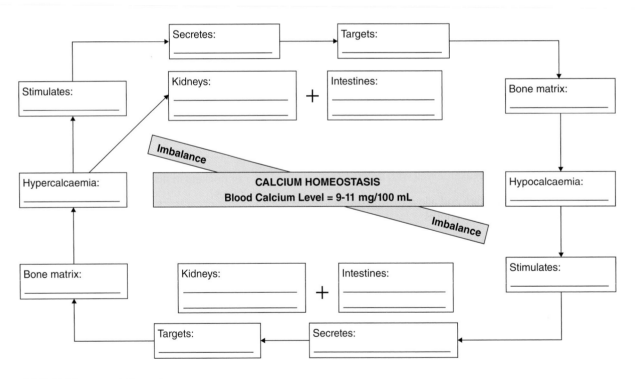

Figure 10.2 Calcium regulation.

1. Complete the calcium regulation feedback loop by filling in the boxes in Fig. 10.2, using the terms provided:

Degraded

Parathyroid hormone (PTH)

Ca^{2+} reabsorption from tubules increases

Thyroid gland

Calcitonin

Blood Ca^{2+} decreases

Osteoblasts in bone

Blood Ca^{2+} increases

Ca^{2+} reabsorption from tubules decreases

Parathyroid glands

Ca^{2+} absorption from food decreases

Ca^{2+} absorption from food increases

Osteoclasts in bone

Deposited

2. Consider the following questions:

a. What are osteoclasts and what is their function?

_____

_____

b. What are osteoblasts and what is their function?

_____

_____

c. Where is parathyroid hormone (PTH) produced and what is its function?

_____

_____

d. Explain what might occur to calcium homeostasis if the parathyroid glands were not functional.

_____

_____

_____

e. Where is calcitonin produced and what is its function?

_____

_____

f. Explain what might occur to calcium regulation if the thyroid gland was not functional.

_____

_____

g. How does the renal system contribute to calcium homeostasis?

_____

_____

h. How does the digestive system contribute to calcium homeostasis?

_____

_____

_____

i. Suggest what might occur in the hypocalcaemia loop if blood calcium regulation is not reached?

_____

_____

_____

_____

j. If calcium regulation is not maintained, how could you determine if the issue was at the bone or glandular level?

_____

_____

_____

_____

Apply the Concepts

1. Explain how hyperparathyroidism can lead to hypercalcaemia.

_____

_____

_____

2. What is bone density, how is it measured and what does it indicate?

_____

_____

_____

3. What is the role of vitamin D in maintaining bone density?

_____

_____

_____

4. What is Paget's disease and how does it occur?

_____

_____

_____

ACTIVITY 10.6: BONE COMPOSITION

Bone originates as either hyaline cartilage or fibrocartilage, which form the organic osteoid portion of bone. The **osteoid** then undergoes ossification with the addition of calcium salts in the form of calcium phosphate, and continues to be remodelled throughout life due to the actions of **osteoblasts**, **osteoclasts** and **osteocytes** under the influence of physical stressors and hormones such as **parathyroid hormone (PTH)** and **calcitonin**. Alterations in the levels of organic and inorganic components in bone will affect the composition and integrity of bone tissue, leading to compromised bone density and strength.

This activity demonstrates the composition of bone.

To conduct this activity, it is important to ensure the following safety precautions:

- *Wear disposable gloves and safety glasses at all times during the activity as the solvents used may cause skin and eye irritation.*
- *Exercise care when handling bleach to avoid damage to clothing and personal belongings.*
- *Exercise care when handling dissecting tools to avoid injury.*
- *Additional precautions, including safe disposal of animal material and solvents, may be required by your demonstrator.*

1. The activity is best conducted in pairs or in groups of four.

2. Obtain a raw chicken wing, dissecting scissors (or kitchen knife), paper towels, two 200 mL beakers, a permanent marker, 1.0 M HCl, household bleach, pH paper and disposable gloves.

3. With the permanent marker, label one beaker HCl, and the other beaker Bleach.

4. To the beaker labelled HCl, add 50 mL HCl.

5. To the beaker labelled Bleach, add 50 mL bleach.

6. Test the pH of each solution with the pH paper and record the pH below:

    a. pH of HCl:_____

    b. pH of bleach: _____

7. Don the disposable gloves and place the raw chicken wing on the paper towels.

8. Using the scissors or kitchen knife, section the wing at the joints so that three sections are obtained.

9. The wing tip section can be discarded, while the remaining two sections may be divided between two groups.

10. Gently remove the skin and flesh from the given wing section to expose the two bones within, and separate both bones from each other.

11. Wash the bones and pat dry with paper towels to ensure that no debris remain.

12. Place one chicken bone into each of the beakers and allow to sit for 30–45 minutes, noting any changes to the bones and the solvents.

    a. Were any changes observed in the bone or solvent in the beaker containing HCl? Explain.

    _____

    _____

    b. Were any changes observed in the bone or solvent in the beaker containing bleach? Explain.

    _____

    _____

13. After the time has elapsed, dispose of the liquid from each beaker carefully and gently pat the bones dry.

14. Gently manipulate each bone between your hands to determine any changes to the bone texture and integrity.

15. Dispose of the bones and solvents as indicated by your demonstrator.

16. Consider the following questions:

    a. Were any changes to the texture and integrity observed in the bone placed in HCl? Explain.

    _____

    _____

    b. Were any changes to the texture and integrity observed in the bone placed in bleach? Explain.

    _____

    _____

    c. Which bone element was removed by the HCl?

    _____

    d. The HCl represents the activity of which structure in bone?

    _____

    e. Which bone element was removed by the bleach?

    _____

    f. The bleach represents the activity of which structure in bone?

    _____

    g. Outline the relationship between pH and osteoclast activity in bone.

    _____

    _____

    _____

    h. Explain why the organic osteoid and inorganic calcium salts are both important to bone integrity.

    _____

    _____

    _____

Apply the Concepts

1. Why is adequate dietary calcium essential for the development of strong bones?

_____

_____

_____

2. What is osteogenesis imperfecta and how does it occur?

_____

_____

_____

3. What is osteomalacia and how does it occur?

_____

_____

_____

4. What is rickets and how does it occur?

_____

_____

_____

5. What is osteoporosis, how does it occur and what are three risk factors for its development?

_____

_____

_____

Additional Activities

For additional activities visit Activity 10D: Bone Fractures and Healing on Evolve˙.

ACTIVITY 10.7: JOINT (ARTICULATION) CLASSIFICATION AND STRUCTURE

A joint, or articulation, is a region of the skeleton where two or more bone ends meet. Joints can be classified structurally, based on the material holding the bone ends together (fibrous, cartilaginous, synovial), and functionally, based on the degree of movement allowed at the joint (immovable, slightly movable, freely movable).

This activity outlines the classification and structure of joints.

Part 1: Joint Classification

Immovable and slightly movable joints tend to be found in the axial skeleton, while freely movable joints tend to be found in the appendicular skeleton (Fig. 10.3). In general, the structural and functional classifications of joints are linked: **fibrous joints** tend to be immovable, **cartilaginous joints** tend to be slightly movable, and **synovial joints** tend to be freely movable (Fig. 10.4).

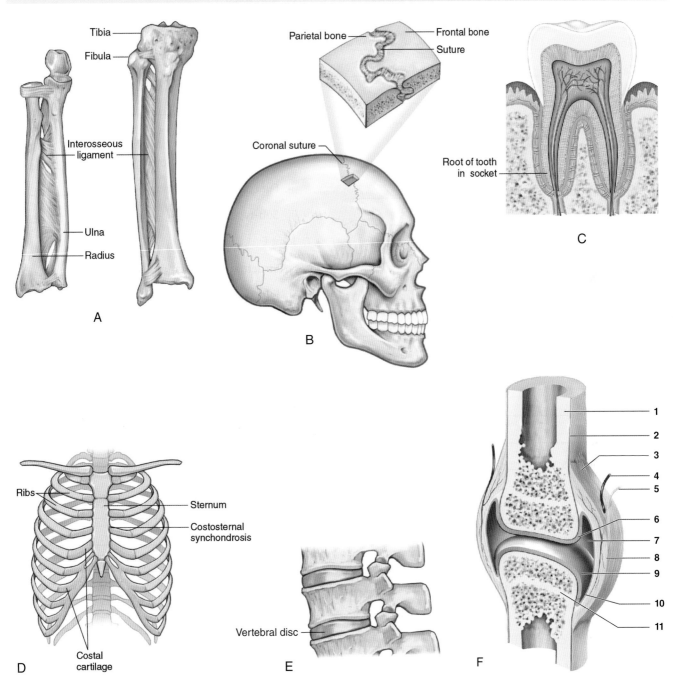

Figure 10.3 Joint classification and structure.
(Source: Patton, K. T., Thibodeau, G. A., & Hutton, A. (2019). Anatomy and physiology. Adapted international edition. Elsevier.)

1. Identify two main functions of joints.

   _____

   _____

2. Explain the following structural classifications relating to joints:

   a. Fibrous: _____

   b. Cartilaginous: _____

   c. Synovial: _____

3. Explain the following functional classifications relating to joints:

   a. Synarthrosis: _____

   b. Amphiarthrosis: _____

   c. Diarthrosis: _____

4. For each of the following joint sub-type classifications, state the functional classification, the structural classification and the connecting tissue involved:

   a. Gomphosis: _____

   _____

   b. Suture: _____

   _____

   c. Symphysis: _____

   _____

   d. Synchondrosis: _____

   _____

   e. Syndesmosis: _____

   _____

5. Consider the joints shown in Fig. 10.3 and identify the structural and functional classifications of each:

   a. Joint A

      i. Structural classification: _____

      ii. Functional classification: _____

      iii. Sub-type: _____

   b. Joint B

      i. Structural classification: _____

      ii. Functional classification: _____

      iii. Sub-type: _____

   c. Joint C

      i. Structural classification: _____

      ii. Functional classification: _____

      iii. Sub-type: _____

   d. Joint D

      i. Structural classification: _____

      ii. Functional classification: _____

      iii. Sub-type: _____

   e. Joint E

      i. Structural classification: _____

      ii. Functional classification: _____

      iii. Sub-type: _____

   f. Joint F

      i. Structural classification: _____

      ii. Functional classification: _____

6. Referring to an articulated skeleton for assistance, identify the structural and functional classification of each of the numbered joints in Fig. 10.4.

   a. Joint 1: _____

   b. Joint 2: _____

   c. Joint 3: _____

   d. Joint 4: _____

   e. Joint 5: _____

   f. Joint 6: _____

   g. Joint 7: _____

   h. Joint 8: _____

   i. Joint 9: _____

   j. Joint 10: _____

   k. Joint 11: _____

7. Consider the following questions:

   a. Which structure/s are common to all joints?

   _____

   _____

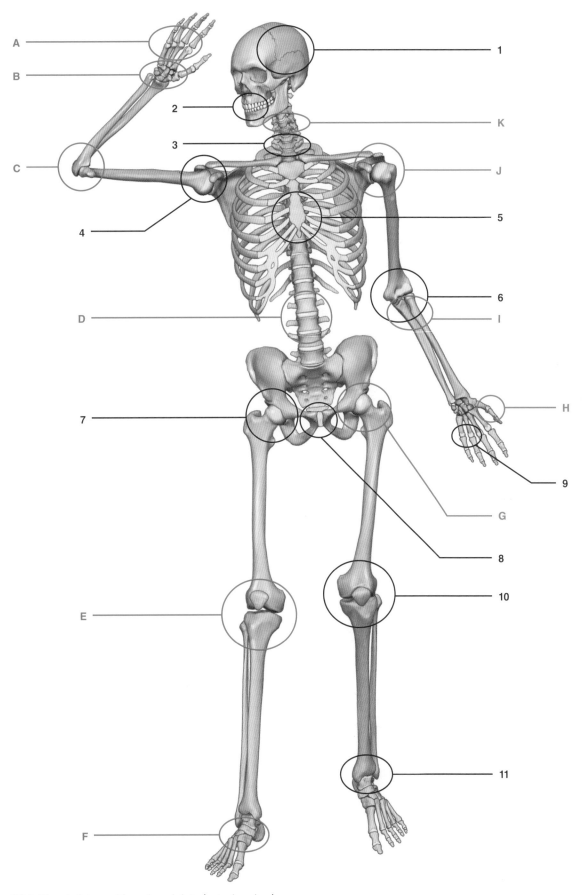

Figure 10.4 The skeleton with various joints (anterior view).
(Source: Solomon, E. P. (2016). Introduction to human anatomy and physiology. Elsevier.)

b. Explain the structural difference between sutures and syndesmoses.

_____

_____

c. Outline the relationship between joint stability and mobility.

_____

_____

d. What is the function of the pubic symphysis?

_____

_____

Part 2: Synovial Joint Structure and Classification

Synovial joints are structurally unique due to the presence of a synovial fluid-filled capsule, and present the most flexibility in terms of movement. Synovial joints are considered freely movable and can be classified into six sub-types, based on the direction of movement allowed by each joint (Fig. 10.5). The location of each synovial joint type within the skeleton is a direct reflection of the type of movement required at that joint.

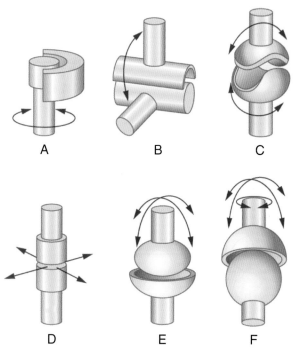

A   B   C

D   E   F

Figure 10.5 Types of synovial joints.
(Source: Hombach-Klonisch, S., Klonisch, T., & Peeler, J. (eds). (2019). Sobotta clinical atlas of human anatomy. Elsevier.)

1. Identify the synovial joint structures in Fig. 10.3F (p. 229):

   a. Structure 1: _____

   b. Structure 2: _____

   c. Structure 3: _____

   d. Structure 4: _____

   e. Structure 5: _____

   f. Structure 6: _____

   g. Structure 7: _____

   h. Structure 8: _____

   i. Structure 9: _____

   j. Structure 10: _____

   k. Structure 11: _____

2. Consider the following questions:

   a. What is found in the joint cavity of synovial joints?

   _____

   b. What is the function of the synovial membrane?

   _____

   _____

   c. Explain the function of the joint capsule and its tissue composition.

   _____

   _____

   _____

   d. What is the function of the articular cartilage?

   _____

   _____

   _____

   e. What is the function of capsular ligaments?

   _____

   _____

   _____

   f. What is a bursa and what is its function?

   _____

   _____

   _____

3. Consider the synovial joints in Fig. 10.5 and identify each joint type:

   a. Joint A: _____

   b. Joint B: _____

   c. Joint C: _____

   d. Joint D: _____

   e. Joint E: _____

   f. Joint F: _____

4. Referring to an articulated skeleton for assistance and noting the shape of the articulating surfaces, identify the type of synovial joint indicated by the letters in Fig. 10.4.

   a. Joint A: _____

   b. Joint B: _____

   c. Joint C: _____

   d. Joint D: _____

   e. Joint E: _____

   f. Joint F: _____

   g. Joint G: _____

   h. Joint H: _____

   i. Joint I: _____

   j. Joint J: _____

   k. Joint K: _____

Apply the Concepts

1. What is dislocation and how does it occur?
   _____
   _____
   _____

2. What is bursitis and how does it occur?
   _____
   _____
   _____

3. If the joint capsule of a synovial joint such as the knee became damaged or diseased, is healing possible? Explain what would occur.
   _____
   _____
   _____

4. What is a herniated (slipped) disc and how does it occur?
   _____
   _____
   _____

5. What are Heberden's and Bouchard's nodes and how do they occur?
   _____
   _____
   _____

ACTIVITY 10.8: SYNOVIAL JOINT SIMULATION

Synovial joints are characterised by the presence of a fibrous connective tissue joint capsule, which is lined by a synovial membrane that secretes synovial fluid into the joint cavity. Synovial fluid is denser than water and has a consistency similar to that of raw egg white. The bone ends are covered in articular (hyaline) cartilage, which lubricates the joint, absorbs shock, distributes pressure evenly over the bone surfaces, and reduces friction at the joint surfaces. Since both the joint capsule and articular cartilage are composed of avascular connective tissue, repair to these structures is not possible in the event of damage. The structure and consistency of both the synovial fluid and articular cartilage are essential in the optimal functioning of synovial joints.

This activity demonstrates the structure and composition of synovial joints.

 To conduct this activity, it is important to ensure the following safety precautions:

- *Wear safety glasses when using the hotplate as heated liquids may superheat and splutter causing permanent eye damage.*

- *Take care when handling and working around hotplates as they heat quickly and retain heat, causing skin burns.*

1. This activity is best conducted in groups of two or three.

2. Obtain 3 party balloons, a permanent marker, plastic funnel, two 200 mL beakers, 100 mL measuring cylinder, water, dry sand, gelatine powder, electronic scale, hotplate (placed on a heat mat) and a popstick.

3. Label the balloons 1 to 3 with the permanent marker.

4. Pour water into the measuring cylinder until 60 mL is measured.

5. Place the funnel into the mouth of one of the balloons, and gently pour the water into balloon 1, tying the end of the balloon to secure. This is joint 1.

6. Place a beaker on the electronic scale and tare the scale to zero.

7. Pour sand into the beaker until 60 g is measured.

8. Place the funnel into the mouth of one of the balloons, and gently pour the sand into balloon 2, tying the end of the balloon to secure. This is joint 2.

9. Place a beaker on the electronic scale and tare the scale to zero.

10. Measure 12 g of gelatine into the beaker, and add 60 mL water with the measuring cylinder. Stir well with a popstick.

11. Place the hotplate on the heat mat and turn the heat setting and the stirrer setting (if available) to high.

12. Place the beaker on the hotplate and heat the gelatine mixture gently until just melted, stirring with the popstick occasionally.

13. Do not overheat the mixture.

14. Place the funnel into the mouth of one of the balloons, and gently pour the gelatine mixture into balloon 3, tying the end of the balloon to secure. This is joint 3.

15. Gently squeeze each balloon in the palm of your hand, noting the consistency and flexibility provided by the contents of each.

16. Making two fists with your hands, place joint 1 between your fists and gently apply pressure to the balloon attempting to touch your hands through the balloon (you may need your laboratory partner to assist with placement).

17. Note how much force is applied and the tension within the balloon.

18. Repeat this process with joints 2 and 3.

19. Push your index finger into joint 3 and note what occurs within the contents of the balloon.

   a. Is the force applied by your finger limited to the point of contact? Explain.

   _____

   _____

   _____

20. Consider the following questions:

    a. Which structure in a synovial joint does the balloon represent?

    _____

    b. Which structure in a synovial joint do the balloon contents represent?

    _____

    c. Which joint contents would be most suitable in a synovial joint and why?

    _____

    _____

    _____

    d. What percentage of water did the gelatine mixture contain and what does this represent physiologically?

    _____

    _____

    _____

    e. How does the composition of articular cartilage across the joint surfaces assist with pressure distribution in the joint?

    _____

    _____

    _____

    f. Which joint contents would be least suitable in a synovial joint and why?

    _____

    _____

    _____

    g. Suggest a condition that the contents in joint 2 may simulate and explain why.

    _____

    _____

    _____

Apply the Concepts

1. What is arthritis and how does it occur?

   _____

   _____

   _____

2. What is osteoarthritis and how does it occur?

   _____

   _____

   _____

3. What is rheumatoid arthritis and how does it occur?

   _____

   _____

   _____

4. What is gout and how does it occur?

   _____

   _____

   _____

Additional Activities

For additional activities visit Activity 10E: Synovial Joint Movement and Range of Motion (ROM) on Evolve˚.

Additional Resources

GetBodySmart: Skeletal System

GetBodySmart presents fully animated, illustrated and interactive eBooks about human anatomy and physiology body systems.

www.getbodysmart.com/skeletal-system

Histology Guide Virtual Microscopy Laboratory: Cartilage and Bone

Histology Guide is an online resource providing a virtual microscopy laboratory experience by allowing users to view microscope slides from professional collections for the purpose of interpreting cellular and tissue structures, as seen through a microscope.

histologyguide.com/slidebox/05-cartilage-and-bone.html

Innerbody Research: Skeletal System

Innerbody Research provides objective, science-based advice to help readers make more informed choices about home health products and services with up-to-date reviews, guides and research, including information about various body systems.

www.innerbody.com/image/skelfov.html

KenHub: Cartilage and Bone

KenHub is an integrated platform that brings together multiple learning tools, such as video tutorials, adaptable quizzes, detailed articles and high-quality atlas images, with information relating to cartilage and bone histology.

www.kenhub.com/en/start/general-histology
www.kenhub.com/en/library/anatomy/histology-of-bone

Michigan Histology: Mature Bone and Bone Formation

A digital microscopy resource for the study of cells, tissues and organs with readings, images and quizzes, provided by the University of Michigan Medical School.

histology.medicine.umich.edu/resources/mature-bone
histology.medicine.umich.edu/resources/bone-bone-formation

Osmosis – Musculoskeletal System

The Musculoskeletal System module of Osmosis provides videos, notes, quiz questions and links to further resources related to the musculoskeletal system.

www.osmosis.org/library/md/foundational-sciences/physiology#musculoskeletal_system

The Histology Guide: Cartilage, Bone and Ossification

The Histology Guide is a virtual experience of using a microscope with zoom features divided into topics and offering histological slides with labels and quizzes for each topic, such as skeletal tissues. It is provided by the University of Leeds.

www.histology.leeds.ac.uk/bone/index.php

VERITAS health

VERITAS health features extensive patient education libraries, including articles, videos and blog posts, as well as a medical glossary and a number of health-related sites such as SPINE-health and ARTHRITIS-health.

www.spine-health.com/
www.arthritis-health.com/

Visible Body: Skeletal System

Visible Body provides interactive and highly accurate visualisations and apps for learning and teaching anatomy and physiology for students and healthcare professionals, including body systems such as the skeletal system.

www.visiblebody.com/learn/skeleton

CHAPTER 11
The Muscular System

Muscle tissue includes skeletal muscle (found attached to skeletal structures and occasionally skin), cardiac muscle (found in the walls of the heart), and smooth muscle (found in the walls of hollow internal organs); however, the muscular system is most commonly associated with skeletal muscle. (Refer to Chapter 7: Tissues and Organs, for information on cardiac and smooth muscle and Chapter 16: The Cardiovascular System, for further information on the heart and cardiac muscle.)

There are over 650 skeletal muscles in the human body, varying in structure, size, shape and location. Among their many functions, skeletal muscles are responsible for body movement and manipulation of the environment, and share a unique relationship with structures of the skeletal system such as bones and articulations (joints). For this reason, both systems are often considered together as forming the musculoskeletal system.

To achieve contraction, skeletal muscles require direct interaction with nervous tissue and are under voluntary control via the somatic nervous system. Biochemical substances such as electrolytes, neurotransmitters and ATP, found within and around the muscle and at the junction between muscle and nervous tissue, are essential in maintaining the structural integrity and functional viability of muscle, as well as facilitating contraction. Conditions affecting the muscular system can arise from damage to the muscle structure, chemical imbalances, stress and trauma.

LEARNING OUTCOMES

On completion of these activities, the student should be able to:

1. identify the functions and characteristics of skeletal muscle tissue
2. classify and name muscles of the muscular system based on structure, function, location and fibre arrangement
3. explain the muscle interactions and lever systems involved in movement
4. identify and describe the macroscopic structures of skeletal muscle
5. identify and describe the microscopic structures of skeletal muscle tissue
6. identify the structures and processes occurring at the neuromuscular junction

LEARNING OUTCOMES—cont'd

7. describe and observe the processes and mechanisms of muscle contraction

8. elicit and observe muscle contraction responses and analyse the factors contributing to muscle fatigue

9. conduct physical assessments for muscle strength and weakness.

KEY TERMS

Actin	Myofibril	Sliding filament mechanism
Agonist	Myofilament	Striations
Antagonist	Myosin	Synergist
Insertion	Neuromuscular junction	T tubule
Isometric	Neurotransmitter	Tendon
Isotonic	Origin	Thick filament
Lever system	Prime mover	Thin filament
Motor unit	Sarcolemma	Tropomyosin
Muscle fibre	Sarcomere	Troponin
Muscle tension	Sarcoplasmic reticulum	
Muscle tone	Skeletal muscle	

ACTIVITY 11.1: MUSCLE INTERACTIONS

Muscles often attach to the surfaces of bones via their outer connective tissue layer, or epimysium, which forms a **tendon**. As muscles contract or shorten, they pull on their bone attachments, causing the **insertion** of the muscle to move towards the **origin** of the muscle. This pulls on the bone associated with the muscle insertion forming a **lever system** (Fig. 11.1). In each movement, certain muscle groups, referred to as **prime movers** or **agonists**, provide the main contractile force and are often assisted by **synergists**, while other muscle groups, or **antagonists**, relax and lengthen (Fig. 11.2).

This activity outlines the interactions of muscles within lever systems, their attachments to bone, and the functional interactions of muscles.

1. For each of the lever systems provided, place the terms load, fulcrum and effort in the correct sequence.

    a. First-class lever: _____

    b. Second-class lever: _____

    c. Third-class lever: _____

2. Identify each of the numbered structures shown in Fig. 11.1, using the terms load, fulcrum and effort.

    a. Structure 1: _____

    b. Structure 2: _____

    c. Structure 3: _____

    d. Structure 4: _____

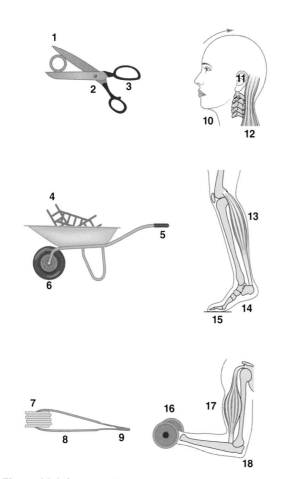

Figure 11.1 Lever systems.
(Source: Hombach-Klonisch, S., Klonisch, T., & Peeler, J. eds). (2019). Sobotta clinical atlas of human anatomy. Elsevier.)

e. Structure 5: _____

f. Structure 6: _____

g. Structure 7: _____

h. Structure 8: _____

i. Structure 9: _____

j. Structure 10: _____

k. Structure 11: _____

l. Structure 12: _____

m. Structure 13: _____

n. Structure 14: _____

o. Structure 15: _____

p. Structure 16: _____

q. Structure 17: _____

r. Structure 18: _____

3. Consider the following questions with reference to Fig. 11.1:

   a. Which structures usually comprise the lever or rigid bar?

   _____

   b. Which structures usually comprise the fulcrum?

   _____

   c. What characteristic do all fulcrums have in common?

   _____

   _____

   d. Which structures usually comprise the load?

   _____

   _____

   e. Which structures usually comprise the effort?

   _____

   f. Explain why the effort is sometimes referred to as a force.

   _____

   _____

   _____

   g. Explain why a power lever operates at a mechanical advantage.

   _____

   _____

   _____

   h. Explain why a speed lever operates at a mechanical disadvantage.

   _____

   _____

   _____

4. Consider the following questions with reference to Fig. 11.2:

   a. Which muscle is indicated at structure B?

   _____

   b. Which muscle is indicated at structure F?

   _____

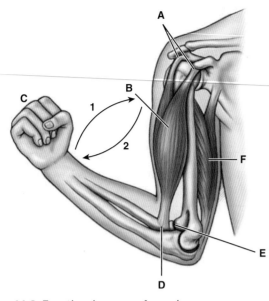

Figure 11.2 Functional groups of muscles.
(Source: Herlihy, B. (2018). The human body in health and illness. Elsevier.)

c. Explain why structure B has two attachments to the shoulder.

_____

_____

d. In the arm movement indicated by the number 1, identify the letters corresponding to the following:

   i. Origin: _____

   ii. Insertion: _____

   iii. Fulcrum: _____

   iv. Load: _____

   v. Prime mover: _____

   vi. Antagonist: _____

e. In the arm movement indicated by the number 2, identify the letters corresponding to the following:

   i. Origin: _____

   ii. Insertion: _____

   iii. Fulcrum: _____

   iv. Load: _____

   v. Prime mover: _____

   vi. Antagonist: _____

f. In each movement, which structure moves towards the other – the origin or the insertion?

_____

_____

_____

g. In each movement, how is the prime mover distinguished from the antagonist?

_____

_____

_____

h. Can a prime mover also perform the function of an antagonist? Explain.

_____

_____

_____

i. What is the function of a synergist?

_____

_____

_____

j. What is the name of the muscle that acts as the synergist to structure B?

_____

k. What is the name of the muscle that acts as the synergist to structure F?

_____

l. Explain why a prime mover may also be called agonist.

_____

_____

m. In each movement, where is the line of force located?

_____

n. Based on the arrangement of structures in Fig. 11.2, what evidence suggests that muscles can pull but not push?

_____

_____

_____

Apply the Concepts

1. Explain why the muscles of the fingers are not able to develop as much force as the muscles of the leg.

   _____

   _____

   _____

2. Explain why there are more tendinous muscle attachments to bone than direct muscle attachments.

   _____

   _____

   _____

3. What is tendonitis and how does it occur?

   _____

   _____

   _____

4. What is compartment syndrome and how does it occur?

   _____

   _____

   _____

5. Which muscles are affected in a pulled groin?

   _____

   _____

   _____

6. What is club foot and how does it occur?

   _____

   _____

   _____

7. What is trigger finger and how does it occur?

   _____

   _____

   _____

8. What is mallet finger and how does it occur?

   _____

   _____

   _____

9. The frequent wearing of shoes with high heels can lead to the development of plantar fasciitis, or high heel syndrome, where pain is experienced when wearing flat shoes or walking barefoot. Explain how this occurs.

_____

_____

_____

Additional Activities

For additional activities visit Activity 11A: Muscles of the Muscular System on Evolve˙.

ACTIVITY 11.2: STRUCTURE OF SKELETAL MUSCLE AND THE NEUROMUSCULAR JUNCTION

Individual muscle groups and their associated structures form the organs of the muscular system (Fig. 11.3). The majority of these structures can be viewed with the unaided eye; however, the banding across muscle fibres, called **striations**, requires viewing with a microscope. The proteins composing the muscle, in the form of **myofilaments**, however, cannot be seen microscopically due to their sub-microscopic size. Skeletal muscles receive impulses from the nervous system at regions referred to as **neuromuscular junctions** (Fig. 11.4).

This activity outlines the structure of skeletal muscles and their association with the nervous system.

Part 1: Skeletal Muscle Structure

Skeletal muscle fibres are bundled together by connective tissues to form organs which comprise the muscular system. Skeletal muscle is associated with and connected to bone, forming the musculoskeletal system.

1. Identify each of the muscle structures shown in Fig. 11.3.

   a. Structure A: _____

   b. Structure B: _____

   c. Structure C: _____

   d. Structure D: _____

   e. Structure E: _____

   f. Structure F: _____

   g. Structure G: _____

   h. Structure H: _____

   i. Structure I: _____

   j. Structure J: _____

   k. Structure K: _____

   l. Structure L: _____

   m. Structure M: _____

   n. Structure N: _____

   o. Structure O: _____

   p. Structure P: _____

   q. Structure Q: _____

   r. Structure R: _____

   s. Structure S: _____

   t. Structure T: _____

   u. Structure U: _____

   v. Structure V: _____

   w. Structure W: _____

   x. Structure X: _____

   y. Structure Y: _____

   z. Structure Z: _____

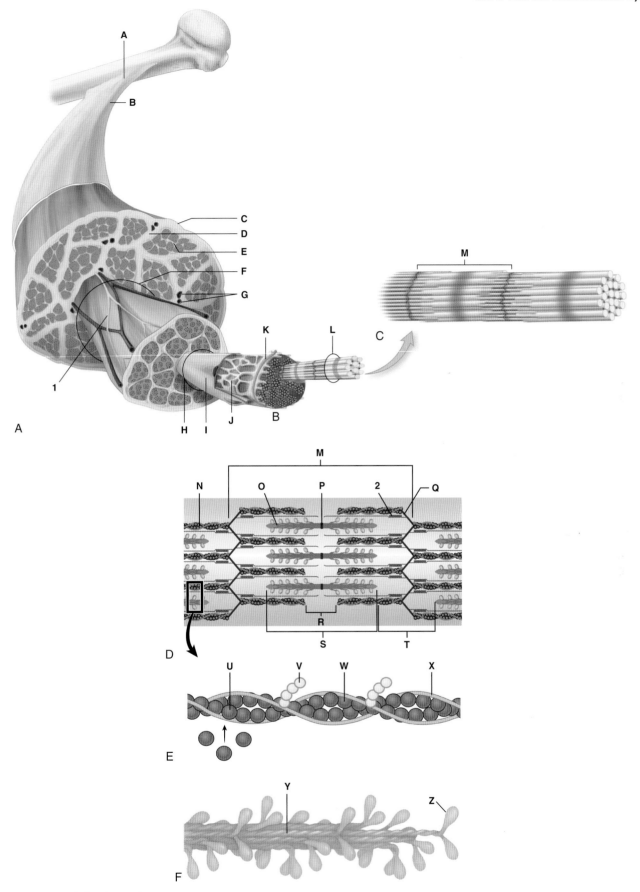

Figure 11.3 Skeletal muscle structure.
*(Source: **B** McCance, K. L., & Huether, S. E. (2019). Pathophysiology: The biologic basis for disease in adults and children. Elsevier.)*

2. Consider the following questions:

a. What is the function of structures C, D, and E? What tissue type are they composed of?

_____

_____

_____

b. What do the prefixes of structures C, D and E refer to in terms of their positions?

_____

_____

_____

c. The collagen content of structures C, D and E increases with age, while the size of structure H decreases. Based on this information, predict whether the muscle of an older animal would be tough or tender.

_____

_____

_____

d. What is the function of the structures labelled G?

_____

_____

_____

e. What is structure I and what is its function?

_____

_____

_____

f. What is the function of structure J?

_____

_____

_____

g. Explain the structural relationship between structure L and structure H.

_____

_____

_____

h. What is the function of structure K?

_____

_____

i. Which of structures I, J or K would contain the highest concentration of calcium ions in a muscle cell and why?

_____

_____

_____

j. What is the function of structure M?

_____

_____

k. What is structure 1 and what is its function?

_____

_____

_____

l. Structures N and O form which structure?

_____

m. What is found in structure P?

_____

_____

_____

n. What is found in structure Q?

_____

_____

_____

o. What is found in structure R?

_____

_____

_____

p. What is found in structure S?

_____

_____

_____

q. What is found in structure T?

_____

_____

r. What is structure 2, what is it composed of, and what is its function?

_____

_____

_____

s. Which structure is shown in Fig. 11.3E?

_____

t. What is the function of structure V?

_____

_____

u. What is the function of structure W?

_____

_____

v. What is the function of structure X?

_____

_____

w. Which structure is shown in Fig. 11.3F?

_____

x. What is the function of structure Z?

_____

_____

Part 2: The Neuromuscular Junction

A series of events at the neuromuscular junction act to convert an electrical impulse delivered by the nervous system via **a motor unit**, into a chemical message in the form of a **neurotransmitter**, to be received by the muscle membrane or **sarcolemma**, initiating contraction.

1. Identify each of the structures associated with the neuromuscular junction shown in Fig. 11.4.

   a. Structure A: _____

   b. Structure B: _____

c. Structure C: _____

d. Structure D: _____

e. Structure E: _____

f. Structure F: _____

g. Structure G: _____

h. Structure H: _____

i. Structure I: _____

j. Structure J: _____

k. Structure K: _____

l. Structure L: _____

m. Structure M: _____

n. Structure N: _____

o. Structure O: _____

p. Structure P: _____

2. Identify each of the events occurring at the neuromuscular junction in Fig. 11.4.

   a. Event 1: _____

   _____

   _____

   b. Event 2: _____

   _____

   _____

   c. Event 3: _____

   _____

   _____

   d. Event 4: _____

   _____

   _____

   e. Event 5: _____

   _____

   _____

   f. Event 6: _____

   _____

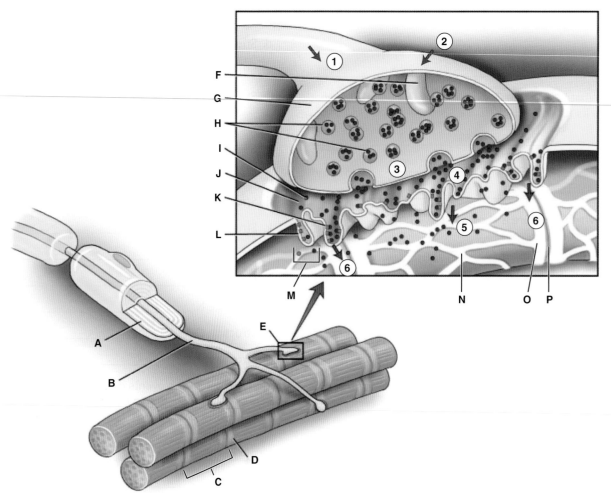

Figure 11.4 The neuromuscular junction.
(Source: VanMeter, K. C., & Hubert, R. J. (2016). Microbiology for the healthcare professional. Elsevier.)

3. Consider the following questions:

a. What is the neuromuscular junction?

_____

_____

b. What is synaptic transmission?

_____

_____

_____

c. Synaptic transmission represents which stage of muscle contraction?

_____

_____

d. Why is synaptic transmission vital to muscle contraction?

_____

_____

_____

e. What type of receptors or channels are located on the post-synaptic membrane?

_____

f. Provide an example of an excitatory neuromuscular junction neurotransmitter.

_____

g. Provide an example of an inhibitory neuromuscular junction neurotransmitter.

_____

h. How are neurotransmitters removed from the synaptic cleft after the impulse has been transferred?

_____

_____

_____

i. What would occur if neurotransmitter remained within the synapse?

_____

j. Event 5 culminates in what type of potential?

_____

k. What constitutes the initial trigger for muscle contraction?

_____

_____

_____

l. What constitutes the final trigger for muscle contraction?

_____

_____

Apply the Concepts

1. Predict the effect on a muscle if its nerve supply is destroyed.

_____

_____

_____

2. What is myofascial pain syndrome and how does it occur?

_____

_____

_____

3. What is myasthenia gravis and how does it occur?

_____

_____

_____

_____

4. Explain the effects that a neurotoxin inhibiting the activity of calcium channels, such as conotoxin, would have on muscle contraction.

_____

_____

_____

5. Explain the effects that a neurotoxin inhibiting synaptic vesicle release, such as botulinum toxin, would have on muscle contraction.

_____

6. Explain the effects that a neurotoxin blocking post-synaptic receptors, such as curare, would have on muscle contraction.

_____

_____

_____

7. Explain why lead (Pb^{2+}) can mimic and interfere with calcium (Ca^{2+}) function in the pre-synaptic membrane.

_____

_____

_____

Additional Activities

For additional activities visit Activity 11B: Identification of Skeletal Muscle Structures on Evolve˙.

For additional activities visit Activity 11C: Microscopic Examination of Skeletal Muscle on Evolve˙.

ACTIVITY 11.3: MECHANISM OF MUSCLE CONTRACTION

Events at the neuromuscular junction lead to the propagation of an action potential down the **T tubules**, causing the release of ionic calcium from the **sarcoplasmic reticulum**. Calcium interacts with **troponin**, affecting the blocking action of **tropomyosin** to initiate muscle contraction. Muscles contract due to the interaction of the protein filaments comprising the **myofibrils**. Referred to as the **sliding filament mechanism** of muscle contraction, the **thick filaments**, or **myosin**, and **thin filaments**, or **actin**, of the **sarcomeres** slide past each other without shortening (Fig. 11.5). This results in the shortening of the sarcomeres and the overall muscle, leading to muscle contraction.

This activity outlines the processes of muscle contraction and the sliding filament mechanism.

1. Outline the stages of skeletal muscle contraction, commencing at the neuromuscular junction and concluding with cross-bridge cycling, and describe the processes that occur in each stage:

a. Stage 1: _____

i. Processes: _____

_____

_____

b. Stage 2: _____

i. Processes: _____

_____

_____

c. Stage 3: _____

i. Processes: _____

_____

_____

d. Stage 4: _____

   i. Processes: _____

      _____

      _____

2. Identify each stage of the sliding filament mechanism (or the cross-bridge cycle) of muscle contraction shown in Fig. 11.5, and outline the events occurring in each stage:

  a. Stage 1: _____

   i. Events: _____

      _____

      _____

b. Stage 2: _____

   i. Events: _____

      _____

      _____

c. Stage 3: _____

   i. Events: _____

      _____

      _____

d. Stage 4: _____

   i. Events: _____

      _____

      _____

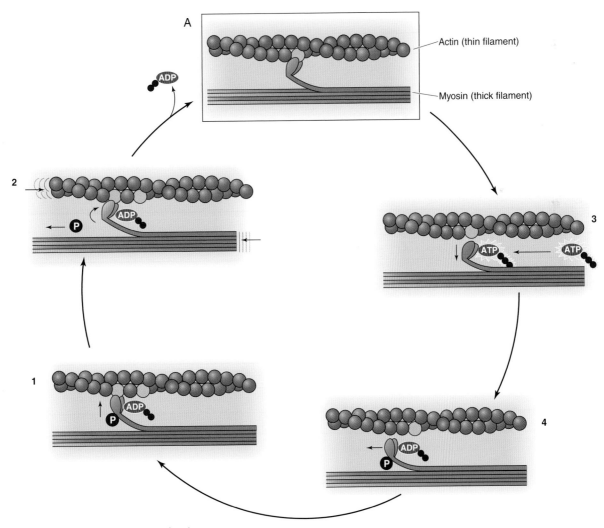

Figure 11.5 The sliding filament mechanism.
(Source: Piano, M. R., & Law, W. R. (2008). Cardiac nursing: A companion to Braunwald's heart disease. Elsevier.)

3. Consider the following questions:

a. Describe the structure of a thin filament.

_____

_____

_____

_____

b. Describe the structure and function of tropomyosin and troponin with reference to the thin filaments.

_____

_____

_____

c. Describe the structure of a thick filament.

_____

_____

_____

d. Which protein is responsible for blocking the binding sites on actin?

_____

e. Calcium interacts with which protein to induce exposure of the binding sites on actin?

_____

f. Where is this calcium stored?

_____

g. ATP is required for muscle contraction but is it also required for muscle relaxation? Explain.

_____

_____

_____

_____

_____

Apply the Concepts

1. What would occur if a muscle fibre ran out of ATP when the sarcomeres had only partially contracted?

_____

_____

_____

2. Which energy-producing pathway is dominant in human muscles?

_____

3. Explain why muscle cells are capable of experiencing gradual fatigue.

_____

_____

_____

ACTIVITY 11.4: EXAMINATION AND CONTRACTION OF SKELETAL MUSCLE FIBRES

A microscopic examination of fresh skeletal muscle provides information relating to the arrangement of the muscle fibres and allows the structural features of the individual fibres, including striations and their sarcomere boundaries, to be seen. Although myofibril proteins cannot be visualised due to their small molecular size, the overall shortening of the fibres can be seen when substances that promote muscle fibre contraction are added.

This activity demonstrates the microscopic structure of skeletal muscle fibres and the factors affecting contraction in chicken muscle.

 To conduct this activity, it is important to ensure the following safety precautions:

- *Wear disposable gloves at all times during the activity as fresh specimens may harbour pathogenic microorganisms.*
- *Methylene blue is a strong stain and can cause irritation.*
- *Exercise care when handling dissection tools.*
- *Additional precautions, including safe disposal of animal material, may be required by your demonstrator.*

1. This activity is best conducted in groups of three.

2. Obtain a small portion of fresh chicken breast or thigh muscle (not frozen), 100 mL beaker, petri dish, 50% glycerine solution, stopwatch, forceps, 2 dissecting needles, methylene blue, dissecting microscope, compound microscope, pencil, 4 microscope slides, coverslips, metric ruler (mm), 3 test tubes, test tube rack, 0.25% ATP in distilled water, 0.05 M KCl, 0.001 M $MgCl_2$, disposable pipettes and disposable gloves.

Part 1: Skeletal Muscle Examination

The preparation of skeletal muscle for microscopic examination provides an understanding of the finer details of muscle structure.

1. Place the chicken muscle in the beaker and pour over enough glycerine solution to completely cover the muscle.

2. Allow the muscle to stand for 5 minutes.

3. Remove the muscle with the forceps and place on the petri dish.

4. Place the petri dish on the stage of a dissecting microscope.

5. Using the dissecting needles, gently tease the chicken muscle apart so that individual fibres can be distinguished (Note: this needs to be done carefully and may take some time.)

6. Ensure that the muscle is well moistened during the process by adding additional glycerine if the muscle is exposed to the microscope lamp for an extended period of time.

7. Place a few fibres onto a clean microscope slide and add 1 drop of methylene blue. (Note: reserve the remaining fibres for Part 2 of this activity.)

8. Gently place a cover slip over the top.

9. View the muscle under low power, focusing on the individual fibres, and gradually move to high power once a section of fibre has been isolated (oil immersion may be required for more detailed viewing).

10. Draw a diagram of what you can see in the space below, and label the structures identified using Fig. 11B.1 to assist (refer to Activity 11B on Evolve).

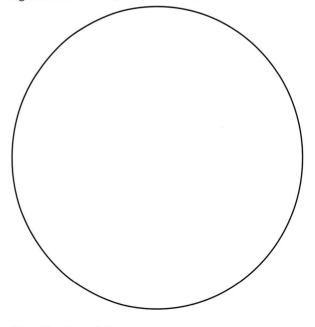

Magnification of diagram: × _____

251

11. Compare and estimate the distance between adjacent light-coloured bands on a single muscle fibre.

   a. Estimated distance: _____

12. Consider the following questions:

   a. What effect does glycerine have on muscle fibres?

   _____

   _____

   b. Were striations visible?

   _____

   c. Which parts of the muscle fibre form the striations?

   _____

   d. Which parts of the muscle fibre form the contractile units?

   _____

   e. What is found in the dark regions of the striations?

   _____

   f. What are the dark regions of the striations called?

   _____

   g. What is found in the light regions of the striations?

   _____

   h. What are the light regions of the striations called?

   _____

Part 2: Skeletal Muscle Contraction

The microscopic observation of skeletal muscle contraction provides an understanding of how sarcomeres function to shorten the entire muscle, pulling on bones to elicit movement.

1. Label the microscope slides 1 to 3 with a pencil.

2. Place the test tubes in a test tube rack and label 1 to 3 with a glass marker.

3. To test tube 1, add 5 drops 0.25% ATP in distilled water. This is solution 1.

4. To test tube 2, add 5 drops 0.25% ATP in distilled water, 5 drops 0.05 M KCl, and 5 drops 0.001 M $MgCl_2$. This is solution 2.

5. To test tube 3, add 5 drops 0.05 M KCl and 5 drops 0.001 M $MgCl_2$. This is solution 3.

6. Place two muscle fibres on each labelled microscope slide with the forceps, keeping them separated. (Note: fibres thicker than 0.2 mm in diameter are too thick to be used.)

7. Place each slide on the dissecting microscope stage and measure the length of each fibre with the ruler, noting your observations in the table provided.

8. To the fibres on slide 1, add the contents of test tube 1 with a pipette.

9. Wait 1 minute, then measure the length of each fibre, noting your observations in the table provided.

10. To the fibres on slide 2, add the contents of test tube 2 with a pipette. (Note: it is important to use a clean pipette for each solution to avoid cross-contamination.)

11. Wait 1 minute, then measure the length of each fibre, noting your observations in the table provided.

12. To the fibres on slide 3, add the contents of test tube 3 with a pipette.

13. Wait 1 minute, then measure the length of each fibre, noting your observations in the table provided.

14. Complete the table based on your observations.

15. Add 1 drop of methylene blue to each slide, and gently place a coverslip over the top of each slide.

16. Observe each of the slides under the compound microscope, noting the distance between adjacent light-coloured bands on the muscle fibres.

17. Once you have completed your examination, dispose of the materials as indicated by your instructor.

Muscle fibre	Solution 1 (ATP + H_2O)	Solution 2 (ATP + KCl + $MgCl_2$)	Solution 3 (KCl + $MgCl_2$)
Muscle fibre 1			
Initial length			
Final length			
Length change[1]			
Muscle fibre 2			
Initial length			

Continued

Muscle fibre	Solution 1 (ATP + H_2O)	Solution 2 (ATP + KCl + $MgCl_2$)	Solution 3 (KCl + $MgCl_2$)
Final length			
Length change[1]			
Average length Change[2]			

Notes:
1. Length change = initial length – final length (mm)
2. Average length change = muscle fibre 1 length change + muscle fibre 2 length change ÷ 2 (mm)

18. Consider the following:

a. Why was it necessary to tease the muscle fibres prior to use?

_____

_____

_____

b. Were any changes in the lengths of the muscle fibres visible?

_____

_____

_____

c. Which solution caused the most noticeable fibre contraction?

_____

_____

_____

d. Which solution caused the least amount of, or no, muscle fibre contraction? Suggest a reason for this.

_____

_____

_____

e. What was the purpose of using solutions 1 and 3?

_____

_____

_____

f. Why was calcium not required to cause contraction in the glycerine-treated muscle fibres?

_____

_____

_____

g. If contraction was not observed, suggest an explanation.

_____

_____

_____

h. Provide an explanation for the roles of ATP, KCl, and $MgCl_2$ in muscle contraction.

_____

_____

_____

_____

_____

_____

i. Predict whether the muscle fibres will remain contracted after adding the ATP solutions.

_____

_____

_____

j. How do the estimated distances between adjacent light-coloured bands on the muscle fibres in solution 2 compare with those observed in Part 1?

_____

_____

_____

Apply the Concepts

1. Provide a reason for the muscle stiffness that occurs with rigor mortis.

_____

_____

_____

ACTIVITY 11.5: MUSCLE STIMULATION AND CONTRACTION

Skeletal muscles are stimulated to contract because their muscle fibres receive electrical impulses via motor units. Skeletal muscle fibre contraction can be studied by observing and palpating the muscles concerned, or by recording and graphing the force or **muscle tension** produced as the muscle contracts and relaxes, by a process called myography (Fig. 11.6). In addition, the degree of stretch within muscles, measured by stretch receptors in the tendons and muscles themselves, results in continual low-level contractions, which contribute to **muscle tone** and produce tension within the muscle (Fig. 11.7). Muscle fibres differ in their characteristics of contraction and fatigue based on their speed (slow or fast) and their method of forming ATP (oxidative or glycolytic). By these criteria, skeletal muscle fibres are classified as slow oxidative, fast oxidative and fast glycolytic fibres.

This activity explores various types of muscle contraction, as well as muscle fatigue.

Part 1A: Muscle Tension and Twitch Contraction

In order to elicit muscle contraction, an electrical stimulus of sufficient intensity, referred to as a threshold stimulus, must be applied to the muscle in order to produce a single, brief, sharp contraction. This contraction is referred to as a twitch contraction. A myograph recording the force generated by a muscle during contraction can provide information on the intensity and velocity of contraction, and on factors affecting muscle activation.

1. What is a muscle twitch?

_____

_____

_____

2. Compare threshold stimulus and maximal stimulus.

_____

_____

_____

_____

_____

3. Identify each of the phases occurring during a muscle twitch contraction in Fig. 11.6A, and describe the events occurring in each stage:

a. Stage A: _____

   i. Events: _____

   _____

   _____

b. Stage B: _____

   i. Events: _____

   _____

   _____

c. Stage C: _____

   i. Events: _____

   _____

   _____

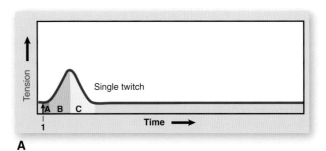

A

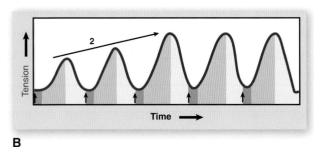

B

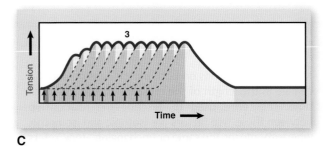

C

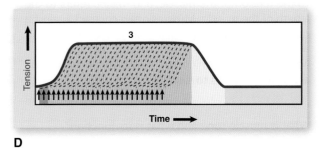

D

Figure 11.6 Myographs of muscle twitch contractions.
(Source: Patton, K. T., & Thibodeau, G. A. (2014). Mosby's handbook of anatomy and physiology, 2nd ed. Elsevier.)

d. What does the back arrow at number 1 indicate?

_____

e. What does the black arrow at number 2 indicate?

_____

f. What does the time difference between numbers 1 and 2 indicate about muscle contraction?

_____

_____

g. What do the black arrows at number 3 indicate?

_____

4. Identify the type of muscle contraction occurring in each of the diagrams in Fig. 11.6, and state the processes in each, based on stimulation, contraction, and relaxation:

a. Diagram A: _____

i. Processes: _____

_____

_____

b. Diagram B: _____

i. Processes: _____

_____

_____

c. Diagram C: _____

i. Processes: _____

_____

_____

d. Diagram D: _____

i. Processes: _____

_____

_____

5. Consider the following questions, with reference to Fig. 11.6:

a. In diagrams A to D, is the size or the frequency of the stimuli changing?

_____

b. What do the muscle contractions in diagrams C and D have in common?

_____

c. What is wave summation as related to muscle contraction?

_____

_____

_____

_____

Part 1B: Muscle Tension and Twitch Contraction (Physiology)

The PowerLab System will be used to demonstrate the relationship between depolarisation and muscle contraction. Depending on the model, coloured clips or electrode pads are placed on the skin, targeting specific muscle groups, to stimulate and record muscle contractions.

1. This activity is best conducted in groups of three.

2. Obtain a PowerLab System, set up the equipment, and test the equipment as directed in the accompanying instructions (your instructor may need to assist).

3. Complete the Twitch Response and Recruitment experiment, following the instructions provided. If headphones are available, the electrical activity of muscle contraction can be heard (the frequency of auditory signals corresponds to the frequency of action potentials stimulating the muscles).

4. Consider the following questions:

   a. Do muscles twitch as observed artificially during normal functioning? Explain.

   _____

   _____

   _____

   b. What is a graded muscle response?

   _____

   _____

   _____

   c. What is recruitment as related to muscle contraction?

   _____

   _____

   _____

   d. Are all motor units of a muscle recruited at the same time? Explain.

   _____

   _____

   _____

   e. How was recruitment achieved in the experiment?

   _____

   _____

   f. Does increasing the size of a stimulus produce a stronger contraction?

   _____

   g. Identify four factors that contribute to the strength of a muscle contraction.

   _____

   _____

   _____

   _____

Part 2A: Isometric and Isotonic Contractions

Muscle tone depends on both muscle tension and the change in the length of the muscle fibres at the same time. The terms used to describe the relationship between these two factors are **isotonic** and **isometric**, where *iso-* means the same or unchanging, *-tonic* refers to the tension of the muscle, and *-metric* refers to the length of the muscle. Muscles often contract against a resistance or load, and their ability to overcome this resistance influences the degree of movement. Movement is determined by the ability of myosin and actin cross-bridges to slide past each other.

1. What is muscle tone and what is its function?

   _____

   _____

   _____

2. What is the meaning of the term isotonic as it applies to muscle contraction?

   _____

   _____

3. What is the meaning of the term isometric as it applies to muscle contraction?

   _____

   _____

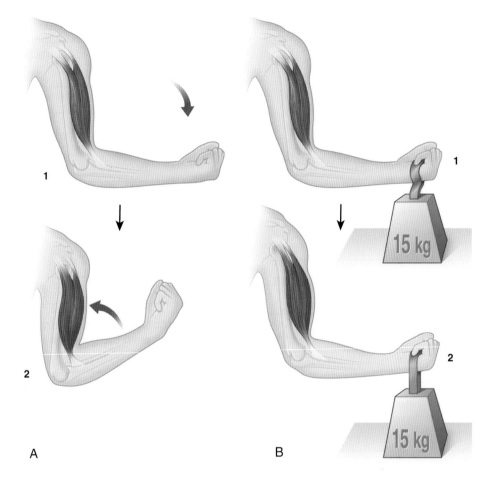

Figure 11.7 Isotonic and isometric contractions.
(Source: Adapted from Klieger, D. M. (2009). Saunders Essentials of Medical Assisting. Elsevier.)

4. Which term is used to describe muscles with less tone than normal?

_____

5. Which term is used to describe muscles with more tone than normal?

_____

6. Consider the following questions with reference to Fig. 11.7:

   a. Diagram A

      i. Type of contraction:

      _____

      ii. Is the muscle at number 1 relaxed or contracted?

      _____

   iii. Is the length of the muscle at number 1 increasing or decreasing?

   _____

   iv. The movement at number 1 indicates what type of contraction?

   _____

   v. Is the muscle at number 2 relaxed or contracted?

   _____

   vi. Is the length of the muscle at number 2 increasing or decreasing?

   _____

   vii. The movement at number 2 indicates what type of contraction?

   _____

viii. Has the muscle tension from number 1 to number 2 increased, decreased or remained the same?

_____

b. Diagram B

i. Type of contraction:

_____

ii. Is the muscle at number 1 relaxed or contracted?

_____

iii. Is the tension of the muscle at number 1 high or low?

_____

iv. Is the muscle at number 2 relaxed or contracted?

_____

v. Is the tension of the muscle at number 2 high or low?

_____

vi. Is any movement indicated from number 1 to number 2?

_____

vii. Has the muscle length from number 1 to number 2 increased, decreased, or remained the same?

_____

Part 2B: Isometric and Isotonic Contractions (Physiology)

The PowerLab System will be used to demonstrate the relationship between depolarisation and muscle contraction. Depending on the model, coloured clips or electrode pads are placed on the skin targeting specific muscle groups in order to stimulate and record muscle contractions.

1. This activity is best conducted in groups of three.

2. Obtain a PowerLab System, set up the equipment, and test the equipment as directed in the accompanying instructions (your instructor may need to assist).

3. Complete the Grip Force experiment, following the instructions provided. If headphones are available, the electrical activity of muscle contraction can be heard (the frequency of auditory signals corresponds to the frequency of action potentials stimulating the muscles).

4. Consider the following questions:

a. Based on the sliding filament mechanism, what is occurring during isotonic contraction?

_____

b. In an isotonic contraction, what happens to muscle length and tension?

_____

c. In an isometric contraction, what happens to muscle length and tension?

_____

d. Concentric and eccentric contractions are associated with which main category of muscle contraction?

_____

e. What happens to muscle length in a concentric contraction?

_____

f. What happens to muscle length in an eccentric contraction?

_____

g. Based on the sliding filament mechanism, what is occurring during isometric contraction?

_____

Part 3: Muscle Fatigue

A muscle undergoes fatigue when it is physiologically unable to contract and produce force, even though it is still receiving stimuli to contract. This prevents indefinite muscle contraction and the subsequent death of muscle cells. Muscle fatigue may be caused by a number of factors, including ionic imbalances within the muscle (Na^+, K^+, Ca^{2+}, inorganic phosphate), decreased ATP (related to glycogen, oxygen, or Mg^{2+} supply), or nervous fatigue. Lactic acid accumulation and lowered pH in the muscle cells, as a result of muscle fatigue, causes the associated sensation of pain.

1. This activity is best conducted in pairs.

2. Obtain an electronic scale, a stopwatch and two objects of differing weight (e.g. 250 g and 500 g).

3. Each person will take turns to act as subject, and to time and record the results.

4. Measure the weight of the first object with the electronic scale, and record this in the table provided.

5. Measure the weight of the second object with the electronic scale, and record this in the table provided.

6. Order the objects in the table from the lowest weight to the highest weight.

7. Ask subject 1 to extend their dominant arm straight out in front of them, and hold that position. This represents no load.

8. Record the time taken for their arm to start shaking or their muscles to start aching. Note this time in the table provided.

9. Repeat this process with the subject's non-dominant arm, recording the results in the table provided.

10. Repeat step 7, but have subject 1 hold object 1 with their dominant arm and record the time taken for their arm muscles to fatigue.

11. Repeat this process with the subject's non-dominant arm, recording the results in the table provided.

12. Repeat step 10, but have subject 1 hold object 2 with their dominant arm and record the time taken for their arm muscles to fatigue.

13. Repeat this process with the subject's non-dominant arm, recording the results in the table provided.

14. Repeat the process for subject 2, while subject 1 times the experiment, and record the results in the table provided.

| | | Time taken to reach fatigue | | | |
| | | Subject 1 | | Subject 2 | |
Load	Weight of load	Dominant	Non-dominant	Dominant	Non-dominant
No load	N/A				
Object 1					
Object 2					

15. Consider the following:

a. Is the dominant arm or non-dominant arm more susceptible to fatigue? Explain why.

_____

_____

_____

_____

b. Suggest a reason for the difference in results between the dominant and non-dominant arm, based on the muscle fibres present in each arm.

_____

_____

_____

_____

c. What do the results indicate about the effect of load on muscle fatigue and why?

_____

_____

d. Explain why fast glycolytic fibres (type IIB) fatigue more readily than slow oxidative fibres (type I).

_____

_____

_____

_____

e. Explain why weight training causes fast glycolytic fibres (type IIB) to hypertrophy, increasing muscle strength.

_____

_____

_____

_____

f. Explain why slow oxidative fibres (type I) have more capillaries and mitochondria than fast glycolytic fibres (type IIB).

_____

_____

_____

_____

g. Explain why slow oxidative fibres (type I) contain less glycogen than fast glycolytic fibres (type IIB).

_____

_____

_____

_____

h. Explain why slow oxidative fibres (type I) contract more slowly than fast glycolytic fibres (type IIB).

_____

_____

_____

_____

Apply the Concepts

1. What is bacterial tetanus and how does it occur?

_____

_____

_____

2. What is a muscle spasm and how does it occur?

_____

_____

_____

3. What is a muscle cramp and how does it occur?

_____

_____

_____

Additional Activities

For additional activities visit Activity 11D: Assessment of Muscle Strength and Weakness on Evolve®.

Additional Resources

BBC Bitesize: Energy Systems in Muscle Cells

BBC Bitesize provides lessons, revision material and tests on a number of human biology-related topics, including muscle cells and energy utilisation during exercise.

www.bbc.co.uk/bitesize/guides/z6fmwty/revision/1

GetBodySmart: Muscular System and Muscle Physiology

GetBodySmart presents fully animated, illustrated and interactive eBooks about human anatomy and physiology body systems.

www.getbodysmart.com/muscular-system
www.getbodysmart.com/muscle-physiology

Gizmos: Muscles and Bones

An interactive simulation with lesson materials where users observe how muscles, bones and connective tissue work together to allow movement, and can construct an arm that can lift a weight or throw a ball.

gizmos.explorelearning.com/index.cfm?method=cResource.dspDetail &resourceID51089

Histology Guide Virtual Microscopy Laboratory: Muscle Tissue

Histology Guide is an online resource providing a virtual microscopy laboratory experience, by allowing users to view microscope slides from professional collections for the purpose of interpreting cellular and tissue structures as seen through a microscope.

histologyguide.com/slidebox/04-muscle-tissue.html

Innerbody Research: Muscular System

Innerbody Research provides objective, science-based advice to help readers make more informed choices about home health products and services with most up-to-date reviews, guides and research, including information about the muscular system.

www.innerbody.com/image/musfov.html

Khan Academy: Muscles

Video tutorials outlining the anatomy of muscle fibres, including the role of the sarcoplasmic reticulum, and how various muscle proteins regulate and cause muscle contraction.

www.khanacademy.org/science/biology/human-biology#muscles

Muscle Atlas

An online atlas containing more than 80 anatomical images of the upper and lower extremities, developed by the Department of Radiology, University of Washington.

rad.washington.edu/muscle-atlas/

Osmosis – Musculoskeletal System

The Musculoskeletal System module of Osmosis provides videos, notes, quiz questions and links to further resources related to the musculoskeletal system.

www.osmosis.org/library/md/foundational-sciences/physiology #musculoskeletal_system

The Histology Guide: Muscle

The Histology Guide is a virtual experience of using a microscope with zoom features divided into topics and offering histological slides with labels and quizzes for each topic, such as muscle tissue. It is provided by the University of Leeds.

histology.leeds.ac.uk/tissue_types/muscle/

Visible Body: Muscular System

Visible Body provides interactive and highly accurate visualisations and apps for learning and teaching anatomy and physiology for students and healthcare professionals, including body systems such as the muscular system.

www.visiblebody.com/learn/muscular

CHAPTER 12
The Nervous System

The nervous system consists of an intricate, interconnected network of highly metabolic tissue whose cells communicate rapidly via electrical signals. There are two types of cells in the nervous system – neurons, which conduct nerve impulses, and neuroglia, which have supporting functions. (Refer to Chapter 7: Tissues and Organs, for further information on nervous tissue.)

The nervous system is divided into the central nervous system (CNS), consisting of the brain and spinal cord, and the peripheral nervous system (PNS), consisting of nerves which innervate body tissues. The chief function of the nervous system is communication. This is achieved through the collection of sensory information in the form of stimuli, the integration and coordination of that information centrally, and the generation of motor activity that brings about a response to the initial stimulus.

The collection and integration of, and response to information is achieved through the actions of neurons by means of action potentials and the release of chemical neurotransmitters. These form the basis for many of the voluntary and automatic reflex actions that regulate locomotion, posture, sensation, balance and chemical parameters, and maintain the homeostatic functions of organs and organ systems.

LEARNING OUTCOMES

On completion of these activities the student should be able to:

1. describe neurons in terms of their types and functions

2. explain resting membrane potentials and the events leading to an action potential in a neuron

3. discuss the characteristics of an action potential and the manner of its propagation along a nerve fibre

4. describe the events involved in the transmission of a nerve impulse from one neuron to another

5. demonstrate familiarity with the organisation of the peripheral nervous system and name the structures innervated by the cranial and spinal nerves

6. explain the mechanisms of a range of spinal and autonomic reflexes

7. examine a range of sensory functions and some of the factors that affect them

LEARNING OUTCOMES—cont'd

8. identify different cell types found in neural tissue and describe the structure of a peripheral nerve

9. identify the major regions of the brain and the structures they contain

10. describe the organisation of the spinal cord and name its structures

11. discuss the functions of the various parts of the brain and spinal cord

12. outline the structures and mechanisms that protect the central nervous system from damage.

KEY TERMS

Action potential

Arbor vitae

Autonomic nervous system (ANS)

Axon

Brain

Brain stem

Central canal

Central nervous system (CNS)

Cerebellum

Cerebral cortex

Cerebral hemisphere

Cerebrospinal fluid (CSF)

Cerebrum

Cranial nerve

Dendrite

Depolarisation

Dermatomes

Effector

Endoneurium

Epineurium

Ganglion

Grey matter

Hyperpolarisation

Hypothalamus

Interneuron

Medulla oblongata

Meninges

Motor (efferent)

Myelin

Nerve

Neuroglia

Neuron

Neurotransmitter

Node of Ranvier

Parasympathetic nervous system

Perineurium

Peripheral nervous system (PNS)

Plexus

Pons

Reflex arc

Repolarisation

Resting membrane potential

Saltatory conduction

Sensory (afferent)

Sensory adaptation

Sensory receptor

Somatic nervous system

Spinal cord

Spinal nerve

Stimulus

Sympathetic nervous system

Synapse

Synaptic transmission

Thalamus

White matter

ACTIVITY 12.1: NEURONS AND IMPULSE CONDUCTION

Neurons, or nerve cells, are specialised cells that conduct messages in the form of electrical impulses throughout the body. They function optimally for a lifetime, are mostly amitotic, and have an exceptionally high metabolic rate, making them especially sensitive to blood oxygen and glucose levels. The neuron cell body, or soma, is the major biosynthetic centre containing all the usual cell organelles except centrioles. Neurons receive impulses via the **dendrites**, and these are then conducted down the length of the **axon** towards the **synapse**. The axon may be either **myelinated** or unmyelinated. In myelinated axons, the speed of nerve impulse conduction is increased by saltatory conduction, where depolarisations "jump" from one node of Ranvier to the next.

Based on their functions, three types of neuron are recognised – **sensory (afferent)** neurons, which conduct impulses toward the CNS from receptors; **motor (efferent)** neurons, which conduct impulses from the **central nervous system (CNS)** to effectors, and **interneurons**, or association neurons, which conduct impulses between sensory and motor neurons or in CNS integration pathways (Fig. 12.1). At rest, neurons experience a **resting membrane potential** (Fig. 12.2), which is converted into an **action potential** and then reverts to a resting membrane potential (Fig. 12.3) through the processes of **depolarisation**, **repolarisation** and **hyperpolarisation**. Once a nerve impulse reaches a synapse, it is converted into a chemical signal in the form of a **neurotransmitter**, enabling the process of **synaptic transmission** (Fig. 12.4).

This activity investigates the structure and functions of the different types of neurons.

1. Examine Fig. 12.1 and use the terms provided to identify each of the labelled structures. (Note: Some terms are used more than once.)

axon	myelin sheath	sensory receptor
dendrite	cell body	

   a. Structure A: _____

   b. Structure B: _____

   c. Structure C: _____

   d. Structure D: _____

   e. Structure E: _____

   f. Structure F: _____

2. Compare axons with dendrites.

   a. In what ways are they similar?

   _____

   _____

   b. In what ways are they different?

   _____

   _____

3. Using arrows, indicate the direction of transmission of a nerve impulse along the axon of each cell.

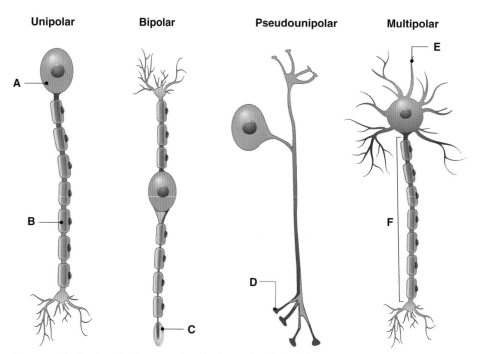

Figure 12.1 Types of neurons (unipolar, bipolar, pseudounipolar and multipolar).

4. Identify the major functions of:

   a. Multipolar neurons _____

   b. Bipolar neurons _____

   c. Unipolar neurons _____

5. Examine Fig. 12.2 and consider the following questions:

   a. What is the resting membrane potential of this neuron?

      _____

   b. On the diagram, indicate the relative concentrations of Na^+ and K^+ ions on each side of the membrane.

   c. List two factors that contribute to the existence of a resting membrane potential in all cells.

      i. _____

      ii. _____

   d. The voltmeter reading suddenly changes to $-60mV$. What is this event called?

      _____

   e. List three factors that can cause a neuron membrane potential to change.

      i. _____

      ii. _____

      iii. _____

   f. What is likely to happen if the membrane potential continues to change in this direction?

      _____

6. Complete the following sentences by filling in the blanks.

   a. Any stimulus reducing the _____ to $-50mV$ will set in action a chain of events in which positive _____ will increase the influx of Na^+ and create an action potential in 0.5 milliseconds.

   b. The stimulus can be _____, _____ or chemical but the result will always be the same.

   c. If a stimulus is strong enough to evoke a response then the response will always be an action potential of $+30$ mV. This is the _____ or _____ rule.

   d. The time interval between stimulation and the action potential starting is the _____ period.

   e. The time interval between the action potential and the return of the neuron sensitivity to another stimulus is the absolute _____ period.

7. Examine Fig. 12.3 and explain the following terms:

   a. Resting potential _____

      _____

   b. Threshold potential _____

      _____

   c. Depolarisation _____

      _____

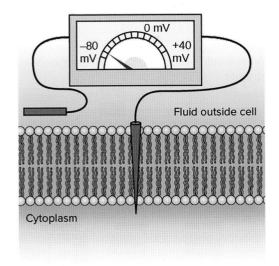

Figure 12.2 Resting membrane potential in a neuron.

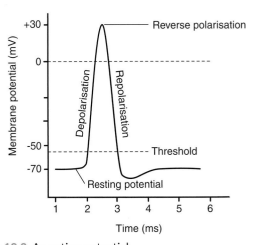

Figure 12.3 An action potential.
(Source: Shiland, B. J. (2020). Medical assistant: Nervous system, law and ethics, psychology and therapeutic procedures—module G. Elsevier.)

265

d. Repolarisation _____

_____

e. Hyperpolarisation _____

_____

8. Describe the ion movements across the cell membrane:

   a. When the cell is at rest _____

   _____

   b. During depolarisation _____

   _____

   c. During repolarisation _____

   _____

9. Explain how the Na$^+$/K$^+$ pumps operate to establish resting membrane potential.

   _____

   _____

   _____

   a. Is the activity of the Na$^+$/K$^+$ pumps considered passive or active transport? Explain.

   _____

   _____

   b. At which point in the conduction of an impulse do the Na$^+$/K$^+$ pumps become active?

   _____

   _____

10. List three factors that determine the rate of conduction of a nerve impulse.

    _____

    _____

    _____

11. Is there a distinction between an action potential and a graded potential? Explain.

    _____

    _____

    _____

12. Examine Fig. 12.4 and identify the labelled structures from the terms provided.

    acetylcholinesterase   presynaptic membrane

    neurotransmitter   synaptic cleft

    neurotransmitter   synaptic vesicle
    reception site

    postsynaptic membrane

    a. Structure A: _____

    b. Structure B: _____

    c. Structure C: _____

    d. Structure D: _____

    e. Structure E: _____

    f. Structure F: _____

    g. Structure G: _____

13. Describe, in sequence, what happens between the arrival of an action potential in the end axon terminal and the generation of an action potential in the post-synaptic membrane.

    _____

    _____

    _____

    _____

    _____

    _____

14. What is the function of acetylcholinesterase?

    _____

    _____

    a. What would occur if acetylcholinesterase was absent?

    _____

    _____

15. Explain the following terms:

    a. Excitatory postsynaptic potential (EPSP)

    _____

    b. Inhibitory postsynaptic potential (IPSP)

    _____

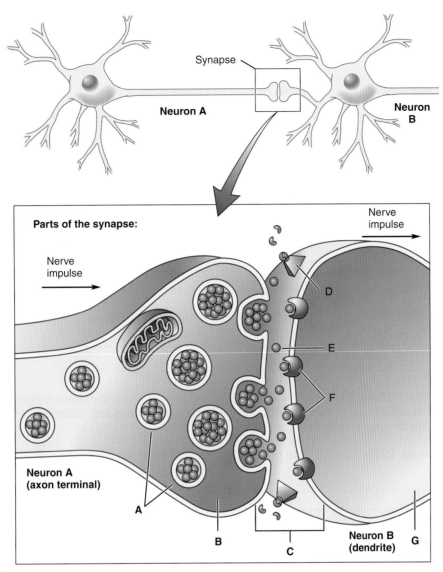

Figure 12.4 Synaptic transmission.
(Source: Fritz, S., & Fritz, L. (2021). Mosby's essential sciences for therapeutic massage: Anatomy, physiology, biomechanics, and pathology. Elsevier.)

c. Temporal summation

_____

d. Spatial summation

_____

16. Explain how spatial summation and temporal summation contribute to the generation of an action potential.

_____

_____

_____

17. What is synaptic delay and what causes it?

_____

_____

_____

18. What is synaptic fatigue and what causes it?

_____

_____

_____

Apply the Concepts

1. Is there a distinction between a voltage-gated channel and a chemically-gated channel? Explain.

   _____

   _____

   _____

   a. Identify one location on the neuron where a voltage-gated channel and one location where a chemically-gated channel can be found.

   _____

   _____

2. Kidney disease can cause the concentration of extracellular K^+ to increase.

   a. Explain the resulting effect on the resting membrane potential of the neurons.

   _____

   _____

3. Multiple sclerosis is a disabling disease of the brain and spinal cord, in which the immune system attacks and degrades the myelin sheaths of nerve fibres. Symptoms may include numbness and weakness in the limbs and loss of coordination of voluntary movement.

   a. Explain why damage to the myelin sheath of nerve fibres could cause these symptoms.

   _____

   _____

   b. What two types of neuroglia lay down myelin sheaths around healthy neurons?

   _____

4. Explain how general anaesthetics operate with reference to impulse conduction.

   _____

   _____

   _____

5. Valium (diazepam) is a drug that is often used to 'quiet the nerves'. One of Valium's actions is to enhance inhibitory postsynaptic potentials.

   a. Explain how this would have a sedative effect.

   _____

   _____

6. For each of the following neurotransmitters, identify the location where it is secreted (CNS or PNS), and explain its effects on neural functioning:

a. Dopamine.

_____

_____

b. Serotonin (5-HT).

_____

_____

c. Histamine.

_____

_____

d. GABA (γ-aminobutyric acid).

_____

_____

7. Explain how sarin achieves its function as a nerve agent.

_____

_____

ACTIVITY 12.2: THE CRANIAL NERVES

The **peripheral nervous system (PNS)** comprises all parts of the nervous system lying outside the **brain** and **spinal cord**. It has two broad divisions – the **somatic nervous system (SNS)** which innervates skeletal muscle and is largely under voluntary control, and the **autonomic nervous system (ANS)** which innervates cardiac muscle, smooth muscle and glands, and is under involuntary control. The autonomic nervous system is further divided into the **sympathetic nervous system** and **parasympathetic nervous system**.

Cranial and **spinal nerves** provide the pathways to and from the CNS for both somatic and autonomic nerves. One important difference between somatic and autonomic pathways is that autonomic nerves are only motor nerves, while somatic pathways may have both sensory and motor fibres. The 12 pairs of **cranial nerves** are part of the peripheral nervous system and primarily serve the head and neck. One pair, the vagus nerves, extend posteriorly through the thoracic and abdominal cavities. Cranial nerves are mostly named after the structures they innervate.

This activity examines the arrangement of the cranial nerves.

1. Examine the ventral surface of a model of the brain and identify the cranial nerves and their origins in the brain.

2. Complete the table below by naming each pair of cranial nerves and the structures they innervate.

Number	Name	Structures innervated
I		
II		
III		
IV		
V		

Number	Name	Structures innervated
VI		
VII		
VIII		
IX		
X		
XI		
XII		

ACTIVITY 12.3: THE SPINAL NERVES AND PLEXUSES

The 31 pairs of human spinal nerves arise from the fusions of the ventral and dorsal roots of the spinal cord. Spinal nerves are named according to their point of issue from the spinal cord. They are classified as cervical, thoracic, lumbar, sacral and coccygeal nerves, and are numbered according to the vertebra from which they emerge. They innervate muscles, glands and organs via functional **plexuses**, and eventually serve the skin, where they form **dermatomes**.

This activity examines the arrangement of the spinal nerves.

1. Using the charts, books or models available, observe the emergence of the paired spinal nerves from the spinal column.

2. Identify each region of the spine on the charts and models, and determine the number of pairs of spinal nerves emerging in that region.

Name of region	Number of pairs of spinal nerves

3. Define a nerve plexus.

_____

_____

_____

4. Using the charts, books or models available, identify the four principal plexuses formed by the spinal nerves and record them in the table below.

5. List the major peripheral nerves that emerge from each plexus and the major structures that they innervate, and record them in the table.

Nerve plexus	Major peripheral nerves	Major structures innervated

Apply the Concepts

1. Explain the effects on bladder and bowel function in an individual that has sustained injury to the nerves in the lumbar spine.

_____

_____

_____

2. Explain why damage to the nerves in the cervical plexus may cause death, and damage to the nerves in the brachial plexus may cause tetraplegia.

_____

_____

_____

3. What is paresthaesia and how does it occur?

_____

_____

4. What are shingles and how do they occur?

_____

_____

5. What is rabies and how does it occur?

_____

_____

6. What is sciatica and how does it occur?

_____

_____

7. What is neuropathy and how does it occur?

_____

_____

ACTIVITY 12.4: SOMATIC REFLEXES

Somatic reflexes are automatic responses that occur in skeletal muscle when a **stimulus** is applied to an appropriate **sensory receptor** (Fig. 12.5). Reflex testing is a standard clinical procedure used to detect damage to intervertebral disks, tumours, polyneuritis, and many other neurological conditions. Stretch reflexes normally act to maintain posture, balance and coordinated movement. They cause contraction of a muscle in response to stretching of the muscle. This involves monosynaptic **reflex arcs**, where a single sensory **neuron** synapses directly onto a single motor neuron in the spinal cord.

This activity demonstrates somatic reflexes in the form of the patellar reflex, the Achilles reflex and the corneal reflex.

Part 1: The Patellar Reflex

Muscles can be stretched by tapping on tendons attached to muscles at the elbow, wrist, ankle and knee joints, such as in the patellar reflex.

1. Examine Fig. 12.5, showing the structures involved in the patellar reflex, which assesses the function of the L2 – L4 level of the spinal cord.

2. Test the patellar (or knee-jerk) reflex by seating a subject on the laboratory bench with legs hanging free or knees crossed.

3. Tap the patellar ligament sharply with the reflex hammer just below the kneecap (Fig. 12.5A). Test both knees noting the response.

   a. What is observed?

   _____

   _____

4. With reference to Fig. 12.5B, describe the events of the patellar reflex at each of the points shown after the hammer strikes the patellar tendon.

   a. Event 1: _____

   _____

   b. Event 2: _____

   _____

   c. Event 3: _____

   _____

   d. Event 4: _____

   _____

   e. Event 5: _____

   _____

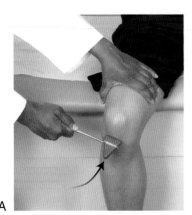

A

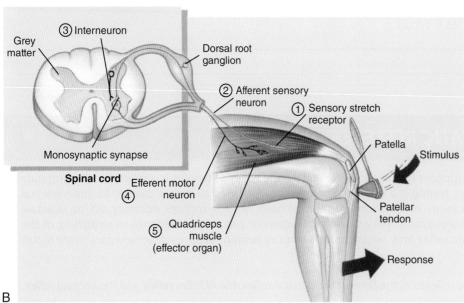

B

Figure 12.5 The patellar reflex. *(Source: **A** Jarvis, C. (2020). Pocket companion for physical examination and health assessment. 8th ed. Elsevier. **B** Heitkemper, M. M., Dirksen, S. R., Bucher, L., & O'Brien, P. G. (2010). Medical–surgical nursing in Canada: Assessment and management of clinical problems. Mosby Elsevier.)*

5. Test the effect of mental distraction on the patellar reflex by asking the subject to add a column of three-digit numbers while the reflex is tested again.

   a. Is the response more or less vigorous than the first response?

   _____

   b. What can be concluded about the ability of higher brain centres to override spinal somatic reflexes?

   _____

6. Now test the effect of muscular activity occurring simultaneously in other areas of the body by asking the subject to clasp the edge of the bench and vigorously attempt to pull it upwards with both hands. At the same time, test the patellar reflex again.

   a. What is observed?

   _____

7. Fatigue also influences the reflex response. Ask the subject to jog on the spot until they are very fatigued. Test the patellar reflex again.

   a. What is observed?

   _____

   b. Can it be concluded that nerve or muscle fatigue is responsible for the changes observed in the patellar reflex? Explain.

   _____

   _____

   _____

Part 2: The Achilles Reflex

The Achilles reflex, or ankle jerk reflex, is a type of stretch reflex that occurs when the Achilles tendon is tapped while the foot is dorsiflexed; the foot, in response, should jerk towards the plantar surface. It tests the function of the gastrocnemius muscle and the nerve that supplies it, the tibial nerve.

1. Test the Achilles (or ankle-jerk) reflex by asking the subject to sit on the bench, remove a shoe (and sock) and dorsiflex the foot slightly to increase the tension on the gastrocnemius muscle.

2. Hold the foot and sharply tap the Achilles tendon with the reflex hammer.

   a. What is observed?

   _____

   b. This is a spinal reflex. Where is the receptor and what is the effector?

   _____

   c. Does the contraction of the gastrocnemius normally result in the response observed? Explain.

   _____

   _____

Part 3: The Corneal Reflex

The corneal reflex is mediated through the trigeminal **nerve**, which is one of the cranial nerves. The absence of this reflex may indicate damage to the **brain stem** resulting from trauma, such as compression of the brain.

1. Stand to one side of the subject. The subject should look away from you towards the opposite wall.

2. Wait a few seconds and then quickly but gently touch the subject's cornea (on the side towards you) with a wisp of absorbent cotton.

   a. What reflexive reaction occurs when something touches the cornea?

   _____

   b. What is the function of this reflex?

   _____

   _____

ACTIVITY 12.5: AUTONOMIC REFLEXES

Autonomic reflexes occur in response to a stimulus that is mediated by the autonomic nervous system (ANS). In the pupillary light reflex and the consensual reflex, the sensory receptors are found in the retina of the eye, the optic nerve is the sensory (afferent) nerve, the oculomotor nerve is the motor (efferent) nerve, and the smooth muscle of the iris is the **effector**. Absence of normal pupillary reflexes is generally an indication of severe trauma or deterioration of brain stem tissue, which includes the **medulla oblongata** and **pons**. The consensual reflex, or any reflex observed on one side of the body when the other side has been stimulated, is called a contralateral response. The patellar reflex, or any reflex occurring on the same side as the stimulus, is an ipsilateral response.

This activity demonstrates autonomic reflexes mediated by cranial nerves.

1. Conduct this experiment in an area where lighting is relatively dim. When the subject is accustomed to the lighting (after about 5 minutes), use a ruler to record the diameter of the subject's pupils to the nearest millimetre.

    Right pupil: _____ mm

    Left pupil: _____ mm

2. Stand to the left of the subject. The subject should shield their right eye by holding a hand vertically between the eye and the right side of the nose.

3. Shine a torch into the subject's left eye.

    a. What is the pupillary response?

    _____

    b. What is the new diameter of the left pupil?

    _____ mm

4. Observe the right pupil.

    a. What is the diameter of the right pupil?

    _____ mm

    b. Has the same change (a consensual response) occurred in the right eye?

    _____

c. What is the benefit of this consensual reflex?

_____

5. Consider the following questions:

    a. When a contralateral response occurs, what does this indicate about the pathways involved?

    _____

    _____

    b. Was the sympathetic or the parasympathetic division of the autonomic nervous system active during testing of these reflexes? Explain.

    _____

    _____

    _____

    c. What is the function of these pupillary responses?

    _____

    _____

Apply the Concepts

1. A nervous disorder called dysautonomia can affect functions like heart rate and blood pressure.

   a. Which part of the peripheral nervous system is affected by this disorder?

   _____

   b. Give examples of other body functions that are likely to be affected.

   _____

   _____

   _____

2. What clinical information can be gained by testing somatic reflexes?

   _____

   _____

3. With reference to spinal nerve function, explain what causes hiccups.

   _____

   _____

4. What are varicosities and where are they located?

   _____

   _____

5. Explain the difference between a cholinergic receptor and an adrenergic receptor.

   _____

   _____

6. What is Horner's syndrome and how does it occur?

   _____

   _____

ACTIVITY 12.6: BASIC AND ACQUIRED REFLEXES

Some reflexes are basic, or inborn, and others are learned, or acquired. If a response involves a specific reflex arc, the synapses are facilitated and response time will be short. Learned reflexes involve a far larger number of neural pathways and many types of higher intellectual activities, lengthening the response time.

This activity demonstrates the time difference between simple and learned reflexes.

1. Using a reflex hammer, elicit the patellar reflex in the subject. Note the fast reaction time of this basic spinal reflex.

2. The subject should now hold out a hand (dorsal surface upwards) with the thumb and index finger extended and slightly apart.

3. The experimenter should hold a ruler vertically above the gap between the subject's thumb and index finger, such that the end of the ruler (0 cm) is exactly 3 cm above the gap.

4. When the ruler is dropped, the subject should be able to grasp it between the thumb and index finger as it passes.

5. Have the subject catch the ruler five times, varying the time between trials.

6. The relative speed of the response can be determined by noting the distance on the ruler at the point of the subject's fingertips.

7. Record the number of centimetres that pass through the subject's fingertips at each trial:

Trial 1: _____ cm

Trial 2: _____ cm

Trial 3: _____ cm

Trial 4: _____ cm

Trial 5: _____ cm

8. Consider the following questions:

   a. What explanation can be provided for the results obtained?

   _____

   _____

   b. Why was the reaction time for the acquired reflex longer than that for the basic reflex?

   _____

   _____

ACTIVITY 12.7: TWO-POINT DISCRIMINATION TEST

Sensory receptors act as transducers, converting stimuli into nerve impulses. As action potentials are essentially identical in all sensory nerves, information about the stimulus is conveyed entirely by the sensory region of the **cerebral cortex** that is stimulated (Fig. 12.6). A single sensory neuron may have a number of sensory receptor structures associated with it, distributed over an area of tissue. This area is termed the receptor field of the neuron, and any stimulus of appropriate modality applied within that field is transmitted via the one neuron to the CNS. Two separate points of stimulation within the same receptor field therefore cannot be distinguished. Sizes of receptor fields vary, being inversely related to the density of sensory innervation and to the sensitivity of the area. The representation of an area in the somatosensory cortex is related directly to its density of sensory innervation; in other words, to the amount of sensory information originating from that area.

This activity employs the two-point discrimination test as a method of measuring the size of receptor fields and therefore the density of sensory innervation.

 To conduct this activity it is important to ensure the following safety precautions:

- *Use an alcohol wipe to sterilise the points after touching lips and tongue.*

1. This activity is best conducted in pairs, with one person as the subject and the other as the experimenter.

2. The experimenter will use a pair of sharp, pointed dividers to apply two separate stimuli to an area of skin. (It is important to apply touch, not pain.)

3. Start with the points several centimetres apart and touch an area of skin – two separate stimuli should be perceived.

4. Instruct the subject to close their eyes while you gradually move the points closer together, touching again each time until the two separate points feel like one. They are now within the same receptor field.

5. Carry out this test on the skin areas listed below, recording the minimum distance at which two distinct stimuli can be felt.

6. Repeat this process three times on a slightly different patch of skin to obtain an average.

Skin area	Average minimum distance for two-point discrimination (mm)
Fingertip	
Back of hand	
Arm	
Shoulder	
Side of nose	
Lips	
Tip of tongue	
Back of neck	
Leg	
Sole of foot	

7. Compare the results with Fig. 12.6B, which shows the cortical representation of somatic structures in the primary sensory area.

a. In which area is the density of sensory receptors the greatest?

_____

b. In which area is the receptor density the lowest?

_____

c. Based on the results, what is the functional significance of the difference in receptor densities between the areas tested?

_____

_____

_____

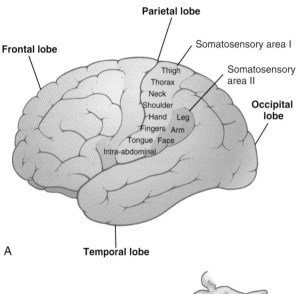

A

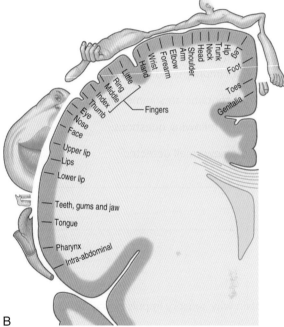

B

Figure 12.6 Sensory centres in the cortex. **A** Location of the somatosensory areas of the parietal lobes of the cortex. **B** Cortical tissue dedicated to each body region.
(Source: **A** Hall, M. E., & Hall, J. E. (2021). Guyton and Hall textbook of medical physiology. (14th ed.). Elsevier. **B** El-Hussein, M. T., Power-Kean, K., Zettel, S., Huether, S. E., & McCance, K. L. (2023). Huether and McCance's understanding pathophysiology, 2nd Canadian edition. Elsevier.)

Additional Activities

For additional activities visit Activity 12A: Modification of Pain Perception on Evolve°.

ACTIVITY 12.8: SENSORY ADAPTATION

When a stimulus persists, sensory receptors adapt – some more rapidly than others – and the frequency of impulses relayed to the CNS declines and may stop altogether. This is a process referred to as **sensory adaptation**. If this did not occur, the nervous system would be continuously bombarded with information on everything occurring in an individual's environment. In general, receptors for a stimulus vital to survival are very slow to adapt, but where a stimulus is non-vital they rapidly adapt so that the individual soon becomes unaware of it.

This activity demonstrates the effect of adaptation on sensory receptors.

1. Place a drop of oil of cloves on a piece of cotton wool.

2. Plug one nostril with clean cotton wool and inhale the odour deeply with the other.

3. Continue until the smell can no longer be detected. At this point, the receptors have adapted.

4. Quickly, before the effect wears off, sniff a piece of cotton wool impregnated with oil of peppermint.

5. Discard all contaminates immediately after use.

6. Consider the following questions:

    a. Was the new smell detected?

    _____

b. What does this suggest about the receptors for these two odours?

    _____

    _____

c. How many primary odours are there? (Note: There is considerable disagreement.)

    _____

d. Provide examples of other rapidly adapting receptors and of some slowly adapting receptors.

    i. Rapid: _____

    ii. Slow: _____

Apply the Concepts

1. Explain why sensory impulses may be hindered or blocked by the application of cold or continuous pressure.

    _____

    _____

2. Suggest what might occur if pain were detected by rapidly adapting receptors.

    _____

    _____

Additional Activities

For additional activities visit Activity 12B: Neural Tissue on Evolve˚.

ACTIVITY 12.9: MICROSCOPIC EXAMINATION OF PERIPHERAL NERVE STRUCTURE

A nerve is a bundle of neuron fibres wrapped in connective tissue (Fig. 12.7). It extends to or from the CNS, connecting the brain and spinal cord to visceral organs, muscles, glands and skin. Nerves carrying both sensory (afferent) and motor (efferent) fibres are called mixed nerves. All spinal nerves are mixed nerves. Other nerves are sensory or motor nerves. Within a nerve, each fibre is surrounded by a thin connective tissue sheath called an **endoneurium**. Groups of fibres are bound by a coarser tissue called the **perineurium** to form bundles of fibres called fascicles. All fascicles are bound together by a tough, white, connective tissue sheath called the **epineurium**, forming the nerve. Blood and lymphatic vessels also travel within a nerve.

This activity examines the microscopic structure of nerves.

1. Obtain prepared slides of a peripheral nerve LS (H&E) and TS (H&E). H&E is a general-purpose stain which normally colours cytoplasm pink and nuclei a darker, more purplish shade.

2. Hold the slide of the TS nerve up to the light.

   a. What is the approximate diameter of the nerve?

   _____

Figure 12.7 Structure of a nerve.
(Source: Winn, H. R. (2022). Youmans and Winn neurological surgery. Elsevier.)

3. Examine the TS specimen under low power. Refer to Fig. 12.7 to assist with identification of the structures examined.

4. Note that the *nerve* consists of several more or less circular bundles of *fibres* (remember, they have been cut across). These fibres are the nerve cell *processes*. A membranous *perineurium* surrounds each bundle, or *fascicle*. Within the fascicle, the *endoneurium* surrounds the individual fibres and the fascicles are held together to form the nerve by a loose network of tissue, the *epineurium*. *Blood vessels* and *lymphatics* travel within these sheaths to supply the nerve.

5. In the space below, draw a diagram of a portion of the nerve and label all the structures you can identify.

6. Identify any *blood vessels* and include these in your diagram (they can often be identified by the presence of *erythrocytes* in the lumen).

Magnification of diagram: × _____

7. Examine the H&E stained LS nerve under low power, to observe that it consists of parallel bundles of fibres.

   a. What are these fibres?

   _____

8. Virtually all peripheral nerves are mixed nerves.

   a. What does this mean about the nature of the fibres and their direction of conduction?

   _____

   _____

   b. Which type of tissue are the endoneurium, perineurium and epineurium composed of?

   _____

   c. Identify the function of the following tissues:

      i. Endoneurium _____

      _____

      ii. Perineurium _____

      _____

      iii. Epineurium _____

      _____

9. Examine the H&E-stained TS nerve at a higher power than used previously and concentrate on a single fascicle.

10. Note the great many nerve fibres (small, round and pink due to their cytoplasmic content). Fatty material does not stain with these dyes and, in fact, is leached out during the mounting process.

    a. What structure is represented by the clear area surrounding many of the fibres?

    _____

11. Obtain a slide of peripheral nerve (H&E), which has been teased to separate the fibres.

12. Examine this initially under low power and then move to high power.

13. The nerve will contain both *myelinated* and *unmyelinated* fibres. Locate a region in which the fibres are well separated and distinct. The myelinated fibres will have a foamy appearance due to the dissolution of the myelin; between the myelin segments *nodes of Ranvier* should be visible.

14. Draw a section of a myelinated fibre, labelling the fibre, its myelin sheath and the nodes of Ranvier.

Magnification of diagram: $\times$ _____

Apply the Concepts

1. What is poliomyelitis and how does it occur?

   _____

   _____

   _____

ACTIVITY 12.10: STRUCTURES OF THE CENTRAL NERVOUS SYSTEM

The central nervous system comprises the brain and spinal cord. The CNS receives and integrates information from the sensory nervous system, and initiates and coordinates motor functions in all parts of the body. The **cerebrum** of the brain consists of a **grey matter** cortex and a **white matter** core (Fig. 12.8), whereas the spinal cord contains a **central canal** containing **cerebrospinal fluid (CSF)**, surrounded by a grey matter core and a white matter exterior (Fig. 12.9).

This activity explores the structures of the central nervous system and their functions.

1. Examine Fig. 12.8 and identify the labelled regions and structures:

   a. Structure A: _____

   b. Structure B: _____

   c. Structure C: _____

   d. Structure D: _____

   e. Structure E: _____

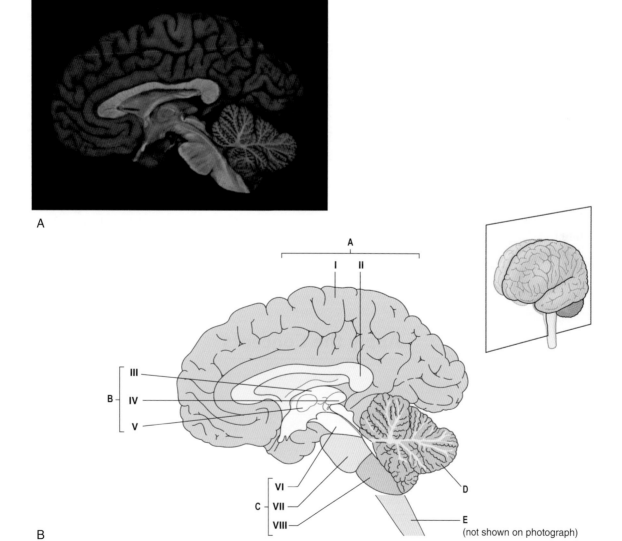

Figure 12.8 Midsagittal section of the human brain. **A** Photograph. **B** Interpretive diagram.
(Source: Waugh, A., & Grant, A. (2014). Ross & Wilson anatomy and physiology in health and illness. Elsevier.)

f. Structure I: _____

g. Structure II: _____

h. Structure III: _____

i. Structure IV: _____

j. Structure V: _____

k. Structure VI: _____

l. Structure VII: _____

m. Structure VIII: _____

2. Examine Fig. 12.9 and identify the labelled structures:

a. Structure A: _____

b. Structure B: _____

c. Structure C: _____

d. Structure D: _____

e. Structure E: _____

f. Structure F: _____

g. Structure G: _____

h. Structure H: _____

i. Structure I: _____

j. Structure J: _____

k. Structure K: _____

l. Structure L: _____

m. Structure M: _____

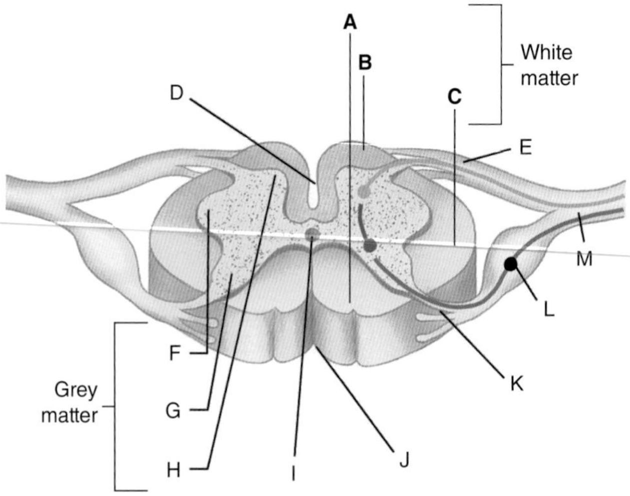

Figure 12.9 Transverse section of the human spinal cord.
(Source: McCourt, T.R. (2020). Trauma nursing: From resuscitation through rehabilitation. Elsevier.)

3. Identify which of the structures in Fig. 12.9 contains:

a. Sensory neuron cell bodies _____

b. Afferent fibres only _____

c. Motor neuron fibres only _____

d. Synapses involved in spinal reflexes _____

e. Cerebrospinal fluid _____

f. Motor neuron cell bodies _____

4. How is the arrangement of white and grey matter in the spinal cord different from that in the brain?

_____

_____

Apply the Concepts

1. What is spina bifida and how does it occur?

_____

_____

_____

2. What is amnesia and how does it occur?

_____

_____

_____

ACTIVITY 12.11: EXTERNAL FEATURES OF THE BRAIN

The brain can be examined based on its four major regions: the **cerebral hemispheres**; the **diencephalon**, consisting of the **thalamus** and **hypothalamus**; the brain stem; and the **cerebellum**, with its distinct arrangement of white matter forming the **arbor vitae**.

This activity examines the external structure of the brain.

1. Obtain a model of the human brain and the diagrams provided to identify each of the major regions listed above.

2. Within each region, locate each of the external structures listed below, and give its functions where indicated:

   a. Cerebral hemispheres

   ☐ Longitudinal fissure

   ☐ Central sulcus

   ☐ Frontal lobe

      i. Functions: _____

      _____

   ☐ Parietal lobe

      ii. Functions: _____

      _____

   ☐ Temporal lobe

      iii. Functions: _____

      _____

   ☐ Occipital lobe

      iv. Functions: _____

      _____

3. Note that the cerebral cortex is a region of grey matter consisting of cell bodies and forms the outer layer of the cerebral hemispheres. The deeper cerebral white matter is composed of fibre tracts carrying impulses to and from the cortex. Along with the cerebral hemispheres, the diencephalon is part of the forebrain.

   a. What is the function of the brain convolutions?

   _____

   _____

4. Turn the model of the brain so that the ventral surface of the brain can be viewed.

5. Locate each of the following and provide their functions:

   a. Diencephalon

      i. Olfactory bulbs _____

      _____

      ii. Optic nerves _____

      _____

      iii. Pituitary gland _____

      _____

6. Continue inferiorly from the *diencephalon* to identify and give the function of the following structures:

   a. Brain stem

      i. Pons _____

      _____

      ii. Medulla oblongata _____

      _____

7. Turn the brain so that the dorsal aspect is uppermost. Identify the large *cerebellum*.

   a. What is the function of the cerebellum?

   _____

   _____

8. What are the similarities and differences between the cerebrum and cerebellum?

   _____

   _____

9. Remove the cerebellum to view the corpora quadrigemina.

   a. What is the function of the corpora quadrigemina?

   _____

   _____

Apply the Concepts

1. Relate the functions of Broca's area and Wernicke's area to the development of aphasia.

_____

_____

_____

2. Suggest a possible consequence of damage to the following areas of the brain:

    a. Primary motor cortex.

    _____

    _____

    b. Premotor cortex.

    _____

    _____

    c. Primary visual cortex.

    _____

    _____

    d. Anterior association area.

    _____

    _____

    e. Posterior association area.

    _____

    _____

3. What is dyslexia and how does it occur?

_____

_____

_____

4. What is autism and how does it occur?

_____

_____

_____

ACTIVITY 12.12: INTERNAL FEATURES OF THE BRAIN

In the brain, the cerebrum and cerebellum have an outer layer of grey matter, which is reduced to scattered grey matter nuclei in the spinal cord. The cavities of the CNS consist of the ventricles of the brain and the **central canal** of the spinal cord. The ventricles are continuous with one another and with the central canal of the spinal cord. They are lined with ependymal cells and are filled with cerebrospinal fluid (CSF).

This activity examines the internal structures of the brain.

1. Take the model of the brain apart to see a median sagittal view of the internal brain structures. In the deeper areas of the *white matter*, observe the large *corpus callosum*.

   a. What is the function of the corpus callosum?

   _____

   _____

2. Identify the *nuclei*, or islands of *grey matter* within the *white matter*. These are clusters of *nerve cell bodies*.

3. Locate the *diencephalon* again. Identify the *thalamus*, consisting of two large *lobes* of *grey matter* that enclose the *third ventricle*.

   a. What is the function of the thalamus?

   _____

   _____

4. The *hypothalamus* makes up the floor of the *third ventricle* and is connected to the *pituitary gland*.

   a. What is the function of the hypothalamus?

   _____

   _____

5. Examine the *cerebellum*. Note that it is composed of two lateral *hemispheres*, each with three *lobes*. The cerebellum has an outer cortex of *grey matter* and an inner area of *white matter*. Locate the tree-like white matter, called the *arbor vitae* (tree of life).

Apply the Concepts

1. What symptoms may be experienced by an individual with hypothalamic damage?

   _____

   _____

2. As well as structural regions, the brain also has two functional systems, the limbic system and the reticular formation. Describe the functions of the:

   a. Limbic system _____

   _____

   b. Reticular formation _____

   _____

3. What are the symptoms of a malfunctioning:

   a. Limbic system _____

   _____

   b. Reticular formation _____

   _____

4. A person falls backwards and receives a heavy blow to the back of the skull. On regaining consciousness, she becomes aware that her movements are jerky and uncoordinated.

   a. Which structure was damaged in the fall?

   _____

5. What is syncope and why does it occur?

   _____

   _____

ACTIVITY 12.13: PROTECTIVE MECHANISMS OF THE BRAIN AND SPINAL CORD

The structures of the CNS, the brain and spinal cord, are protected against damage in a number of ways. Bone, in the form of the skull and vertebrae, protect against compressive forces, cerebrospinal fluid bathes the brain and spinal cord both internally and externally to provide cushioning, and the **meninges** are three connective tissue layers that envelop the brain and spinal cord like a sheath to provide both cushioning and physical protection.

This activity tests knowledge of the structures and mechanisms that protect the central nervous system from physical and chemical damage.

1. Complete the following sentences by filling in the blanks.

   a. The brain is protected by a bony case called the

   _____, and the spinal cord by bones called

   _____.

   b. The brain and spinal cord are also protected by three connective tissue membranes collectively called

   _____. The outermost of these is

   the _____, consisting of two layers called

   the _____ layer and the _____ layer.

   c. The middle membrane is the _____,

   separated from the outermost membrane by the

   _____ space. The innermost membrane is

   the _____, which clings tightly to the

   surface of the _____.

   d. The brain is also protected by the selective permeabilities of the capillaries supplying blood to the brain. This mechanism is called the

   _____.

   e. Protection from physical trauma is provided by the

   cushioning effect of the fluid called _____,

   which circulates in the _____ of the

   brain and the _____ of the spinal cord.

2. Consider the following questions:

    a. What is the function of the CSF?

_____

_____

    b. Describe the composition of CSF.

_____

_____

    c. Describe how the CSF is transported throughout the nervous system.

_____

_____

Apply the Concepts

1. In their correct order, identify all the tissue layers that a brain surgeon cuts through from the skin to the brain.

_____

_____

2. A victim of a car accident arrives in hospital, conscious but finding it difficult to speak and experiencing severe muscle weakness in the right limbs. A CT scan of the head showed an acute subdural haematoma and extensive subarachnoid bleeding.

    a. Which region of the brain was affected by the injury?

_____

    b. Damage to what specific parts of this region has caused the symptoms described?

_____

    c. Which side of the brain was damaged in the accident?

_____

    d. What is meant by subarachnoid bleeding?

_____

_____

    e. Why is bleeding likely to occur there after a head injury?

_____

_____

3. What is meningitis and how does it occur?

_____

_____

_____

Additional Activities

For additional activities visit Activity 12C: Examination of Brain Structure (Brain Dissection) on Evolve.

Additional Resources

Anatomy Zone: Neuroanatomy Anatomy Tutorials

AnatomyZone provides numerous video tutorials and interactive 3D models on various regions of the human body, such as the nervous system.

anatomyzone.com/neuroanatomy/

Functional Neuroanatomy

An interactive resource covering regions of the brain, cross sections, videos, interactive modules and MRIs, created by the University of British Columbia.

www.neuroanatomy.ca/

GetBodySmart: Nervous System

GetBodySmart presents fully animated, illustrated and interactive eBooks about human anatomy and physiology body systems.

www.getbodysmart.com/nervous-system

Histology Guide Virtual Microscopy Laboratory: Nervous Tissue

Histology Guide is an online resource providing a virtual microscopy laboratory experience, by allowing users to view microscope slides from professional collections for the purpose of interpreting cellular and tissue structures as seen through a microscope.

histologyguide.com/slidebox/06-nervous-tissue.html

Innerbody Research: Nervous System

Innerbody Research provides objective, science-based advice to help readers make more informed choices about home health products and services with most up-to-date reviews, guides and research, including information about the nervous system.

www.innerbody.com/image/nervov.html

Interactive Neuroanatomy Atlas

Interactive Neuroanatomy Atlas is an online multimedia project developed by Columbia University where learners can select from a number of lab activities and interact with the gallery of images provided.

www.columbia.edu/itc/hs/medical/neuroanatomy/neuroanat/

Learn Biology: Neurons and the Nervous System

The Learn Biology site provides a number of interactive anatomy and physiology tutorials for students at various levels of learning.

https://learn-biology.com/ap-biology/module-28-neurons-and-the-nervous-system/

Osmosis – Nervous System

The Nervous System module of Osmosis provides videos, notes, quiz questions and links to further resources related to the nervous system.

www.osmosis.org/library/md/foundational-sciences/physiology#nervous_system

Sumanas Animated Tutorials: Neurobiology

Sumanas Animated Tutorials provide an animation gallery relating to neuronal development, action potentials and synaptic transmission, and reflex arcs.

www.sumanasinc.com/webcontent/animations/neurobiology.html

The Brain from Top to Bottom

A free resource blog covering a number of topics related to the brain and brain function, provided according to topic, level of explanation (beginner, intermediate and advanced), level of organisation, module, and offering guided tours.

thebrain.mcgill.ca/index.php

The Histology Guide: Nervous System

The Histology Guide is a virtual experience of using a microscope with zoom features divided into topics and offering histological slides with labels and quizzes for each topic. It is provided by the University of Leeds.

www.histologyguide.com/slidebox/06-nervous-tissue.html

The McGill Physiology Virtual Lab: Resting Membrane Potential

A series of interactive tutorials on a variety physiology topics created for students enrolled in introductory physiology courses at McGill University.

www.medicine.mcgill.ca/physio/vlab/rmp/vlabmenurmp.htm

Visible Body: Nervous System

Visible Body provides interactive and highly accurate visualisations and apps for learning and teaching anatomy and physiology for students and healthcare professionals, including body systems such as the nervous system.

www.visiblebody.com/learn/nervous

CHAPTER 13
The Special Senses

The special senses are those senses for which specialised sense organs exist and which incorporate specific sensory receptors into their structure. The special senses are vision, hearing, equilibrium (balance), gustation (taste) and olfaction (smell). Sensory receptors in the special sense organs detect specific stimuli and, via neural pathways, relay this information to the sensory cortex in the brain. (Refer to Chapter 12: The Nervous System, for further information on nervous tissue and the brain). The process whereby we are made aware of a stimulus is referred to as sensation, while perception refers to the interpretation of the stimulus in the brain. Disorders of the special senses can lead to impaired perception of a particular sense. To determine the extent of impairment, a variety of tests have been devised which often feature in diagnostic assessments for certain conditions.

LEARNING OUTCOMES

On completion of these activities, the student should be able to:

1. discuss the macroscopic and microscopic structure of the eyes
2. describe the cellular structure of the retina
3. explain how photoreceptors process light stimuli
4. discuss the macroscopic and microscopic structure of the ears
5. describe the structure of the cochlea
6. explain how the stereocilia process sound stimuli
7. describe the macroscopic and microscopic structure of the vestibular apparatus
8. explain how balance and equilibrium are maintained
9. describe the macroscopic and microscopic structure of the tongue, tastebuds and olfactory structures, and how these contribute to the sense of taste
10. conduct a series of tests associated with the processes of vision, hearing, balance, smell and taste.

KEY TERMS

Auditory ossicles
Auricle (pinna)
Blind spot
Cochlea
Cochlear nerve
Colour blindness
Conductive hearing
Cones
Ear
Endolymph
Eye
Fovea centralis
Hair cells (stereocilia)

Inner ear
Macula lutea
Middle ear
Olfactory epithelium
Optic chiasma
Optic disc
Optic nerve
Organ of Corti
Outer ear
Oval window
Photoreceptors
Phototransduction
Proprioception

Retina
Rods
Semicircular canals
Sensorineural hearing
Sensory receptors
Sound transduction
Stereoscopic vision
Tastebuds (papillae)
Tympanic membrane
Vestibular apparatus
Vestibule
Visual field

ACTIVITY 13.1: SENSORY RECEPTORS

Sensory receptors convey information about stimuli or changes in their environment. This information is sent via afferent or sensory pathways to the central nervous system, where it is processed in the sensory cortex of the brain. Sensory receptors are often named according to their location or their function; that is, the type of stimulus they respond to.

This activity highlights the functions of various sensory receptors in the body.

1. For each of the categories of sensory receptors below, identify the type of stimulus detected and provide an example.

   a. Exteroceptors: _____

   _____

   b. Proprioceptors: _____

   _____

   c. Visceroceptors (interoceptors): _____

   _____

   d. Mechanoreceptors: _____

   _____

   e. Chemoreceptors: _____

   _____

   f. Thermoreceptors: _____

   _____

   g. Photoreceptors: _____

   _____

   h. Baroreceptors: _____

   _____

2. Describe the difference between sensation and the perception of sensation.

   _____

   _____

3. Which system in the brain decides if perception occurs?

   _____

   _____

ACTIVITY 13.2: STRUCTURES OF THE EYE

The **eyes** are the special sense organs of vision. They are paired, spherical structures approximately 2.5 centimetres in diameter. The eyes contain a number of structures which help to direct and focus light onto the back of the eye, where specialised **photoreceptors** are located (Fig. 13.1). In addition, accessory structures of the eyes help to move, cleanse and protect the eyes from damaging stimuli and foreign objects.

This activity examines the structures of the eye and associates each structure with its function.

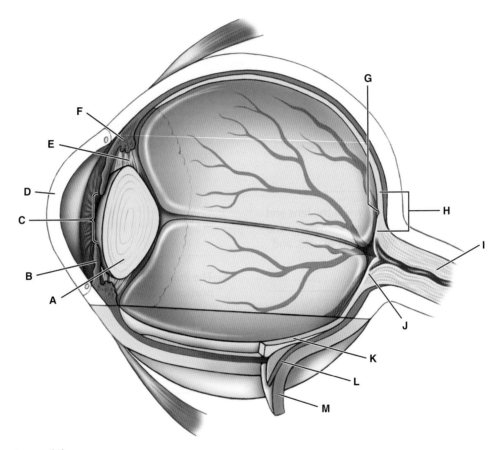

Figure 13.1 Structures of the eye.
(*Source: Herlihy, B. (2022). The human body in health and illness. Elsevier.*)

1. Identify the structures of the eye shown in Fig. 13.1 by inserting the matching letter next to each of the terms listed:

   a. Choroid: _____

   b. Ciliary body: _____

   c. Cornea: _____

   d. Fovea centralis: _____

   e. Iris: _____

   f. Lens: _____

   g. Macula lutea: _____

   h. Optic disc: _____

   i. Optic nerve: _____

   j. Pupil: _____

   k. Retina: _____

   l. Sclera: _____

   m. Suspensory ligament: _____

2. Match the structures of the eye with the functions provided, by inserting the matching number below each of the explanations that follow.

1. Aqueous humour	7. Lens
2. Choroid	8. Optic nerve
3. Conjunctiva	9. Pupil
4. Cornea	10. Retina
5. Fovea centralis	11. Sclera
6. Iris	12. Vitreous humour

a. The light-sensitive layer in the eye composed of photoreceptors (rods and cones) and sensory neurons.

_____

b. The fibrous, transparent frontal portion of the sclera that admits light into the eye.

_____

c. A plasma-like liquid in the space between the lens and the cornea in the eye. Helps maintain the shape of the eye, supplies nutrients and oxygen to its tissues, and disposes of wastes.

_____

d. Cranial nerves that arise from the retina and carry visual information to the thalamus and other parts of the brain.

_____

e. An eye's centre of focus and the place on the retina where photoreceptors are highly concentrated.

_____

f. A jelly-like substance that fills the space behind the lens in the eye. Helps to maintain the shape of the eye.

_____

g. A thin, dark pigmented layer in the eye that prevents light from scattering within the eye; surrounded by the sclera.

_____

h. The structure in the eye that focuses light rays onto the retina.

_____

i. Thin, protective mucous membrane that helps keep the eye moist. Lines the inner surface of the eyelids and covers the front of the eyeball, except the cornea.

_____

j. Opening in the iris that admits light into the interior of the eye. Muscles in the iris regulate its size.

_____

k. The coloured part of the eye formed by the anterior portion of the choroid.

_____

l. A layer of connective tissue forming the outer surface of the eye.

_____

Apply the Concepts

1. What is a stye and how does it occur?

_____

_____

_____

2. What is blepharitis and how does it occur?

_____

_____

_____

3. What are cataracts and how do they occur?

_____

_____

_____

Additional Activities

For additional activities visit Activity 13A: Microscopic Examination of the Eye on Evolve˙.

ACTIVITY 13.3: PHYSIOLOGY OF VISION

Light entering the eye is focused towards the back of the eye onto the **retina**, where the photoreceptors, the **rods** and **cones**, are located (Fig. 13.2). The process whereby the rods and cones are stimulated by incident light, which is converted to and conveyed as electrical sensory information to the brain, is referred to as **phototransduction**.

This activity considers the structures, processes and pathways involved in vision.

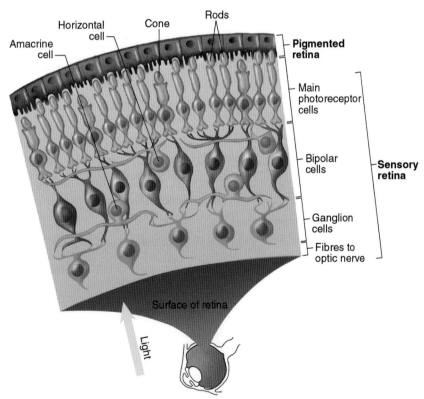

Figure 13.2 Structure of the retina.
(*Source: Herlihy, B. (2022). The human body in health and illness. Elsevier Health Sciences.*)

Part 1: Structure of the Retina

Light passes through air to enter the eye through the cornea, aqueous humour, lens and vitreous humour. As light passes through these structures towards the retina, it is refracted due to loss of speed, and is further adjusted by the condition of the lens and the activity of the ciliary muscles acting on the lens. The image received by photoreceptors in the retina is converted into electrical impulses and sent to the brain via the **optic nerve**.

1. Consider the following questions with reference to Fig. 13.2:

    a. Trace the pathway of light starting from the yellow arrow until the point at which it reaches the fibres to the optic nerve.

    _____

    _____

    b. Where are the receptors for the sense of vision located?

    _____

    c. What are the two types of photoreceptors called?

    _____

    d. What quality of light does each photoreceptor respond to?

    _____

    _____

    e. How does the light stimulate the photoreceptor cells?

    _____

    _____

Part 2: Visual Acuity and Astigmatism

The ability of the eye to focus an image on the retina is assessed by use of the Snellen chart, which is composed of lines of letters arranged in decreasing size. The person to be tested is placed at a distance 6 metres away from the chart and is asked to cover one eye and read a line of letters. In Australia, the test is conducted in metres, based on the 6/6 principle, while in the United States the test is conducted in feet, based on the 20/20 principle.

Astigmatism is often diagnosed with an eye examination, but can be detected simply through the use of an astigmatism mirror chart, which assesses refractive error resulting in bending or disappearance of lines along various planes. This is caused by altered curvature of the cornea or the lens.

1. This activity is best conducted in pairs.

2. Obtain a human subject and a Snellen eye chart and follow the instructions for set-up and usage.

3. Follow the instructions for using the chart to test for visual acuity.

4. Note your observations based on the following scores:

    • 6/6 – indicates normal vision.

    • 6/12 – indicates less than normal vision.

    • 6/60 – indicates severely impaired vision (considered legally blind).

    a. Were any visual disturbances detected in the subject?

    _____

5. Obtain a subject and an astigmatism mirror chart and follow the instructions for set-up and usage.

6. Follow the instructions for using the chart to test for astigmatism.

7. Note your observations.

    a. Was astigmatism detected in the subject?

    _____

Apply the Concepts

1. What is presbyopia and how does it occur?

   _____

   _____

   _____

2. What is myopia and how does it occur?

   _____

   _____

   _____

3. What is hyperopia and how does it occur?

   _____

   _____

   _____

4. What is astigmatism and how does it occur?

   _____

   _____

   _____

ACTIVITY 13.4: STEREOSCOPIC (BINOCULAR) VISION

Humans have **stereoscopic vision**; that is, the visual fields of both eyes largely overlap and, due to the **optic chiasma**, are integrated in the visual cortex of the brain to give a three-dimensional image (Fig. 13.3). The position of the eyes within the head affects the **visual field**. Animals that hunt prey, such as cats, hawks and primates, have eyes at the front of their heads and experience stereoscopic vision to assist with locating objects and judging their distance, while animals that are hunted, such as rabbits, doves and mice, have eyes at the sides of their heads and experience panoramic vision to improve detection of potential threats.

This activity demonstrates the visual field in humans with an emphasis on stereoscopic vision.

1. This activity is best conducted in pairs.

2. Obtain a pencil and hold it upright at arm's length (or have a partner hold it).

3. With both eyes open, bring your hand smartly up from your side and touch the top of the pencil with your fingertip.

   a. Were you successful?

   _____

4. Repeat the process again, but this time with one eye closed or covered.

   a. How successful were you this time?

   _____

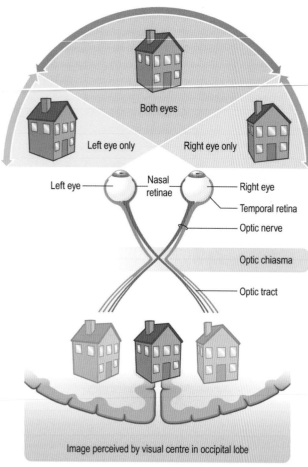

Figure 13.3 Visual fields.
(Source: Waugh, A., & Grant, A. (2018). Ross & Wilson anatomy and physiology in health and illness. Elsevier.)

5. Obtain a table-tennis ball and with both eyes open, have a partner throw the ball to you while trying to catch it. Repeat the process again with one eye closed or covered.

a. Does it make a difference?

_____

_____

b. What aspect of the visual sense is lost when only one eye is used?

_____

6. Consider the following questions with reference to Fig. 13.3:

a. How is sensory information from the eyes relayed to the brain and what effect can be expected if these pathways are compromised?

_____

_____

_____

b. How would vision be affected by pressure on the optic chiasma and why?

_____

_____

c. How would vision be affected by damage to the left optic tract?

_____

_____

d. How would vision be affected by damage to the visual cortex?

_____

_____

Apply the Concepts

1. What is glaucoma and how does it occur?

_____

_____

_____

2. What is strabismus and how does it occur?

_____

_____

_____

3. What is motion sickness and how does it occur?

_____

_____

_____

ACTIVITY 13.5: VISUAL RECEPTORS OF THE RETINA

The retina is the layer of the eye associated with vision and is composed of visual receptors, or photoreceptors, that respond to colour (cones) and monochromatic or dim light (rods). These photoreceptors are distributed in a specific pattern across the retina. The cones are concentrated towards the centre of the retina in the region called the **macula lutea**, and are most densely packed at the centre of the macular lutea in the **fovea centralis**, while the rods are distributed through the rest of the retina (Fig. 13.4a).

This activity demonstrates the arrangement and function of rods and cones across the retina based on the location of focus on the retina.

1. This activity is best conducted in pairs.

2. Obtain a penlight torch and a stopwatch.

3. Stare directly at the torch for 10 seconds and then close your eyes.

   a. What can you see?

   _____

   _____

b. Suggest an explanation for this visual afterimage.

   _____

   _____

4. Obtain a piece of brightly coloured card (red, green or blue is best).

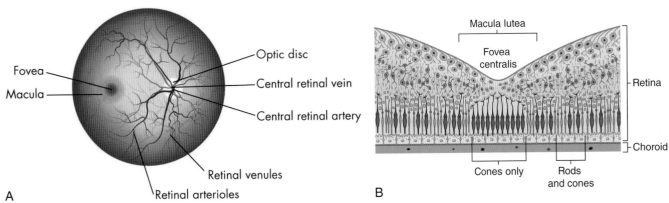

A

B

Figure 13.4 The retina. **A** Macroscopic structure of the retina. **B** Microscopic structure of the retina showing distribution of rods and cones.
(_Source:_ **A** _Craft, J., Gordon, C., Huether, S. E., McCance, K. L., Brashers, V. L., & List, S. (2019). Understanding pathophysiology Australia and New Zealand edition. Elsevier._ **B** _Waugh, A., & Grant, A. (2018). Ross & Wilson anatomy and physiology in health and illness. Elsevier._)

5. Hold the card at arm's length and look directly at the card without diverting your gaze for 30 seconds.

   a. How does the colour appear?

   _____

   b. On what part of the retina is the image of the card focused?

   _____

   _____

   c. What is this region called and what is found there?

   _____

   _____

6. Without diverting your gaze, and still holding the card at arm's length, move the card around to the periphery of the visual field where you can still see it.

   a. How does the colour appear?

   _____

   b. On what part of the retina is the image focused now?

   _____

   c. What type of receptors predominate in this part of the retina?

   _____

7. Obtain brightly coloured red and yellow cards, a white piece of paper and a stopwatch.

8. Stare intently at the red card for 30 seconds and then look at the white piece of paper.

   a. What is the colour of the afterimage?

   _____

9. Repeat the process with the yellow card.

   a. What is the colour of the afterimage?

   _____

   b. How can the colours of the afterimages be explained?

   _____

   _____

   c. What is the relationship between each colour and its afterimage?

   _____

   _____

   _____

Apply the Concepts

1. Relate the arrangement of cones in the retina to the visual disturbances experienced in macular degeneration.

   _____

   _____

   _____

2. What is retinopathy and how does it affect vision?

   _____

   _____

   _____

ACTIVITY 13.6: TESTING FOR COLOUR BLINDNESS

Colour vision occurs due to stimulation of the cones (photoreceptors) in the retina of the eye; however, occasionally deficiencies in their function may occur, resulting in **colour blindness**. Doctor Shinobu Ishihara developed a test for detecting red–green colour blindness in 1917. The Ishihara test consists of a series of 38 plates which contain a number or pattern among dots of randomised size and colour. Generally, four plates are enough to determine colour blindness. The plates are designed to test for deficiencies in the cones and this remains the most well-known test for colour blindness.

This activity demonstrates the ability to discern red and green colours, highlighting the functionality of cones in the retina.

1. This activity is best conducted in pairs.

2. Examine the Ishihara plates in Figs 13.5A–D below.

3. Have one person view each plate in bright light or sunlight while holding the plates about 0.5 metres away and at a right angle to the line of vision.

4. Take no longer than 3 seconds to view each plate, recording your observations below.

   a. What do you see in plate number 2?

   _____

   b. What is an individual with red-green colour blindness likely to see?

   _____

   c. What do you see in plate number 9?

   _____

   d. What is an individual with red-green colour blindness likely to see?

   _____

   e. What do you see in plate number 12?

   _____

   f. What is an individual with red-green colour blindness likely to see?

   _____

   g. What do you see in plate number 23?

   _____

   h. What is a red-blind individual likely to see?

   _____

   i. What is a green-blind individual likely to see?

   _____

5. Have the other person in your pair repeat the procedure.

   a. Is there any indication that you have some degree of colour blindness? If so, what type?

   _____

   _____

   b. How does red-green colour blindness occur?

   _____

   _____

   c. Which individuals are more likely to have red-green colour blindness and why?

   _____

   _____

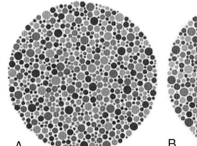 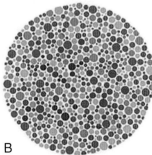 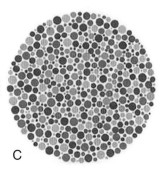 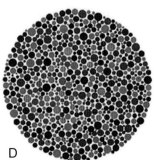

Figure 13.5 **A** Ishihara plate number 2. **B** Ishihara plate number 9. **C** Ishihara plate number 12. **D** Ishihara plate number 23. (*Source: https://www.color-blindness.com*)

d. Cones have one of three different visual pigments. What colour wavelengths do these respond to?

_____

_____

e. Explain how we are able to see a wide array of colours if cones have only one of three different visual pigments.

_____

_____

Apply the Concepts

1. Based on the structure of the retina, how can staring at the sun cause blindness?

_____

_____

_____

2. Based on the functions of the rods and cones, explain how light adaptation and dark adaptation occur.

_____

_____

_____

ACTIVITY 13.7: THE BLIND SPOT

The optic nerve leaves the retina at a region called the **optic disc** (Fig. 13.4A). The optic disc contains no light-detecting photoreceptor cells, hence the corresponding portion of the field of vision is invisible. The point at which this occurs is called the **blind spot** (scotoma).

This activity demonstrates the presence of the blind spot in the field of vision.

1. This activity is best conducted individually.

2. Close or cover your left eye and hold the page at arm's length.

3. With your right eye, look directly at the cross below (you should be able to see the dot as well).

+   •

4. Slowly move the page towards you, continuing to focus on the cross.

5. Continue to do this until you reach a point at which the dot disappears.

a. Why did the dot disappear?

_____

_____

b. Why are we not aware of the blind spot as creating a gap in our visual field?

_____

_____

6. Rule a line right across the page through the cross and the spot with a ruler.

7. Repeat the exercise above.

a. When the spot disappears are you aware of a break in the line?

_____

b. Why not?

_____

ACTIVITY 13.8: STRUCTURES OF THE EAR

The **ears** are the special sense organs of hearing. They are paired organs that contain a number of structures which help to direct sound-waves towards specialised hearing receptors deep within the ear. The ears consist of three regions: the **outer ear** funnels external sound-waves into the ear by way of the **auricle (pinna)**. Sound-waves entering the outer ear strike the **tympanic membrane**, causing it to vibrate. These vibrations are conducted towards the **oval window** in the **middle ear** via three small bones called the **auditory ossicles**. These vibrations are then conducted into the **inner ear**, where they are detected by specialised receptor cells for hearing contained within the **cochlea**.

This activity examines the structures of the ear and associates each structure with its function.

1. Identify the structures of the ear shown in Fig. 13.6, by inserting the letters next to each of the terms listed:

   a. Auricle (pinna): _____

   b. Auditory canal: _____

   c. Cochlea: _____

   d. Cochlear nerve: _____

   e. Eustachian tube: _____

   f. External ear: _____

   g. Incus: _____

   h. Inner ear: _____

   i. Malleus: _____

   j. Middle ear: _____

   k. Semicircular canals: _____

   l. Stapes: _____

   m. Tympanic membrane: _____

   n. Vestibular nerve: _____

   o. Vestibule: _____

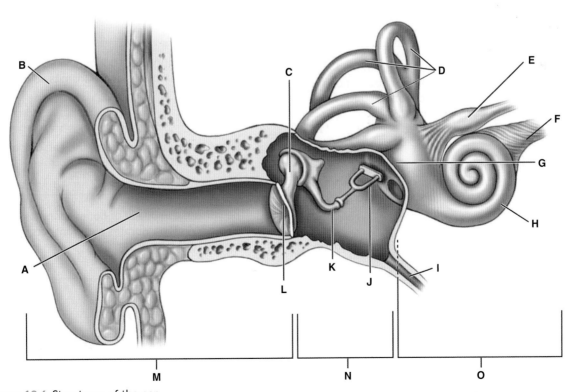

Figure 13.6 Structures of the ear.
(*Source: Herlihy, B. (2018). The human body in health and illness. Elsevier.*)

2. Consider the following questions with reference to Fig. 13.6:

a. What are the receptor cells for the sense of hearing called?

_____

b. Where are they located?

_____

c. Outline the mechanism by which the receptor cells for hearing are stimulated by sound-waves.

_____

_____

_____

3. Match the structures of the ear with the functions listed.

1. Auditory canal
2. Cochlea
3. Eustachian tube
4. Incus
5. Inner ear
6. Malleus
7. Middle ear
8. Outer ear
9. Round window
10. Semicircular canals
11. Stapes
12. Tympanic membrane

a. One of the three main regions of the ear; includes the cochlea, organ of Corti and semicircular canals.

_____

b. Three hollow canals in the inner ear positioned at anterior, posterior and lateral planes that respond to angular movements of the head; contain thick fluid (endolymph) and cilia for balance detection.

_____

c. One of the three main regions of the ear; a chamber containing three small bones (hammer, anvil, stirrup) that convey vibrations from the eardrum to the inner ear.

_____

d. An air passage between the middle ear and throat that equalises air pressure on either side of the eardrum.

_____

e. Part of the outer ear that channels sound-waves from the pinna or outer body surface to the eardrum.

_____

f. Opening surrounded by the secondary tympanic membrane; vibrates in opposition to vibrations entering cochlea through the oval window; allows fluid in the cochlea to move and convey sound-waves.

_____

g. A coiled tube in the inner ear that contains the hearing organ, the organ of Corti; contains fluid (endolymph) which conveys sound-waves to the auditory nerve.

_____

h. A sheet of connective tissue separating the outer ear from the middle ear, which vibrates when stimulated by sound-waves and transmits the waves to the middle ear.

_____

i. The hammer; composed of bone; connects the tympanic membrane to the incus; vibrates and transmits sound-waves to the incus.

_____

j. The anvil; composed of bone; connects the malleus to the stapes; vibrates and transmits sound-waves to the stapes.

_____

k. One of three main regions of the ear; made up of the auditory canal and the pinna.

_____

l. The stirrup; composed of bone; connects the incus to the oval window; vibrates and transmits sound-waves through to the inner ear.

_____

Apply the Concepts

1. What is otitis media and how does it occur?

_____

_____

_____

2. What is labyrinthitis and how does it occur?

_____

_____

_____

3. Explain how ear infections are caused.

_____

_____

_____

Additional Activities

For additional activities visit Activity 13B: Microscopic Examination of the Ear on Evolve.

ACTIVITY 13.9: PHYSIOLOGY OF HEARING

Vibrations conducted towards the inner ear are conveyed into the cochlea via movement of the **endolymph**, located in the membranous labyrinth of the cochlea. Movement of the endolymph causes the **hair cells (stereocilia)** embedded in the **organ of Corti** within the cochlea to deflect. This deflection of the stereocilia, based on the frequency of the incoming sound-waves, generates nerve impulses which travel towards and along the **cochlear nerve**, a process referred to as **sound transduction**. These nerve impulses are eventually interpreted as sound in the auditory cortex of the brain.

This activity considers the structures, processes and pathways involved in hearing.

1. Consider the following questions with reference to Fig. 13.7:

   a. Trace the pathway of sound from the point at which it enters the outer ear until the point at which it reaches the fibres to the auditory nerve.

   _____

   _____

   _____

   b. What is the function of the oval window?

   _____

   _____

   c. What is the function of the round window?

   _____

   _____

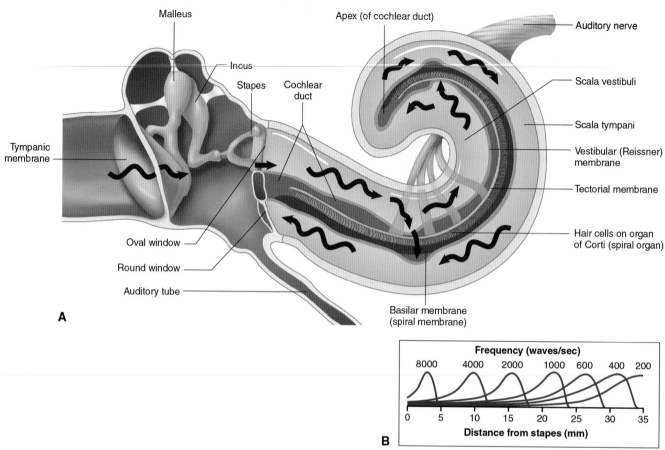

Figure 13.7 Structure of the cochlea. **A** The pathway of sound through the cochlea. **B** The degree of hair cell stimulation based on sound frequency.
(Source: Thibodeau, G. A., & T Patton, K. (2012). Anthony's textbook of anatomy and physiology. Mosby, Elsevier.)

d. What is the organ of hearing called and where is it located?

_____

_____

e. Compare the locations of the perilymph and endolymph in the inner ear.

_____

_____

f. Explain, with reference to Fig. 13.7B, how sounds of different frequencies stimulate the hair cells.

_____

_____

_____

Apply the Concepts

1. What is tinnitus and how does it occur?

_____

_____

_____

2. What is otosclerosis and how does it occur?

_____

_____

_____

ACTIVITY 13.10: LOCALISATION OF SOUND

The intensity and timing of sound-waves reaching the ears assist the brain in determining the direction of the sound. The direction of sounds reaching the ears at the same time can be difficult to determine as the intensity and timing of the sound is identical for both ears; however, when one ear receives the sound earlier and more vigorously due to proximity, the direction of the sound is easier to determine.

This activity demonstrates the ability to determine the direction of sound based on proximity to the ears.

1. This activity is best conducted in pairs.

2. Obtain a blindfold, a ticking clock and cotton wool.

3. The subject should have their eyes closed or blindfolded.

4. Hold the ticking clock about 1 metre from the subject's left ear and ask them to point to the source of sound.

5. Repeat the process holding the clock about 1 metre from the subject's right ear and ask them to point to the source of the sound.

6. Try this several times with the sound source in different positions.

   a. How well is the subject able to identify the direction of the sound?

   _____

   b. Are there any positions in which this is more difficult than others?

   _____

   _____

7. Block the external meatus of one ear with a piece of cotton wool and repeat the exercise above.

   a. How good is the subject at recognising the direction of the sound now?

   _____

   b. Explain how receiving sound-waves through two ears enables the direction of the sound source to be located.

   _____

   _____

Additional Activities

For additional activities visit Activity 13C: Sound Conduction via Bone and Air on Evolve.

For additional activities visit Activity 13D: Balance and Equilibrium on Evolve.

ACTIVITY 13.11: PHYSICAL EXAMINATION OF THE TASTEBUDS

The **tastebuds** are the sensory receptors for taste and are mostly distributed across the tongue, while some are scattered throughout the mouth. They are chemoreceptors, detecting chemicals in solution, a process often facilitated through the actions of saliva. The tastebuds are housed within **papillae**, small peg-like projections of the tongue mucosa which create a slightly abrasive surface. There are four types of papillae, with three of these housing tastebuds. Filiform papillae are distributed across the tongue and do not house tastebuds, but sense the texture of food; foliate papillae form ridges on the sides at the back of the tongue and contain tastebuds that reduce with age; fungiform papillae appear slightly mushroom-shaped and respond to taste and texture; and vallate papillae are arranged in a V-shape at the back of the tongue and have tastebuds around their bases.

This activity provides a physical examination of the tastebuds to determine their location and structure.

1. This activity is best conducted in groups of three.

2. Obtain a tongue depressor, penlight torch, magnifying glass and disposable gloves.

3. Don a pair of disposable gloves.

4. Place the tip of the tongue depressor gently but firmly on the tip of the subject's tongue to prevent the tongue from moving.

5. The penlight torch may be used to illuminate the oral structures.

6. With the magnifying glass, carefully examine the surface of the tongue and, using Fig. 13.10A as a guide, take note of the location and structure of the filiform, foliate, fungiform and vallate papillae.

7. Note also the location of the lingual tonsils. The palatine tonsils may also be present if they have not been surgically removed (tonsillectomy).

8. Consider the following questions:

   a. Where are the vallate papillae located, and approximately how many are visible?

   _____

   _____

   b. How does the number of foliate papillae and their colour relate to their function?

   _____

   _____

   _____

   c. How does the number of filiform papillae compare to that of the fungiform papillae, and how does this relate to their function?

   _____

   _____

   _____

   d. How does the size of the fungiform papillae compare to that of the filiform papillae, and how does the term 'fungiform' relate to the shape of these papillae?

   _____

   _____

   _____

ACTIVITY 13.12: DISTRIBUTION OF PRIMARY TASTE RECEPTORS

The olfactory and gustatory receptors are considered chemical receptors (chemoreceptors) as both respond to the presence of certain types of chemicals, which must be in solution to be tasted (one of the functions of saliva is to dissolve substances so that they can be tasted) or in a gaseous state to be smelled. The olfactory receptors are located in the **olfactory epithelium** in the roof of the nasal cavity, while the gustatory receptors are found in the tastebuds (papillae) distributed over the surface of the tongue and parts of the lining of the oral cavity (Fig. 13.8).

This activity demonstrates the distribution of primary taste receptors over the surface of the tongue.

⚠ To conduct this activity, it is important to ensure the following safety precautions:

- *Notify the instructor of any food allergies before commencing the activity.*

1. This activity is best conducted in pairs.

2. Obtain four taste solutions (sweet, salty, sour, bitter), disposable pipettes, cotton swabs, potable water, disposable cups and disposable gloves.

3. The four solutions represent the four primary taste modalities.

4. Taste a few drops of each solution and record your results in the table provided.

5. Rinse the mouth between solutions with the potable water and cup, and after the final solution is tasted.

Taste	Solution number
Sweet	
Salty	
Sour	
Bitter	

6. Using cotton swabs, brush each of the four solutions in turn on the tip, sides and back of your partner's tongue.

7. Rinse the mouth between solutions with the potable water and cup, and use a fresh cotton swab with each application.

8. Discard used cotton swabs immediately after use, as indicated by your demonstrator.

9. On Fig. 13.8A, map where the sensory receptors for each taste are located.

   a. Is there any overlap in taste regions?

   _____

   _____

   b. What area of the tongue seems to lack taste receptors?

   _____

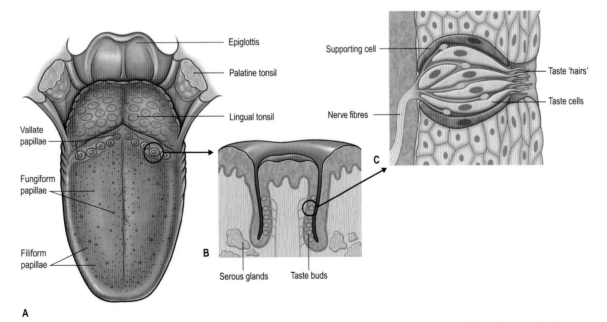

Figure 13.8 The tongue and tastebuds. **A** Surface of the tongue with papillae. **B** Section of a papilla with tastebuds located in its walls; **C** Structure of a taste bud (enlarged).
(*Source: Waugh, A., & Grant, A. (2018). Ross & Wilson anatomy and physiology in health and illness. Elsevier.*)

10. Compare your taste map to that of other students.

    a. Is it possible to definitely assign types of tastebud to a specific location?

_____

_____

11. Consider the following questions with reference to Fig. 13.8B and 13.8C:

    a. What are the receptors for the sense of taste called and what are they structurally?

_____

_____

    b. How do these receptor cells detect taste?

_____

_____

_____

12. Suggest an explanation for how tastebuds are chemically able to detect:

    a. Sour taste _____

_____

_____

    b. Salt taste _____

_____

_____

    c. Sweet taste _____

_____

_____

    d. Bitter taste _____

_____

_____

Apply the Concepts

1. What is ageusia and why is this more likely to occur during a severe cold?

_____

_____

_____

2. What is hypogeusia and why is this more likely to occur in older adults?

_____

_____

_____

Additional Activities

For additional activities visit Activity 13E: Microscopic Examination of the Taste Buds on Evolve.

ACTIVITY 13.13: OLFACTION AND TASTE PERCEPTION

The organ of smell is located in the roof of the nasal cavity and is referred to as the olfactory epithelium (Fig. 13.9). As air enters the nasal cavity, it circulates around the nasal conchae and comes into contact with the olfactory receptors. Much of the taste, and hence flavour, of food and drink comes from the contribution of the olfactory sense. If this is removed (e.g. by a heavy cold), our ability to discriminate flavours is largely removed and only the gustatory sense remains.

This activity demonstrates the role of olfaction on taste perception by removing the sense of smell.

 To conduct this activity, it is important to ensure the following safety precautions:

- *Notify the instructor of any food or scent allergies before commencing the activity.*

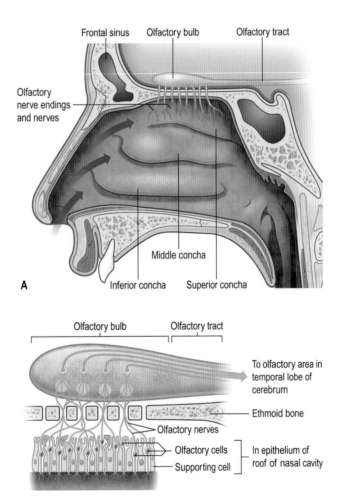

Figure 13.9 The sense of smell. **A** Structures of olfaction. **B** Microscopic structure of the olfactory epithelium (enlarged). *(Source: Waugh, A., & Grant, A. (2018). Ross & Wilson anatomy and physiology in health and illness. Elsevier.)*

1. This activity is best conducted in pairs.

2. Obtain four different fruit juices, safety glasses, aluminium foil, disposable pipettes, potable water, disposable cup, disposable gloves, nose clip and ice cubes.

3. Ask a subject to wear the safety glasses covered with aluminium foil (or have them close their eyes).

4. Don a pair of disposable gloves and check the subject's ability to distinguish the juices supplied.

5. Test by placing a few drops in the mouth from a disposable pipette using a new pipette with each juice to avoid contamination.

6. Rinse the mouth with potable water between samples.

7. Discard used pipettes immediately after use, as indicated by your demonstrator.

8. Record your results in the control column of the table provided.

9. Now ask the subject to apply a nose clip (or pinch their nostrils) and repeat the exercise this time changing the order of the juices tested.

10. Record your results in column 3 of the table provided.

11. Remove the nose clip and have the subject hold some ice on their tongue for 1 minute. Repeat the exercise again changing the order of the juices tested.

12. Record your results in column 4 of the table provided.

Juice tested	Subject's identification (control)	Subject's identification (nose clip)	Subject's identification (ice)

13. Consider the following questions:

    a. How has the subject's ability to identify flavours been altered by the nose clip?

    _____

    b. Can you suggest a reason for this outcome?

    _____

    _____

    c. Has the subject's ability to identify favours been altered by the temperature change? In what way?

    _____

    d. Can you suggest a reason for this outcome?

    _____

    _____

    _____

14. Consider the following questions with reference to Fig. 13.9:

    a. What are the receptors for the sense of smell called, and what can be found at their surface?

    _____

    _____

    b. How do these receptor cells detect smell?

    _____

    _____

Apply the Concepts

1. How does sniffing intensify the sense of smell?

_____

_____

_____

2. What is anosmia and how does it occur?

_____

_____

_____

Additional Activities

For additional activities visit Activity 13F: Microscopic Examination of the Olfactory Receptors on Evolve®.

Additional Resources

3D Virtual Imaging Core

3D virtual models of the visible ear, temporal bone, round window and incudostapedial joint anatomy in humans available for download and developed by Eaton-Peabody Laboratories.

www.masseyeandear.org/research/otolaryngology/eaton-peabody-laboratories/imaging-core

Atlas of Ophthalmology

The Atlas of Ophthalmology is a public multimedia database providing pictorial documentation of eye diseases, and is edited by specialists in the field.

www.atlasophthalmology.net/

Colblindor

Colblindor addresses issues associated with colour vision deficiency, and includes tests, tools, animations and simulations relating to colour blindness, which can be conducted online.

www.color-blindness.com/

Gizmos: Senses

An interactive simulation with lesson materials where users explore how stimuli are detected by specialised cells, transmitted through nerves and processed in the brain.

gizmos.explorelearning.com/index.cfm?method=cResource.dspDetail&resourceID=1069

Histology Guide Virtual Microscopy Laboratory: Organs of Special Sense

An online resource providing a virtual microscopy laboratory experience, by allowing users to view microscope slides from professional collections for the purpose of interpreting cellular and tissue structures, as seen through a microscope.

histologyguide.com/slidebox/20-organs-of-special-sense.html

Know Your Noise

Provides information about noise exposure and its impact on hearing health, allowing individuals to take hearing tests online provided by the National Acoustic Laboratories and funded by the Australian Government Department of Health.

knowyournoise.nal.gov.au/

Osmosis – Special Senses

The Special Senses module of Osmosis provides videos, notes, quiz questions and links to further resources related to the special senses.

www.osmosis.org/library/md/foundational-sciences/physiology#eyes,_ears,_nose_and_throat

Otoscopy Atlas

This site provides otoscopic images of common and rare lesions of the middle ear in children with rationale for treatment.

atlasotoskopii.pl/language/en/diseases/

Physclips: Eye and Colour Vision

Online tutorials and experiments addressing optics, eye anatomy, accommodation, complementary colours, after-images, retinal fatigue, colour mixing and eye performance. It is provided by the University of New South Wales.

www.animations.physics.unsw.edu.au/light/eye-colour-vision/

Retina Gallery

A resource for teaching and learning through exchange of interesting retina cases and the sharing of high-quality images of retinal diseases.

retinagallery.com/

CHAPTER 14
The Endocrine System

The nervous system and endocrine system act together to control and integrate the activity of all the body's cells. While the nervous system acts rapidly by using electrochemical signals, the endocrine system is mostly involved in long-term regulation of body functions such as metabolism, reproduction, growth and development, and water and solute balance. The autonomic nervous system and the endocrine system both work to maintain homeostasis and involuntary body functions. (Refer to Chapter 8: Body Orientation and Homeostasis, for further information on homeostasis and feedback mechanisms.)

Endocrine glands are ductless glands which secrete hormones directly into the blood. This distinguishes them from exocrine glands such as sweat glands, whose secretions are carried out of the body through ducts. (Refer to Chapter 9: The Integumentary System, for further information on exocrine glands.) All hormones circulate in the blood to all parts of the body, but have effects only on those cells (target cells) which are receptive to them. Hormones are constructed from either amino acids or steroid lipids and act by causing changes in the metabolic activity of the target cells. These can include changes in cell membrane permeability, stimulation of protein synthesis, activation or deactivation of enzymes, induction of secretory activity and stimulation of mitosis. (Refer to Chapter 18: The Lymphatic System, for further information on the structure and function of the thymus gland and Chapter 22: The Reproductive System and Heredity, for further information on the structure and function of the ovaries and testes.)

LEARNING OUTCOMES

On completion of these activities, the student should be able to:

1. list the endocrine glands and their major hormones
2. distinguish between true endocrine glands, secondary endocrine glands and mixed glands
3. explain the differences between, and give examples of, negative and positive feedback control of endocrine secretion
4. describe, with examples, the function of trophic hormones
5. explain why hormones are only effective in target organs
6. discuss the structure and functions of the pituitary gland and its hormones

LEARNING OUTCOMES—cont'd

7. describe the arrangement of the thyroid and parathyroid glands and the roles of their hormones

8. discuss the differences between the adrenal cortex and adrenal medulla and compare the functions and chemistry of their hormones

9. explain the complementary functions of insulin and glucagon and describe the pancreatic structures that secrete them.

KEY TERMS

Adrenal glands
Adrenal medulla
Adrenaline
Alpha cells
Anterior pituitary
Beta cells
Catecholamines
Control mechanism
Corticosteroids
Endocrine gland
Exocrine gland
Feedback mechanism

Follicular tissue
Glandular tissue
Glucagon
Hormone
Hormone receptor
Hypophyseal portal system
Hypothalamus
Insulin
Islets of Langerhans
Melatonin
Mixed gland
Noradrenaline

Pancreas
Parathyroid glands
Parathyroid hormone
Pineal gland
Pituitary gland
Posterior pituitary
Second messenger
Target cell
Target organ
Thyroid gland
Thyroid hormone

ACTIVITY 14.1: ENDOCRINE GLANDS AND THEIR HORMONES

The **endocrine glands** are ductless glands that secrete **hormones** into the bloodstream via the extracellular space (Fig. 14.1). They are transported throughout the body to act on specific **target organs** via interaction with the cell's **hormone receptors**. Thus, endocrine glands typically have a rich supply of blood and lymphatic capillaries. The body's **target cells** must also be close to blood capillaries. Some organs have a secondary endocrine function; that is, hormone production has a minor or secondary role in their activities.

This activity examines the major and secondary endocrine glands and identifies their hormones.

1. Identify each of the glands labelled in Fig. 14.1.

   a. Gland A: _____

   b. Gland B: _____

   c. Gland C: _____

   d. Gland D: _____

   e. Gland E: _____

   f. Gland F: _____

   g. Gland G: _____

   h. Gland H: _____

   i. Gland I: _____

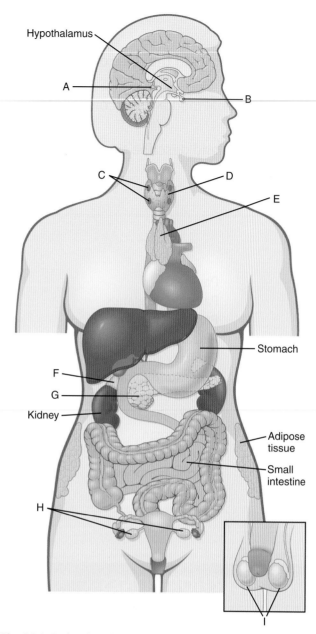

Fig. 14.1 Endocrine glands in the human.
(Source: Hall, M. E., & Hall, J. E. (2016). Guyton and Hall textbook of medical physiology. (14th ed.). Elsevier.)

2. Identify and explain the three stimuli which cause hormone release.

_____

_____

_____

3. The table below lists the organs of the endocrine system. Next to each organ, write the name(s) of the hormone(s) it secretes.

Endocrine organ	Hormone(s) secreted
Anterior pituitary gland	
Posterior pituitary gland	
Pineal gland	
Thyroid gland	
Parathyroid glands	
Thymus	
Pancreas	
Adrenal cortex	
Adrenal medulla	
Ovaries	
Testes	

4. Define the following terms:

a. Hormone _____

b. Target organ _____

c. Endocrine gland _____

d. Exocrine gland _____

e. Mixed gland _____

5. Identify three organs with a secondary endocrine function and the hormones they secrete.

_____

_____

_____

Apply the Concepts

1. Explain why nervous system signalling is much faster than endocrine system signalling.

   _____

   _____

2. Explain why autocrines and paracrines are not technically considered part of the endocrine system.

   _____

   _____

ACTIVITY 14.2: HORMONE FUNCTION

Hormones are highly specific in their action. They have effects only in target organs with receptors for that hormone and their secretion is regulated by **feedback mechanisms**. The ability or inability of a hormone to enter a cell determines the need for a **second messenger** system.

This activity examines hormone targets and their responses, as well as the mechanisms which regulate hormone secretion.

1. What is a hormone?

   _____

   _____

   _____

2. Distinguish between a target organ and a target cell.

   _____

   _____

   _____

3. In the table below, identify the source of each hormone, its target organ(s) and the physiological response(s) triggered by the hormone.

Hormone	Source gland	Target organ(s)	Response(s)
Adrenaline			
Parathyroid hormone (PTH)			
Luteinising hormone (LH)			
Adrenocorticotrophic hormone (ACTH)			
Antidiuretic hormone (ADH)			
Cortisol			

Continued

Hormone	Source gland	Target organ(s)	Response(s)
Glucagon			
Testosterone			
Thyroid stimulating hormone (TSH)			
Oestrogen			
Melatonin			
Thyroid hormone (TH)			
Growth hormone (GH)			

4. Consider the following questions:

   a. Give two locations where hormone receptors can be found in cells.

   _____

   _____

   b. What types of hormones bind to these receptors?

   _____

   c. Describe the mechanism by which amino acid-based hormones exert their effects on target cells.

   _____

   _____

   _____

   d. Explain why amino acid-based hormones operate in this manner.

   _____

   _____

   _____

   e. Describe the mechanism by which steroid-based hormones exert their effects on target cells.

   _____

   _____

   _____

   f. Explain why steroid-based hormones operate in this manner.

   _____

   _____

   _____

Apply the Concepts

1. Explain why not all tissues respond to hormones distributed by the bloodstream.

_____

_____

2. Explain how first messengers differ from second messengers.

_____

_____

3. Based on chemical structure, explain why adrenaline remains in the bloodstream longer than cortisol.

_____

_____

4. Explain how anabolic steroids can assist in building muscle tissue when skeletal muscle is largely composed of protein.

_____

_____

_____

ACTIVITY 14.3: FEEDBACK CONTROL OF HORMONE SECRETION

Homeostasis refers to the body's ability to maintain relatively constant internal conditions through the involvement of negative feedback mechanisms (Fig. 14.2). In all animals, homeostasis involves a dynamic range of responses that act to maintain physiological quantities not perfectly constant, but within relatively narrow limits or tolerances. Many of these responses are mediated by hormones.

Homeostatic **control mechanisms**, including those involving hormones, almost always involve negative feedback, where a stimulus (such as increased body temperature) triggers a response (such as sweating), which has the effect of reducing the intensity of the stimulus (by cooling the body down). A negative feedback mechanism always includes a variable (the quantity being regulated), a receptor or detector (a structure sensitive to the variable), a control centre capable of responding to the information from the receptor, and an effector which carries out the response (Fig. 14.3).

This activity explores examples of endocrine feedback mechanisms.

1. Normal arterial blood pressure is maintained by adjustment of peripheral resistance vessels, arteries which can be dilated to lower blood pressure or constricted to elevate it. When blood pressure rises, stretch receptors in the walls of the aorta and carotid sinus send signals to the vasomotor centre in the medulla, which causes smooth muscle in the walls of peripheral blood vessels to relax, resulting in lower blood pressure.

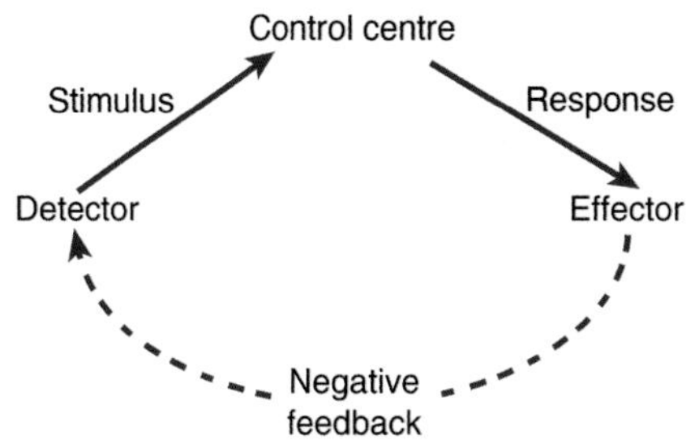

Fig. 14.2 A generalised negative feedback loop.
(Source: Watson, R. (2018). Anatomy and physiology for nurses. Elsevier.)

   a. Why is this type of feedback loop referred to as 'negative'?

   _____

   _____

   _____

   _____

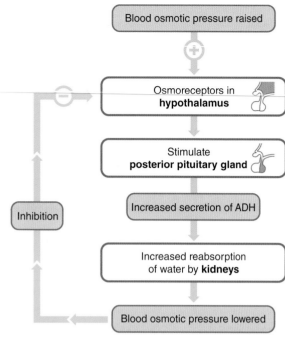

Fig. 14.3 Negative feedback regulation of the secretion of antidiuretic hormone (ADH).
(Source: Waugh, A., & Grant, A. (2018). Ross & Wilson anatomy and physiology in health and illness. Elsevier.)

2. As it relates to control of arterial blood pressure, in the negative feedback loop in Fig. 14.2, identify the:

   a. Variable _____

   b. Receptor _____

   c. Control centre _____

   d. Effector _____

   e. Negative feedback _____

3. Explain the negative feedback regulation of ADH secretion in Fig. 14.3.

   _____

   _____

   _____

   _____

4. In the response of the pituitary gland to dehydration shown in Fig. 14.3:

   a. What is the stimulus?

   _____

b. What is the response?

   _____

c. Where is the control centre?

   _____

d. Where is the sensory organ?

   _____

e. What is the effector?

   _____

5. An individual ingests a large volume of water and sometime later starts excreting increased volumes of dilute urine. Complete the following sentences by filling in the blanks.

   a. Ingestion of water caused the concentration of

      _____ in the blood to _____ (stimulus).

   b. This was detected by the _____, (receptor and control centre) which caused the _____ (endocrine gland) to _____ its production of _____.

   c. This caused the _____ (effector) to _____ its production of urine.

   d. As a result, the concentration of the solutes in the blood _____ and the intensity of the stimulus _____.

   e. This is an example of _____ feedback.

6. Oxytocin secretion in childbirth is a rare example of a positive feedback mechanism in the body.

   a. Which organ secretes oxytocin?

      _____

   b. What is the stimulus for its secretion?

      _____

   c. What is the uterine response to oxytocin?

      _____

   d. Which receptor organ detects this response?

      _____

e. How does the receptor react to this information?

_____

_____

f. Why is positive feedback required in this situation?

_____

_____

7. What are trophic hormones?

_____

_____

_____

8. In the table provided, give the full name of each trophic hormone shown and indicate the gland from which it is secreted, the target gland, and the hormones regulated by the trophic hormone.

Trophic hormone	Full name	Source gland	Target gland	Hormone(s) regulated
TSH				
ACTH				
LH				

Apply the Concepts

1. Explain what is meant by up-regulation and down-regulation.

_____

_____

_____

ACTIVITY 14.4: THE PITUITARY GLAND

The **pituitary gland**, or hypophysis, is connected to the hypothalamus and is divided structurally and functionally into an anterior lobe and a posterior lobe (Fig. 14.4). The **anterior pituitary**, or adenohypophysis (also known as the pars anterior), is derived from an upgrowth of embryonic pharyngeal tissue known as Rathke's pouch. The **posterior pituitary** or neurohypophysis (also known as the pars posterior and pars nervosa) is a down growth of nervous tissue from the hypothalamus, to which it remains joined via a connecting stalk called the hypothalamic hypophyseal tract.

This activity investigates the structure and the many functions of the pituitary gland.

1. Examine Fig. 14.4 and identify the structures labelled from the terms provided.

Anterior pituitary gland
Collecting vein
Endocrine cells
Hypophyseal portal system
Inferior hypophyseal artery
Infundibulum

Neurons of the ventral hypothalamus
Posterior pituitary gland
Primary capillary plexus
Secondary capillary plexus
Superior hypophyseal artery
Supraoptic and paraventricular nuclei

a. Structure 1: _____

b. Structure 2: _____

c. Structure 3: _____

d. Structure 4: _____

e. Structure 5: _____

f. Structure 6: _____

g. Structure 7: _____

h. Structure 8: _____

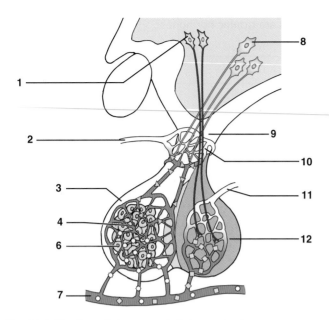

Fig. 14.4 The hypothalamus and pituitary gland.
(Source: Cottrell, J. E., & Patel, P. (2017). Cottrell and Patel's neuroanesthesia. Elsevier.)

   i. Structure 9: _____

   j. Structure 10: _____

   k. Structure 11: _____

   l. Structure 12: _____

2. Consider the following questions:

   a. Identify the two hormones secreted from the posterior pituitary gland.

   _____

   b. Describe the chemical nature of these hormones.

   _____

   c. Which hormone is under negative feedback control?

   _____

   d. Strictly speaking, the posterior pituitary is not an endocrine gland. Explain why.

   _____

   _____

   e. Identify the six hormones of the anterior pituitary gland.

   _____

   _____

   _____

   f. The anterior pituitary has sometimes been called the 'master gland' of the endocrine system. Explain why.

   _____

   _____

   _____

   g. The hypothalamus controls the secretions of both the anterior and posterior pituitary glands but in different ways. How and why are they different?

   _____

   _____

   _____

Apply the Concepts

1. What is acromegaly and how does it occur?

_____

_____

2. What is pituitary dwarfism and how does it occur?

_____

_____

3. What is a hypophysectomy and why is it performed?

_____

_____

4. What is diabetes insipidus and how does it occur?

_____

_____

5. What is syndrome of inappropriate ADH (SIADH) secretion and how does it occur?

_____

_____

6. What is hyperprolactinaemia and how does it occur?

_____

_____

ACTIVITY 14.5: MICROSCOPIC EXAMINATION OF THE PITUITARY GLAND

The anterior pituitary lobe contains many glandular epithelial cells and forms the glandular portion of the pituitary. A system of blood vessels, known as the **hypophyseal portal system**, connects the anterior lobe with the **hypothalamus**. Hormones from the hypothalamus travel through the hypophyseal portal system to the anterior pituitary where they stimulate or inhibit the secretion of hormones manufactured there. Hormones in the posterior pituitary are synthesised in one of two hypothalamic nuclei: the paraventricular nucleus and the supraoptic nucleus. They then move down nerve axons to the posterior pituitary, where they are secreted into blood capillaries.

This activity examines the microscopic structure of the pituitary gland.

1. Obtain a prepared slide of a pituitary gland LS (H&E) and examine it under low power to observe its general structure.

2. Distinguish the glandular _anterior pituitary_ from the _posterior pituitary_. The visible granules have been stained with eosin and methylene blue. Refer to Fig. 14.5 to assist with identification of the structures seen.

3. Change to high power and focus on the _anterior pituitary_.

   a. Attempt to identify the following cell types:

   • _Chromophobes_
   These cell have no distinct dye affinity in the cytoplasm. They appear in clusters in the central regions of groups of cells between sinusoids (blood capillaries) and are smaller than chromophils. Chromophobes are considered to be resting or reserve cells which will become chromophils and develop granules in their cytoplasm.

   • _Chromophils_ are subdivided into two sub-groups:
     ○ _Acidophils_
     These are larger than chromophobes and their cytoplasm is packed with small granules that stain with acidic dyes. Acidophils are responsible for the secretion of human growth hormone and prolactin.

   ○ _Basophils_
   These cells are larger than acidophils but with smaller and fewer granules than acidophils. Groups of basophils secrete ACTH, TSH, FSH and LH.

   b. How do cells in the hypothalamus control the secretions of the cells of the anterior pituitary?

   _____

   _____

4. Examine the posterior pituitary under high power.

5. Observe the nerve fibres (axons) that comprise most of this portion of the pituitary.

6. Also observe the pituicytes, glial cells that are randomly distributed among the nerve fibres.

   a. Where are the hormones of the posterior pituitary produced and how do they get to the posterior pituitary?

   _____

   _____

   _____

Chromophobe Acidophil   Basophil

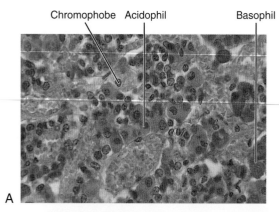

A

Nerve
fibres

Pituicytes

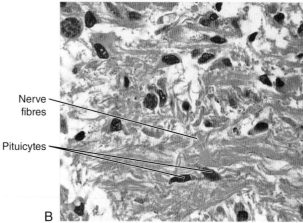

B

Fig. 14.5 **A** Cells of the anterior pituitary. **B** Cells of the
posterior pituitary.
*(Source: **A** Patton, K. T., Bell, F. B., Matusiak, D. J., & Wood, S. R. (2021).
Anatomy and physiology laboratory manual. Elsevier. **B** Lowe, J. S., &
Stevens, A. P. (2020). Stevens and Lowe's human histology. Elsevier.)*

b. How do the cells of the hypothalamus control the
secretion of the cells of the posterior pituitary?

_____

_____

7. Use the space below for a low-power diagram of the
pituitary gland. Label the posterior and anterior lobes
and any other structures that can be identified.

Magnification of diagram: × _____

Apply the Concepts

1. A 6-year-old boy is brought to a clinic complaining of headaches and joint pains. It is observed that he is very tall
for his age and he is sent for a CT scan which reveals a large non-malignant pituitary tumour.

a. Which hormone is being secreted in excessive amounts? _____

b. What condition will result if no treatment is undertaken? _____

c. What further symptoms could develop without treatment?

_____

_____

2. What is Cushing's disease and how does it occur?

_____

_____

   a. Explain how Cushing's disease is treated with surgery.

   _____

   _____

   b. Why might this treatment be considered necessary?

   _____

   _____

ACTIVITY 14.6: THE PINEAL GLAND

The **pineal gland** is a small gland found in the brain of most vertebrate animals. The French philosopher René Descartes believed it to be 'the seat of the soul', but most of his contemporaries disagreed. They thought it was just a tiny neuroanatomical structure without metaphysical qualities and whose function was yet to be discovered. Today the function of the pineal gland is still not completely understood, but it is known to secrete at least one hormone, **melatonin**.

This activity examines the structure and function of the pineal gland.

1. In what region of the brain is the pineal gland located?

_____

2. What name is given to the secretory cells of the pineal gland?

_____

3. Which hormone is secreted by the pineal gland?

_____

   a. Chemically, what type of hormone is this?

   _____

4. This hormone is thought to control circadian rhythms. Explain what this means.

_____

_____

_____

5. In humans the pineal gland cannot directly sense light intensity. How does it receive this information?

_____

_____

6. The suprachiasmatic nucleus in the hypothalamus is richly supplied with receptors for this hormone.

   a. What does this indicate about the function of the nucleus?

   _____

   _____

   _____

7. Consider the following questions regarding the hormone produced by the pineal gland:

   a. When do peak levels of secretion occur?

   _____

   b. When do reduced levels of secretion occur?

   _____

   c. List two other roles that this hormone is thought to play in the human body.

   _____

   _____

Apply the Concepts

1. Synthetic melatonin supplements are now available from pharmacists without prescription.

   a. What conditions might these supplements be used for?

   _____

   b. Explain how these supplements may assist in the regulation of mood and circadian rhythm.

   _____

   _____

ACTIVITY 14.7: THE THYROID AND PARATHYROID GLANDS

The **thyroid gland** is located on the trachea, just below the larynx. It is comprised of two lateral lobes connected by an isthmus of thyroid tissue and secretes **thyroid hormone** (Fig. 14.6). There are usually four **parathyroid glands** located on the posterior aspect of the thyroid gland, but which are occasionally distributed throughout the thorax. These secrete **parathyroid hormone**.

This activity examines the structure and function of the thyroid and parathyroid glands.

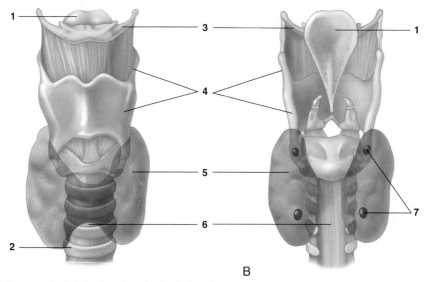

A   B

Fig. 14.6 Structures of the throat. **A** Anterior view. **B** Posterior view.
(Source: Patton, K. T., Thibodeau, G. A., & Douglas, M. M. (2012). Essentials of anatomy and physiology. Elsevier.)

1. Based on Fig. 14.6, showing anterior and posterior views of some structures in the throat, identify the structures labelled from the terms provided.

   Epiglottis   Thyroid gland
   Hyoid bone   Trachea
   Parathyroid glands   Tracheal cartilage
   Thyroid cartilage

   a. Structure 1: _____

   b. Structure 2: _____

   c. Structure 3: _____

   d. Structure 4: _____

   e. Structure 5: _____

   f. Structure 6: _____

   g. Structure 7: _____

2. Consider the following questions:

   a. Thyroid hormone consists of two amine hormones, T3 and T4. What are their full names?

   _____

   _____

   b. To what do the numbers 3 and 4 refer?

   _____

3. In the table below, list the effects of hyposecretion and hypersecretion of thyroid hormone on the body's functions and structures shown.

Function or structure	Effects of hyposecretion	Effects of hypersecretion
Metabolic rate		
Cardiovascular system		
Gastrointestinal system		
Skin		
Skeletal system		
Eyes		
Muscular system		

4. Complete the following sentences by filling in the blanks:

   a. The third hormone secreted by the thyroid gland is

   _____.

   b. It is secreted in response to a rise in blood _____ levels and has its effect by targeting the skeleton, where it inhibits the activity of _____ cells which break down _____ tissue.

   c. The parathyroid gland secretes _____, which is the most important hormone regulating blood _____ levels.

   d. Its release is triggered by _____ levels of _____ ions in the blood and its target organs include the _____, _____ and small intestine.

   e. This hormone is antagonistic to the hormone _____.

Apply the Concepts

1. What is myxoedema and how does it occur?

   _____

   _____

2. What is Graves' disease and how does it occur?

   _____

   _____

3. Explain why hypoparathyroidism can lead to tetany.

   _____

   _____

   _____

4. Explain why hyperparathyroidism leads to hypercalcaemia.

_____

_____

5. Explain what is meant by a thyroid storm.

_____

_____

ACTIVITY 14.8: MICROSCOPIC EXAMINATION OF THE THYROID AND PARATHYROID GLANDS

The thyroid gland is located on the anterior surface of the trachea, and the parathyroid glands are located on the posterior aspect of the thyroid gland. These glands share a unique relationship, particularly in the regulation of blood calcium. The thyroid gland is rich in **follicular tissue** associated with the secretion of colloids that form the basis of the thyroid hormones, whereas follicular tissue is absent in the parathyroid glands, which contain **glandular tissue** (Fig. 14.7).

This activity examines the microscopic structure of the thyroid and parathyroid glands.

1. Examine the prepared slides of thyroid and parathyroid tissues LS (H&E) under low power. Refer to Fig. 14.7 to assist with identification of the structures examined.

2. Note the arrangement of the *glandular epithelium* and the presence of pink-stained *thyroid colloid* in the sac-like *thyroid follicles.*

3. Stored T3 and T4 hormones are attached to the colloidal protein in the follicles and are released gradually into the blood. Active *follicles* tend to be small with less colloid present. Their cuboidal *follicular cells*, which form the walls of each follicle and secrete the colloid are relatively tall, reflecting active hormone secretion and synthesis. Less active follicles are distended by stored *colloid* and their follicular cells appear flattened.

4. Look for *parafollicular cells*, which are found in the spaces between the *follicles*. These cells are larger than typical follicular cells and have a clear cytoplasm. Parafollicular cells secrete calcitonin, which lowers the levels of circulating calcium.

   a. Calcitonin has an antagonistic hormone, which raises the levels of circulating calcium. What is it and where is it secreted?

   _____

   _____

5. Use the space below for a high-power diagram of two or three thyroid follicles.

Magnification of diagram: × _____

6. Examine a slide of parathyroid tissue under low and high power and compare it to Fig. 14.7B. Note the absence of follicles and the presence of densely packed glandular cells. Chief cells, often found in rows, are thought to be the main producers of parathyroid hormone. The function of the larger oxyphil cells is not known.

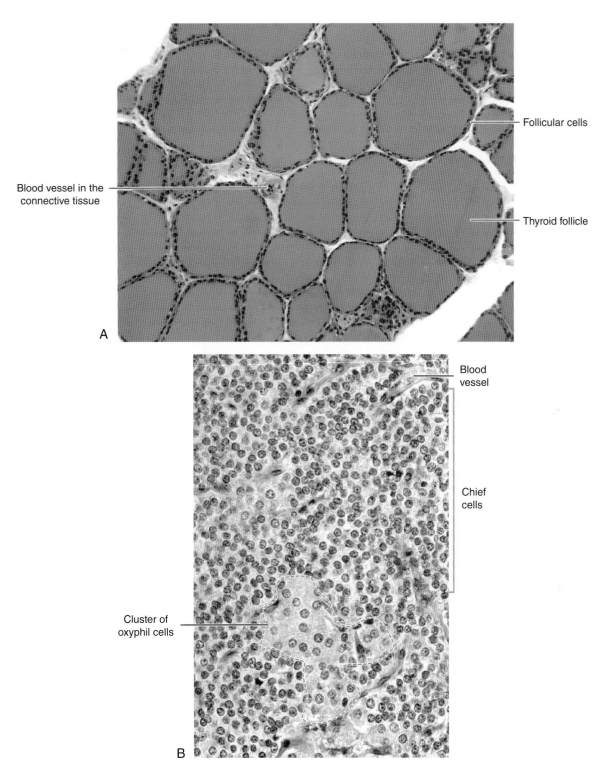

Fig. 14.7. A Thyroid and **B** parathyroid tissues.
(Source: Kierszenbaum, A. L., & Tres, L. L. (2016). Histology and cell biology: An introduction to pathology, 5th ed. Elsevier.

Apply the Concepts

1. A young woman presents at a clinic with constant fatigue, weight gain, dry skin and hair, facial puffiness and intolerance to cold. These symptoms have been developing for some years. After tests are performed, she is prescribed a drug called levothyroxine and the symptoms slowly decline in severity.

   a. What condition was she suffering from? _____

   b. Could this condition have been prevented (i.e. was it a lifestyle problem)? Explain.

   _____

   _____

   c. Can she expect to discontinue use of the drug when she has recovered? Explain.

   _____

   _____

2. What is a goitre and how does it occur?

   _____

   _____

   a. Historically, goitre was much more common in inland regions than in coastal areas. Suggest a reason for this.

   _____

   _____

   b. How can goitre now be easily prevented?

   _____

ACTIVITY 14.9: ADRENAL GLANDS AND THEIR HORMONES

The **adrenal glands** are situated at the superior poles of each kidney and a connective tissue capsule surrounds each gland. The glandular tissue is organised into an outer cortex and an inner medulla. The **adrenal cortex** and the **adrenal medulla** are distinctly different glands that are controlled by different mechanisms, even though one gland encases the other. The hormones produced by each adrenal gland, **catecholamines** and **corticosteroids**, are also chemically different.

This activity examines the functions of the adrenal gland and its hormones.

1. The adrenal cortex and medulla are both involved in the response to what type of situation?

   _____

2. Consider the following questions:

   a. Which two hormones are produced by the adrenal medulla?

   _____

b. What type of chemical compound are these hormones?

   _____

c. Which of these is also a neurotransmitter in the autonomic nervous system?

   _____

d. Which organ controls the secretion of these hormones and how is control effected?

_____

_____

e. How are the hormones of the adrenal cortex chemically different from those of the medulla?

_____

_____

f. Which two organs are involved in controlling secretion from the adrenal cortex?

_____

3. Complete the table below for hormones produced by the adrenal glands:

4. Identify the hormones listed in the table which are examples of a:

a. Glucocorticoid _____

b. Mineralocorticoid _____

c. Catecholamine _____

5. Describe the chemical structure of a:

a. Glucocorticoid _____

_____

b. Mineralocorticoid _____

_____

c. Catecholamine _____

_____

Hormone	Released in response to	Effect(s) of hormone
Aldosterone		
Cortisol		
Adrenaline		
Noradrenaline		

6. Hormonal responses to stimuli are normally gradual, taking place over hours or days, but the 'fight or flight' response mediated by adrenaline secretion takes only seconds. Explain why.

_____

_____

_____

Apply the Concepts

1. What is aldosteronism and how does it occur?

_____

_____

2. What is Addison's disease and how does it occur?

_____

_____

3. Is there a distinction between Cushing's syndrome and Cushing's disease? Explain.

_____

_____

_____

ACTIVITY 14.10: MICROSCOPIC EXAMINATION OF THE ADRENAL GLANDS

The tissues of the adrenal gland are histologically distinct (Fig. 14.8). The adrenal cortex shows three morphologically distinct areas from the periphery inwards – the zona glomerulosa with a whorl-like arrangement of cells; the zona fasciculata, consisting of cells arranged in columns; and the zona reticularis, containing anastomosing (freely connecting) rows of cells. The adrenal medulla is the smaller middle portion of the gland, consisting of irregular masses of cells separated by thin-walled sinusoids. Cells of the medulla are morphologically similar to the postganglionic neurones of the sympathetic nervous system and are innervated by preganglionic neurones. Stimulation of the splanchnic nerve leads to the secretion of **adrenaline** and **noradrenaline** from the medulla into the bloodstream.

This activity examines the microscopic structure of the adrenal gland.

1. Obtain a slide of an adrenal gland LS (H&E) and hold it up to the light to see the outer cortex and inner medulla.

   a. Are these easily distinguished?

   _____

2. Examine the cortex under low power and identify the areas of the cortex indicated. Refer to Fig. 14.8 to assist with identification of the structures examined.

   ☐ Zona glomerulosa

   ☐ Zona fasciculata

   ☐ Zona reticularis

3. Identify the hormones produced within the:

   a. Zona glomerulosa

   _____

   b. Zona fasciculata

   _____

   c. Zona reticularis

   _____

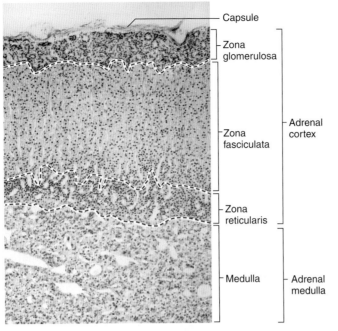

Fig. 14.8 Tissues of the adrenal gland.
(*Source: Patton, K. T., Bell, F. B., Matusiak, D. J., & Wood, S. R. (2021). Anatomy and physiology laboratory manual. Elsevier.*)

4. Observe the large, lightly stained cells of the adrenal medulla beneath the zona reticularis. Notice their clumped arrangement.

5. In the space below make a labelled sketch of your slide, showing the boundaries and relative sizes of the three cortical zones and the medulla.

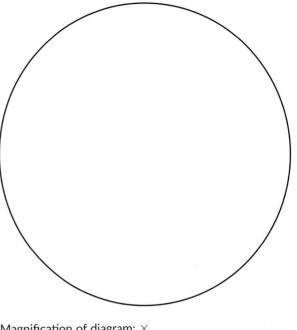

Magnification of diagram: × _____

Apply the Concepts

1. What is adrenogenital syndrome and how does it occur?

_____

_____

2. Explain how a pheochromocytoma can lead to uncontrolled sympathetic nervous system activity.

_____

_____

ACTIVITY 14.11: HORMONES OF THE PANCREAS

The organ chiefly responsible for the maintenance of blood glucose levels, which must be kept within relatively narrow limits, is the **pancreas**. The pancreas secretes two antagonistic hormones, **insulin** and **glucagon**. The pancreas lies partly behind the stomach and also produces bicarbonate ions and digestive enzymes, which are carried to the small intestine via the pancreatic duct. Thus, the pancreas is a **mixed gland** undertaking both endocrine and **exocrine** functions.

This activity explores the function of the endocrine portion of the pancreas.

1. Obtain relevant charts or models and locate the pancreas.

   a. Which organs are adjacent to the pancreas?

   _____

2. The pancreas secretes which two hormones?

   _____

   a. These hormones are what type of chemical compound?

   _____

3. Complete the following sentences by filling in the blanks with the terms provided. (Note: Some terms may be used more than once or not at all).

Amino acids	Glycogenolysis	Liver
Fall	Hyperglycaemic	Parasympathetic
Gluconeogenesis	Hypoglycaemic	Rise
Glucose	Insulin	Sympathetic
Glycogen	Lipids	

   a. Glucagon causes blood _____ levels to _____ and is a powerful _____ agent.

   b. It does this mainly by targeting the _____, where it causes the breakdown of the storage carbohydrate _____ to _____, a process known as _____.

   c. It also causes the synthesis of _____ from non-carbohydrate molecules, a process called _____.

   d. Glucagon secretion is inhibited by rising levels of blood _____ and by its antagonistic hormone, _____.

   e. Insulin causes blood _____ levels to _____ and is a powerful _____ agent.

   f. Insulin achieves this by stimulating the uptake of _____ by the body's cells, inhibiting the breakdown of _____ to _____ in the liver, and inhibiting the conversion of _____ and _____ to glucose.

   g. Insulin secretion can be stimulated by the _____ nervous system and inhibited by the _____ nervous system.

4. Consider the following questions:

   a. Which medical condition results from the hyposecretion of insulin?

   _____

   b. What are the symptoms of this condition?

   _____

   _____

Apply the Concepts

1. What is insulin resistance?

   _____

   _____

2. Explain how hyperinsulinaemia can lead to hypoglycaemia.

   _____

   _____

3. Explain why individuals with type 2 diabetes are at risk of developing ketoacidosis.

   _____

   _____

ACTIVITY 14.12: MICROSCOPIC EXAMINATION OF THE PANCREAS

The pancreas is a major exocrine gland as well as an endocrine gland (Fig. 14.9). The exocrine portion of the gland, which makes up 99% of its mass, is composed of serous acinar cells. The exocrine secretory cells have a round nucleus near the cell base. The pancreatic islets, or **islets of Langerhans**, form the endocrine portion of the pancreas. Islets may be up to 3 mm in diameter, and they number about one million in total, being most numerous in the tail of the pancreas. They consist of clusters of pale cells of two major types – **alpha cells** constituting 20% of the islet cells, and **beta cells** constituting 70% of the islet cells.

This activity examines the microscopic structure of the pancreas.

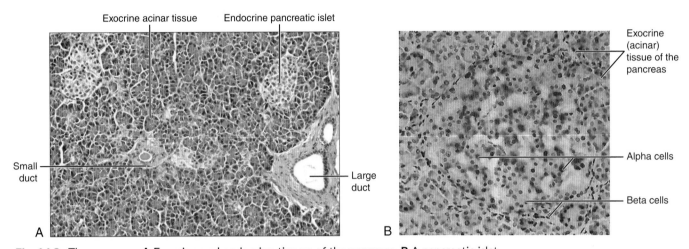

Fig. 14.9. The pancreas. **A** Exocrine and endocrine tissues of the pancreas. **B** A pancreatic islet.
(Source: A Standring, S. (ed.). (2021). Gray's anatomy: The anatomical basis of clinical practice. Elsevier. B Marieb, E. N., Mitchell, S. J., & Zao, P. Z. (2008). Human anatomy and physiology laboratory manual. Pearson.)

1. Examine the prepared slide of the pancreas TS (H&E) under low power.

2. Observe the roughly circular and lightly coloured *pancreatic islets* scattered among the excretory *acinar cells*. Refer to Fig. 14.9 to assist with identification of the structures examined.

3. Focus on an *islet* and examine its cells under high power.

4. Note that their arrangement is more irregular than that of the *acinar cells*, which are organised around *secretory ducts*. Within an *islet*, identify the *alpha cells* around the periphery of the islet, with their bright pink cytoplasm, and the *beta cells*, which stain a paler pink. Refer to Fig. 14.9 to assist with identification of the structures examined.

5. Draw a diagram of a single *pancreatic islet of Langerhans* in the space on the right. Label the *alpha* and *beta* cells of the *islet* and the exocrine *acinar cells*.

6. Identify the hormone secreted by the:

   a. Alpha cells _____

   b. Beta cells _____

7. Which of the alpha and beta cells are more numerous?

_____

Magnification of diagram: × _____

Apply the Concepts

1. A man is brought to hospital with rapid and irregular breathing and excessive sweating. His breath smells of acetone and he is found to have very high blood glucose levels.

   a. What condition is he suffering from? _____

   b. Which hormone should be administered by injection? _____

   c. Why can this hormone not be taken orally?

   _____

   _____

2. Diabetes mellitus and diabetes insipidus are both caused by the absence of a hormone.

   a. Which hormone is absent in diabetes mellitus? _____

   b. Which hormone is absent in diabetes insipidus? _____

   c. What symptom do these two types of diabetes have in common?

   _____

   d. Which substance would you expect to find in the urine of a person suffering diabetes mellitus, and would not be present in the urine of a person suffering diabetes insipidus? _____

3. Approximately 85–90% of all cases of diabetes are type 2 diabetes.

   a. How does type 2 diabetes differ from type 1 diabetes?

   _____

   _____

   b. What is thought to cause type 2 diabetes?

   _____

   _____

   c. While there is no cure for type 2 diabetes, it can be managed. Explain how.

   _____

   _____

   _____

Additional Resources

Histology Guide Virtual Microscopy Laboratory: Endocrine Glands
Histology Guide is an online resource providing a virtual microscopy laboratory experience, by allowing users to view microscope slides from professional collections for the purpose of interpreting cellular and tissue structures, as seen through a microscope.

histologyguide.com/slidebox/13-endocrine-glands.html

Innerbody Research: Endocrine System
Innerbody Research provides objective, science-based advice to help readers make more informed choices about home health products and services, with most up-to-date reviews, guides and research, including information about the endocrine system.

www.innerbody.com/image/endoov.html

Lumen Learning: Overview of the Endocrine System

Lumen Learning provides a number of online courses and modules related to the anatomy and physiology of a variety of body systems, including the endocrine system and endocrine glands.

courses.lumenlearning.com/boundless-ap/chapter/overview-of-the-endocrine-system/courses.lumenlearning.com/boundless-ap/chapter/hormones/

courses.lumenlearning.com/boundless-ap/chapter/mechanisms-of-hormone-action/

NursesLabs: Endocrine System Anatomy and Physiology

NursesLabs is an educational resources for student nurses covering care plans, exams, test banks, and study notes on a variety of health-related topics.

nurseslabs.com/endocrine-system/

Osmosis – Endocrine System

The Endocrine System module of Osmosis provides videos, notes, quiz questions and links to further resources related to the endocrine system.

www.osmosis.org/library/md/foundational-sciences/physiology#endocrine_system

Teach Me Physiology: Endocrine

Teach Me Physiology provides basic information on physiological subjects and systems, with reference to the clinical relevance of the system being reviewed.

teachmephysiology.com/endocrine-system/

The Histology Guide: Glandular Tissue

The Histology Guide is a virtual experience of using a microscope with zoom features divided into topics and offering histological slides with labels and quizzes for each topic, such as glandular tissue. It is provided by the University of Leeds.

www.histology.leeds.ac.uk/glandular/index.php

Visible Body: Endocrine System

Visible Body provides interactive and highly accurate visualisations and apps for learning and teaching anatomy and physiology for students and healthcare professionals, including body systems such as the endocrine system.

www.visiblebody.com/learn/endocrine

CHAPTER 15
Blood

Blood is unique as it is the only liquid tissue in the body. Its fluid nature allows for a number of unique functions that are not possible with fixed tissues. Whole blood is composed of a number of different cells, referred to as formed elements. These cells possess specialised characteristics and functions. Erythrocytes, or red blood cells, are vital in gas transport through the function of haemoglobin; leukocytes, or white blood cells, have a chief role in immunity, and thrombocytes or platelets are instrumental in blood clotting.

Since blood is a connective tissue, it consists of a matrix in the form of liquid plasma, and rather than fibrous proteins, it contains soluble proteins that become fibrous when a blood vessel is damaged. This event signals the beginning of haemostasis, or blood clotting, which involves the combined actions of thrombocytes and clotting factors, and initiates the process of tissue repair. In addition, erythrocytes have antigens on their cell membranes, which form the basis of the ABO system of blood grouping. The corresponding absence of blood plasma antibodies prevents the immune system from attacking blood cells with those antigens. (Refer to Chapter 22: Reproductive System and Heredity, for further information on the genetic basis of blood groups.)

LEARNING OUTCOMES

On completion of these activities, the student should be able to:

1. list and describe the main functions of blood

2. describe the composition of whole blood

3. identify and describe the formed elements of blood

4. describe the structure, function and development of erythrocytes

5. describe the structure and function of haemoglobin

6. describe the structure, function and development of leukocytes

7. describe the structure, function and development of thrombocytes

8. identify and describe the stages of haemostasis

9. explain the basis for ABO blood types and how cross-matching reactions occur

10. undertake simple laboratory tests that highlight the characteristics of blood.

KEY TERMS

Agranulocyte

Antibody

Antigen

Blood

Erythrocyte

Erythropoiesis

Erythropoietin

Formed elements

Granulocyte

Haematocrit (Hct)

Haemoglobin

Haemostasis

Leukocyte

Leukopoiesis

Plasma

Platelet

Red blood cell

Thrombocyte

Thrombopoiesis

White blood cell

ACTIVITY 15.1: COMPOSITION OF WHOLE BLOOD

Blood is a viscous, colloidal, homogenous liquid containing both fluid and cellular components. As with other connective tissues, it consists of a non-living matrix called **plasma**, which is fluid, and the cellular portion containing the **formed elements** or blood cells (Fig. 15.1). Centrifugation of whole blood causes the denser, heavy elements to sink to the bottom, while less dense, lighter elements remain at the top, thereby separating the cellular and liquid components of blood.

This activity examines the composition of whole blood.

1. Consider the following questions, with reference to Fig. 15.1:

    a. How does centrifugation separate the components of blood?

    _____

    _____

    _____

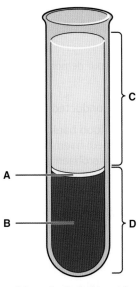

Figure 15.1 Composition of whole blood (centrifuged).
(Source: Herlihy, B. (2018). The human body in health and illness. Elsevier.)

b. What is the term for layer A?

_____

c. What is found in layer A?

_____

d. What is found in layer B?

_____

e. What is found in layer C?

_____

f. What is found in layer D?

_____

g. What percentage of whole blood does layer C comprise?

_____

h. What percentage of whole blood does layer D comprise?

_____

i. What are the three main components of blood plasma?

_____

j. Identify three proteins found in blood plasma.

_____

k. Identify three solutes found in blood plasma.

_____

Apply the Concepts

1. What is a blood fraction?

_____

_____

_____

2. Why might transfusion of a blood fraction be preferred over a whole blood transfusion?

_____

_____

_____

Additional Activities

For additional activities visit Activity 15A: Functions of Blood on Evolve®.

ACTIVITY 15.2: HAEMATOCRIT OR PACKED CELL VOLUME (PCV)

A **haematocrit (Hct)** is the proportion of the blood volume that is occupied by the **erythrocytes** or **red blood cells**. It is determined by centrifuging whole blood in glass haematocrit or capillary tubes to pack down the cells. The length of the column of cells in relation to the total blood column is then measured and compared to normal reference ranges and can provide valuable physiological information of clinical importance (Fig. 15.2). Abnormal haematocrit values can be due to abnormalities of erythrocyte numbers, size, or changes in plasma volume; however, further clinical testing is necessary to identify specific causes.

This activity examines the components of whole blood based on haematocrit or packed cell volume (PCV).

⚠️ To conduct this activity, it is important to ensure the following safety precautions:

- _Bodily fluids and sharps will be used in this laboratory, exercise caution at all times._
- _Wear disposable gloves, disposable apron and safety glasses at all times during the activity as blood may harbour biological hazards._
- _Exercise care when handling haematocrit tubes as the ends may be sharp._
- _Additional precautions including safe disposal of blood materials may be required by your demonstrator._

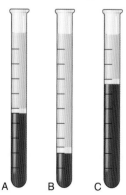

Figure 15.2 Haematocrit (Hct) tubes. **A** Normal haematocrit. **B** Anaemia. **C** Polycythaemia.

(Source: Cooper, K., & Gosnell, K. (2022). Adult health nursing. Elsevier.)

1. This activity is best conducted individually.

2. Obtain a sample of blood bank blood (or horse's blood), a plain (not heparinised) haematocrit tube, haematocrit sealing compound, microhaematocrit centrifuge, haematocrit reader, disposable gloves, disposable apron and safety glasses.

3. Partly fill the haematocrit tube with blood to about three-quarters full.

4. Seal the clean end of the haematocrit tube by pressing firmly into the sealing compound provided.

5. Place the sealed tube into a microhaematocrit centrifuge with the sealed end facing outwards from the centre of the machine.

6. Screw down the lid on the centrifuge and spin for 5 minutes.

7. Determine the haematocrit either by using the haematocrit reader or by measuring:

   a. Length of column of red cells (mm):

   _____

   b. Total length of column of blood (mm):

   _____

   c. Haematocrit (HCt) $= \dfrac{\text{Length of column of red cells (mm)}}{\text{Total length of column of blood (mm)}}$

   _____

d. Haematocrit is not expressed in units, but is sometimes expressed as a percentage. Multiply the answer to (c) by 100%.

   _____

8. Consider the following questions, with reference to Table 15.1:

   a. What is meant by the term packed cell volume (PCV)?

   _____

   _____

Table 15.1 Haematological variable ranges

Reference variable	Reference range
Haematocrit (male)	37–47%
Haematocrit (female)	40–54%
Haemoglobin concentration (male)	130–170 g/L*
Haemoglobin concentration (female)	115–155 g/L
Mean cell haemoglobin (MCH)	29–33 pg*
Mean cell haemoglobin concentration (MCHC)	320–360 g/L
Mean cell volume (MCV) (male)	82–98 fL*
Mean cell volume (MCV) (female)	81–98 fL
Erythrocytes (male)	4.4–5.9×10^{12}/L
Erythrocytes (female)	4.1–5.5×10^{12}/L
Reticulocytes	0.7–3.2%
Leukocytes	4.0–10.0×10^{9}/L
Neutrophils	2.0–7.5×10^{9}/L
Lymphocytes	1.5–4.0×10^{9}/L
Monocytes	0.2–0.8×10^{9}/L
Eosinophils	0.04–0.4×10^{9}/L
Basophils	0.01–0.1×10^{9}/L
Thrombocytes	150–400×10^{9}/L

*fL = femtolitre; g/L = gram/litre; pg = picogram

b. Is a thin white layer on top of the red column visible?

_____

c. What is this thin white layer and what does it contain?

_____

d. What colour is the plasma layer?

_____

e. Which other colour might the plasma be and why?

_____

_____

f. Why is plasma sometimes clear and sometimes cloudy?

_____

_____

g. Does your result fall within the reference haematocrit range? Explain.

_____

_____

h. Assuming that the average person's blood volume is 5 litres, how many of the following will be present?

i. Erythrocytes: _____

ii. Leukocytes: _____

iii. Platelets: _____

9. Consider the following questions, with reference to Fig. 15.2:

a. The haematrocrit that you produced resembles which of the tubes in Fig. 15.2?

_____

b. Tube B in Fig. 15.2 indicates anaemia. Explain why Tube B shows anaemia.

_____

_____

c. Tube C in Fig. 15.2 indicates polycythaemia. Explain why Tube C shows polycythaemia.

_____

_____

Apply the Concepts

1. What is polycythaemia and how does it occur?

_____

_____

_____

2. Why is it necessary to use a heparinised tube for fresh blood, but not for blood bank blood?

_____

_____

_____

3. What conditions might an increased haematocrit value indicate?

_____

_____

_____

4. What conditions might a decreased haematocrit value indicate?

_____

_____

_____

5. What is anaemia and how does it occur?

_____

_____

_____

6. Why are blood studies so important in the diagnosis of disease?

_____

_____

_____

Additional Activities

For additional activities visit Activity 15B: Osmotic Resistance in Erythrocytes on Evolve.
For additional activities visit Activity 15C: Formed Elements of Blood on Evolve.
For additional activities visit Activity 15D: Microscopic Examination of Blood Cells on Evolve.

ACTIVITY 15.3: ERYTHROPOIESIS

Erythropoiesis refers to the process of erythrocyte or red blood cell production. It is the homeostatic regulation pathway for erythrocyte production and occurs in response to the reduced oxygen-carrying capacity of the blood (hypoxia). Erythrocyte development occurs under the regulating influence of erythropoietin (Fig. 15.3). **Erythropoietin** acts on the red bone marrow to stimulate the production of erythrocyte precursors (Fig. 15.4).

This activity outlines the process of erythropoiesis and the developmental pathway of erythrocytes.

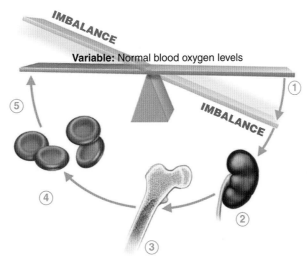

Figure 15.3 Erythropoiesis (role of erythropoietin).
(Source: Marieb, E. N., & Hoehn, K. (2010). Human anatomy and physiology. Pearson Education.)

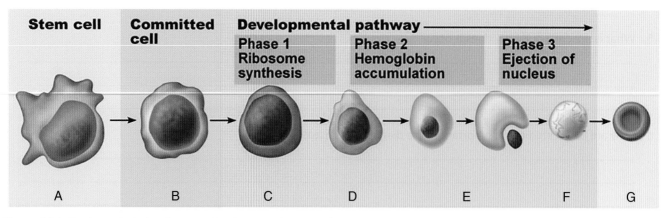

Figure 15.4 Erythropoiesis (erythrocyte developmental pathway).
(Source: Marieb, E. N., & Hoehn, K. (2010). Human anatomy and physiology. Pearson Education.)

1. Consider the following questions with reference to Fig. 15.3:

   a. What is the stimulus for erythropoiesis?

   _____

   b. Which structure is the receptor?

   _____

   c. Which structure is the control centre or integrator?

   _____

   _____

   d. Which structure is the effector?

   _____

   _____

2. Explain the processes occurring in each of the stages in Fig. 15.3, using the terms stimulus, receptor, control centre and effector in your response.

   a. Stage 1: _____

   _____

   _____

   b. Stage 2: _____

   _____

   _____

   c. Stage 3: _____

   _____

   _____

   d. Stage 4: _____

   _____

   _____

   e. Stage 5: _____

   _____

   _____

3. If blood oxygen levels are not increased after the process indicated is complete, what will occur?

   _____

   _____

   _____

4. Identify the cells in the erythrocyte developmental pathway shown in Fig. 15.4, using the terms provided.

   Reticulocyte   Early erythroblast

   Late erythroblast   Normoblast

   Erythrocyte   Haemocytoblast

   Proerythroblast

   a. Cell A: _____

   b. Cell B: _____

   c. Cell C: _____

   d. Cell D: _____

   e. Cell E: _____

   f. Cell F: _____

   g. Cell G: _____

5. Consider the following questions with reference to Fig. 15.4:

a. What is a stem cell and where do these originate?

_____

_____

b. What does the term 'committed cell' refer to?

_____

_____

c. At which stage in the erythrocyte developmental pathway does a cell become committed?

_____

_____

d. Which substance is responsible for initiating erythropoiesis, what does this act on, and where is it produced?

_____

_____

e. What is the significance of ribosome synthesis?

_____

_____

f. At what stage does haemoglobin synthesis and accumulation occur?

_____

g. What is the significance of the reduction in nucleus size?

_____

_____

h. What is the significance of nucleus ejection in the developing erythrocyte?

_____

_____

i. What is a reticulocyte?

_____

j. How does a reticulocyte develop into the characteristic erythrocyte shape?

_____

_____

k. At which developmental stage do erythrocytes enter the blood stream?

_____

_____

l. Explain what happens to erythrocytes at the end of their lifecycle.

_____

_____

m. What shape are sickle cell erythrocytes and how does this affect their function?

_____

_____

Apply the Concepts

1. What is hypoxia and how does it occur?

_____

_____

_____

2. Why might individuals with kidney disease suffer from anaemia?

_____

_____

3. What is bilirubin and where does it originate?

_____

_____

_____

4. How would you expect blood levels of bilirubin to change in an individual that has severe liver disease?

_____

_____

_____

ACTIVITY 15.4: BLOOD DOPING

Erythropoietin (EPO), although essential in erythropoiesis and the production of erythrocytes, can be utilised by competition athletes to enhance performance in the process referred to as blood doping. The result is an increased blood oxygen carrying capacity as indicated by an altered haematocrit (Fig. 15.5), which assists muscles in the aerobic production of ATP.

Consider a fictitious case in which four Olympic athletes have recently won medals, and the Olympic Medal Committee has received information that these athletes have engaged in blood doping, giving them a competitive advantage over other athletes. If the athletes are found to have used illegal substances, their medals will be stripped from them. An investigation is launched, and blood and urine samples from the winners are obtained for testing.

This activity simulates the effect of blood doping on haematocrit values.

 To conduct this activity, it is important to ensure the following safety precautions:

- *Wear UV protective eyewear at all times when using the black light as light wavelengths below 410 nm may cause damage to the cornea and retina.*

- *Wear disposable gloves at all times during the activity to prevent contamination.*

1. This activity is best conducted in pairs.

2. Obtain 4 test tubes containing simulated haematocrit samples (athletes 1, 2, 3, 4), 4 test tubes containing simulated urine samples (athletes 1, 2, 3, 4), test-tube rack, disposable pipettes, filter paper, black light, disposable gloves and UV protective eyewear.

3. Place the samples in the test-tube rack, arranging them so that they match the sample order in the table provided.

4. To test the haematocrit samples for the possible presence of EPO, hold each sample against the haematocrit reader chart provided in Fig. 15.5 to determine the packed cell volume (PCV).

5. Repeat for the remaining haematocrit samples, recording your data in the table provided and indicating whether the EPO level for each sample was high, low or normal.

6. To test the urine samples for the presence of EPO, place 2 drops of each urine sample on a clean piece of filter paper.

7. Wearing UV protective eyewear, view each filter paper sample under black light. The sample should fluoresce if EPO is present.

8. Repeat for the remaining urine samples, recording your data in the table provided and indicating whether the EPO level for each sample was high, low or normal.

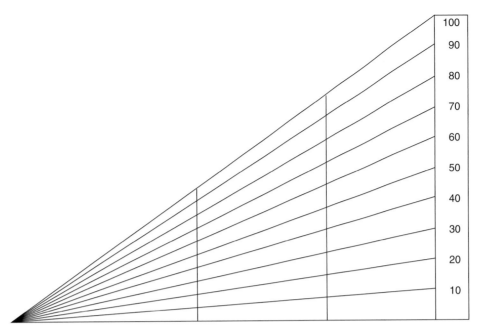

Figure 15.5 Haematocrit reader chart.

9. Based on the results, determine the possible health or doping status of each athlete in the table provided.

	Athlete 1	Athlete 2	Athlete 3	Athlete 4
Haematocrit level (blood)				
EPO level (urine)				
Health/ doping state				

10. Consider the following questions:

   a. What is blood doping?

   _____

   _____

   _____

   b. How is blood doping achieved?

   _____

   _____

   _____

c. Explain the results for athlete 2.

_____

_____

_____

d. Explain the results for athlete 3.

_____

_____

_____

e. Explain the results for athlete 4.

_____

_____

_____

Apply the Concepts

1. How does the blood doping practised by some athletes enhance performance?

_____

_____

_____

2. Identify a possible health risk factor for athletes engaging in blood doping.

_____

_____

_____

Additional Activities

For additional activities visit Activity 15E: Haemoglobin on Evolve˙.

ACTIVITY 15.5: LEUKOCYTES (WHITE BLOOD CELLS) AND LEUKOPOIESIS

Leukocytes, or white blood cells, are the body's chief immune cells and are active in mediating immune functions. There are five types of leukocytes – neutrophils, lymphocytes, monocytes, eosinophils and basophils – which are grouped into two main classes, granulocytes and agranulocytes. Each leukocyte has a specific immune function and is normally produced in predetermined quantities or in increased quantities in the presence of infection. Leukocytes are produced through the process of leukopoiesis, which occurs within the red bone marrow (Fig. 15.6).

This activity outlines the characteristics of leukocytes and the process of leukopoiesis.

1. Complete the table based on the characteristics of leukocytes.

Leukocyte	Granulocyte/ agranulocyte	Nucleus characteristics	Number of cells/μL of blood

2. Consider the following questions:

a. On average, how many leukocytes are present per microlitre of whole blood.

_____

b. Suggest a reason for the varying nucleus morphology of leukocytes.

_____

_____

_____

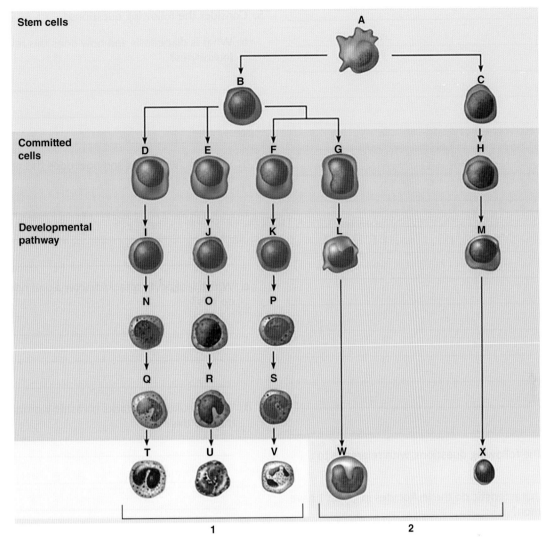

Stem cells

A

B

C

Committed cells

D E F G H

Developmental pathway

I J K L M

N O P

Q R S

T U V W X

1 2

Figure 15.6 Leukopoiesis (leukocyte developmental pathway).
(Source: Marieb, E. N., & Hoehn, K. (2010). Human anatomy and physiology. Pearson Education.)

c. Suggest a reason for the higher number of neutrophils compared with other leukocytes.

_____

_____

_____

3. Identify the cells in the leukocyte developmental pathway shown in Fig. 15.6, using the terms provided. (Note: some terms are used more than once).

Basophil	Monocyte	Myeloid stem cell
Promyelocyte	Eosinophilic band cells	Prolymphocyte
Neutrophilic myelocyte	Basophilic band cells	Basophilic myelocyte
Neutrophil	Promonocyte	Lymphoblast

Eosinophilic myelocyte	Haemocytoblast	Eosinophil
Myeloblast	Lymphocyte	Lymphoid stem cell
Neutrophilic band cells	Monoblast	

a. Cell A: _____

b. Cell B: _____

c. Cell C: _____

d. Cell D: _____

e. Cell E: _____

f. Cell F: _____

g. Cell G: _____

h. Cell H: _____

i. Cell I: _____

j. Cell J: _____

k. Cell K: _____

l. Cell L: _____

m. Cell M: _____

n. Cell N: _____

o. Cell O: _____

p. Cell P: _____

q. Cell Q: _____

r. Cell R: _____

s. Cell S: _____

t. Cell T: _____

u. Cell U: _____

v. Cell V: _____

w. Cell W: _____

x. Cell X: _____

4. Consider the following questions, with reference to Fig. 15.6:

a. What characteristic do the leukocytes in group 1 have in common?

_____

b. What characteristics do the leukocytes in group 2 have in common?

_____

c. Which substances are responsible for initiating leukopoiesis and what do these act on?

_____

_____

d. Differentiate between a myeloid stem cell and a lymphoid stem cell.

_____

_____

e. What is a band cell?

_____

_____

_____

5. Consider the following questions:

a. What is diapedesis and how does this relate to leukocytes?

_____

_____

_____

b. What is chemotaxis and how does this relate to leukocytes?

_____

_____

_____

c. Which leukocyte attacks bacteria and how do they do this?

_____

_____

_____

d. Which leukocyte attacks parasitic worms and how do they do this?

_____

_____

_____

e. Which leukocyte produces histamine and what is the function of histamine?

_____

_____

_____

f. Which leukocyte forms T cells and B cells and what is their function?

_____

_____

_____

g. Which leukocyte is an active phagocyte and what does it defend against?

_____

_____

_____

Apply the Concepts

1. What is leukocytosis and how does it occur?

_____

_____

_____

2. What is leukaemia and how does it occur?

_____

_____

_____

3. What is septicaemia and how is it managed?

_____

_____

_____

Additional Activities

For additional activities visit Activity 15F: Leukocyte Count on Evolve˙.

ACTIVITY 15.6: THROMBOCYTES (PLATELETS) AND THROMBOPOIESIS

Thrombocytes, or **platelets**, are the smallest of the blood cells and are actually cellular fragments rather than complete cells. They do not contain nuclei or organelles and are produced in the red bone marrow through a process called **thrombopoiesis** (Fig. 15.7). Their main function is **haemostasis**, or blood clotting, which occurs when a blood vessel is damaged.

This activity outlines the process of thrombopoiesis and the developmental pathway of thrombocytes.

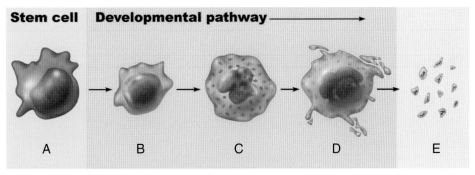

Figure 15.7 Thrombopoiesis (thrombocyte developmental pathway).
(Source: Marieb, E. N., & Hoehn, K. (2010). Human anatomy and physiology. Pearson Education.)

1. Identify the cells in the thrombocyte developmental pathway shown in Fig. 15.7, using the terms provided.

Promegakaryocyte   Megakaryocyte

Megakaryoblast   Platelets

Haemocytoblast

a. Cell A: _____

b. Cell B: _____

c. Cell C: _____

d. Cell D: _____

e. Cell E: _____

2. Consider the following questions with reference to Fig. 15.7:

a. Which substance is responsible for initiating thrombopoiesis, what does this act on, and where is it produced?

_____

_____

_____

b. What processes occur at the cell B stage?

_____

_____

_____

c. What processes occur at the cell C stage?

_____

_____

_____

d. What processes occur at the cell D stage?

_____

_____

_____

e. What are the structures at E?

_____

f. What is the function of the structures at E?

_____

g. What do the structures at E contain and what is their function?

_____

_____

Apply the Concepts

1. What is thrombocytopaenia and how does it occur?

_____

_____

_____

ACTIVITY 15.7: HAEMOSTASIS (BLOOD CLOTTING)

Connective tissues generally contain high proportions of structural proteins such as collagen and elastic fibres, which provide flexibility and strength. Blood does not contain these proteins, but instead contains the protein fibrin, which is normally soluble within circulating blood, but forms fibres when blood vessels become injured. This marks the beginning of the process known as haemostasis or blood clotting (Fig. 15.8). Blood clotting involves a number of processes where specific clotting factors are converted chemically to form the clot. This may occur via intrinsic or extrinsic pathways.

This activity outlines the processes of haemostasis (blood clotting).

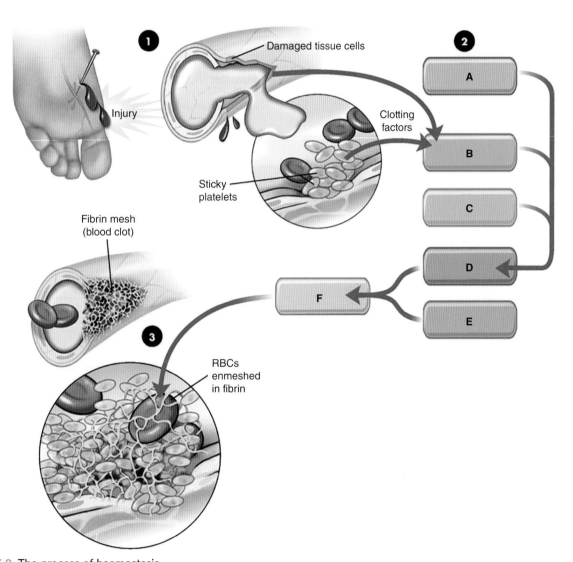

Figure 15.8 The process of haemostasis.
(Source: Craft, J., Gordon, C., Huether, S. E., McCance, K. L., Brashers, V. L., & List, S. (2019). Understanding pathophysiology. Australia and New Zealand edition. Elsevier.)

1. Identify the stages of haemostasis as shown in Fig. 15.8, and briefly outline the events occurring in each stage.

   a. Stage 1:

      i. Identification: _____

      ii. Events: _____

      _____

      _____

   b. Stage 2:

      i. Identification: _____

      ii. Events: _____

      _____

      _____

   c. Stage 3:

      i. Identification: _____

      ii. Events: _____

      _____

      _____

2. Haemostasis is not concluded with blood clot formation. Explain the additional processes of:

   a. Clot retraction

      _____

      _____

   b. Fibrinolysis

      _____

      _____

3. Why is fibrinolysis crucial?

   _____

   _____

   _____

4. Identify the clotting factors outlined in Stage 2 of Fig. 15.8, using the terms provided:

Calcium	Fibrin
Thrombin	Prothrombin activator
Fibrinogen	Prothrombin

   a. Factor A: _____

   b. Factor B: _____

   c. Factor C: _____

   d. Factor D: _____

   e. Factor E: _____

   f. Factor F: _____

5. Consider the following questions:

   a. Distinguish between fibrinogen and fibrin.

      _____

      _____

      _____

   b. Compare a platelet plug with a blood clot.

      _____

      _____

      _____

   c. What are the differences between the intrinsic and extrinsic coagulation pathways?

      _____

      _____

      _____

   d. What is an anticoagulant?

      _____

   e. What is the body's natural anticoagulant?

      _____

   f. Why does the body require a natural anticoagulant?

      _____

      _____

Apply the Concepts

1. Are heparin and warfarin used in the same manner? Explain.

_____

_____

_____

2. Is a blood thinner the same as an anticoagulant? Explain.

_____

_____

_____

3. What is haemophilia and how does it affect haemostasis?

_____

_____

_____

4. What is a haematoma?

_____

_____

_____

Additional Activities

For additional activities visit Activity 15G: Bleeding and Clotting Time on Evolve®.

ACTIVITY 15.8: BLOOD TYPING AND BLOOD COMPATIBILITY

All normal erythrocytes appear identical under a microscope; however, different **antigens** may be present on the surfaces of their cell membranes and different **antibodies** may also be present within the blood plasma. It is the antigens that are recognised by the body's defence system as belonging to 'self' so that they are not destroyed. These antigens include those that form the basis of the ABO blood typing system. The most significant antigens are the A and the B antigens. Cells may have only A antigens (blood type A), only B antigens (blood type B), both A and B antigens (blood type AB), or no antigens (blood type O).

This activity demonstrates the process of blood typing using simulated blood.

Part 1: Blood Typing

Blood type is determined through the use of anti-serum which contains antibodies that may react with antigens on the erythrocyte surface (Fig. 15.9). For example, anti-A serum contains anti-A antibodies which causes agglutination or clumping of a blood sample containing A antigens.

 To conduct this activity, it is important to ensure the following safety precautions:

- *Wear disposable gloves, disposable apron, and safety glasses at all times during the activity as blood samples may harbour biological hazards.*
- *Additional precautions including safe disposal of blood materials may be required by your demonstrator.*

1. This activity is best conducted individually.

2. Obtain a dimple tile, toothpicks, 4 samples of simulated blood, anti-A serum, anti-B serum, anti-AB serum, anti-D serum, disposable pipettes, disposable apron, safety glasses and disposable gloves.

3. Don the protective equipment.

4. Using the table provided as a guide, dispense 2 drops of each of the 4 blood samples to be tested in separate dimples on the dimple tile. You should have 4 columns and 4 dimples for each sample, giving a total of 16 samples.

5. Using the table provided as a guide, place a drop of anti-serum in each dimple together with the blood samples.

6. Mix the blood with the anti-serum in each dimple gently, using the tip of a toothpick. (Note: use a new toothpick each time to prevent contamination of samples.)

7. Observe each sample for agglutination or clumping of cells.

8. Record your results in the table provided.

Anti serum	Blood sample 1	Blood sample 2	Blood sample 3	Blood sample 4
Anti-A serum[1]				
Anti-B serum[2]				
Anti-AB serum[3]				
Anti-D serum[4] (Rh+ or Rh−)				
Blood type identified				

Notes:
1. Anti-A serum contains anti-A antibodies. Agglutination indicates presence of A antigens
2. Anti-B serum contains anti-B antibodies. Agglutination indicates presence of B antigens
3. Anti-AB serum is a combined anti-serum used as a check against anti-A and anti-B serums
4. Anti-D serum contains anti-Rh antibodies. Agglutination indicates presence of Rh antigens

9. Consider the following questions:

a. What caused agglutination in some of the blood samples?

_____

b. Why was agglutination not indicated in some of the blood samples?

_____

c. What is the difference between coagulated and agglutinated blood?

_____

_____

_____

d. Antibodies are composed of which type of organic molecule?

_____

_____

e. Where are antibodies made?

_____

f. Explain how erythrocyte antigens and plasma antibodies cause agglutination.

_____

_____

_____

_____

g. Which blood types have A antigens?

_____

h. Which blood types have A antibodies?

_____

i. Which blood types have Rh antigens?

_____

Part 2: ABO Blood Types

Careful cross-matching of blood types between donor and recipient is crucial in the event of blood transfusion. It identifies either a compatible combination of donor-recipient blood causing no agglutination, or an incompatible combination causing agglutinated blood (Fig. 15.9).

1. Consider the following questions, with reference to Fig. 15.9:

a. Where are blood antigens found?

_____

b. Where are blood antibodies found?

_____

c. What other term is used to refer to blood antibodies?

_____

d. What is the difference between serum and plasma?

_____

2. Consider the following questions, with reference to Fig. 15.9. In each case, indicate whether the following combinations between potential blood donors and recipients are compatible, and provide an explanation:

a. A type A donor donates blood to a type B recipient.

i. Compatibility: _____

ii. Explanation: _____

_____

b. A type AB recipient receives blood from a type B donor.

i. Compatibility: _____

ii. Explanation: _____

_____

Recipient's blood		Reactions with donor's blood			
RBC antigens	Plasma antibodies	Donor type O	Donor type A	Donor type B	Donor type AB
None (Type O)	Anti-A Anti-B				
A (Type A)	Anti-B				
B (Type B)	Anti-A				
AB (Type AB)	(None)				

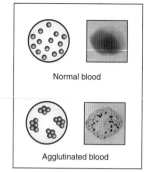

Normal blood

Agglutinated blood

A

	Type A	Type B	Type AB	Type O
	Antigen A	Antigen B	Antigens A and B	Neither antigen A nor B
Red blood cells				
	Antibody B	Antibody A	Neither antibody A nor antibody B	Antibodies A and B
Plasma				

B

Figure 15.9 ABO blood types. **A** Cross-matching compatibility. **B** ABO antigens and antibodies.
(*Source: Patton, K. T., Thibodeau, G. A., & Hutton, A. (2019). Anatomy and physiology. Adapted international edition. Elsevier.*)

c. A type O donor donates blood to a type B recipient.

   i. Compatibility: _____

   ii. Explanation: _____

   _____

d. A type O recipient receives blood from a type A donor.

   i. Compatibility: _____

   ii. Explanation: _____

   _____

e. A type AB donor donates blood to a type B recipient.

   i. Compatibility: _____

   ii. Explanation: _____

   _____

f. A type A recipient receives blood from a type AB donor.

   i. Compatibility: _____

   ii. Explanation: _____

   _____

Apply the Concepts

1. Explain why someone who is Rh D negative cannot be described as Rh negative.

   _____

   _____

   _____

2. Based on the interactions of plasma antibodies, explain how haemolytic disease of the newborn occurs.

   _____

   _____

   _____

3. Suggest a reason why typed blood may still be unsafe to transfuse.

   _____

   _____

   _____

4. Which donor blood type can be used in an emergency when the blood type of the recipient is unknown and why?

   _____

   _____

   _____

5. The genetic basis of blood type is a form of multiple allele inheritance, including codominance. Explain what this means.

   _____

   _____

   _____

Additional Resources

Access Virtual Learning: Blood Types
A short virtual lesson addressing the basis of blood types, including a blood typing simulation relating to blood transfusions.

accessdl.state.al.us/AventaCourses/access_courses/anatomy_ua_v17/04_unit/04-05/04-05_introduction.htm

Histology Guide Virtual Microscopy Laboratory: Peripheral Blood and Haematopoiesis
Histology Guide is an online resource providing a virtual microscopy laboratory experience, by allowing users to view microscope slides from professional collections for the purpose of interpreting cellular and tissue structures as seen through a microscope.

histologyguide.com/slidebox/07-peripheral-blood.html
histologyguide.com/slidebox/08-hematopoiesis.html

Human Bio Media: Hematocrit Lab
An open-source resource providing illustrations, animations, activities, simulations and lessons on human anatomy and physiology topics.

www.humanbiomedia.org/hematocrit-lab-simulation/

Lab Tests Online: Blood Film Examination
Lab Tests Online provides information relating to a number of blood pathology tests managed by the Australasian Association for Clinical Biochemistry and Laboratory Medicine and supported by the Royal College of Pathologists of Australasia.

www.labtestsonline.org.au/learning/test-index/blood-film

MedPics: Hematology
MedPics provides an image library accompanied by lessons for medical education on pathophysiology, pathology, haematology and histology. It is provided by the University of California.

medpics.ucsd.edu/index.cfm?curpage5main&course5heme

Osmosis – Haematological System
The Haematological System module of Osmosis provides videos, notes, quiz questions and links to further resources related to the haematological system.

www.osmosis.org/library/md/foundational-sciences/physiology#hematological_system

The Blood Typing Game

The Blood Typing game, which outlines the basics of blood types, typing and transfusions, is based on the 1930 Nobel Prize in Physiology or Medicine, which was awarded for the discovery of human blood groups in 1901.

https://educationalgames.nobelprize.org/educational/medicine/bloodtypinggame/

The Histology Guide: Blood

The Histology Guide is a virtual experience of using a microscope with zoom features divided into topics and offering histological slides with labels and quizzes for each topic. It is provided by the University of Leeds.

www.histology.leeds.ac.uk/blood/

CHAPTER 16

The Cardiovascular System

The cardiovascular system comprises the heart (cardio) and the blood vessels (vascular). These structures contain and propel blood throughout the body, forming a closed delivery system approximately 10,000 kilometres in length.

The heart acts as a muscular pump and is composed of three tissue layers, the chief layer, or myocardium, comprising cardiac muscle tissue. (Refer to Chapter 7: Tissues and Organs, for further information on cardiac muscle structure.) The myocardium provides contractile force for the propulsion of blood through the heart and throughout the vascular system. The vascular system forms a diverging and converging transport network, delivering blood to and from the heart. Arteries distribute blood throughout the body towards the capillaries, while veins return blood from the capillaries to the heart. The smallest blood vessels, the capillaries, serve the direct needs of the tissues by allowing exchange of nutrients and metabolic wastes between the tissue cells and the blood.

Transporting blood throughout the cardiovascular system presents unique challenges. Blood is a connective tissue composed of formed cellular elements and a fluid medium of dynamic composition. (Refer to Chapter 15: Blood, for further information on blood composition.) The composition and concentration of the blood, the condition of the blood vessels, and the factors affecting heart contraction all have an overall effect on blood flow and pressure. These factors are in turn influenced by physical, neural and chemical stimuli, which can exert combined effects on cardiovascular functioning. (Refer to Chapter 12: The Nervous System, for further information on nervous tissue and the brain.) An inability of the cardiovascular system to meet the body's demands for oxygen may indicate an underlying cardiovascular condition, which can often be detected by a number of physical assessments.

LEARNING OUTCOMES

On completion of these activities, the student should be able to:

1. outline the pathway of blood circuits and circulation throughout the body
2. describe the structure and function of the heart
3. conduct an examination of the heart and its associated structures
4. describe the structure and function of the different categories of blood vessels

LEARNING OUTCOMES—Cont'd

5. identify, describe, and examine the microscopic structures of the heart and blood vessels

6. outline the structures comprising the cardiac conduction system and describe their functions

7. conduct an electrocardiogram (ECG) and analyse an ECG tracing

8. describe the events of the cardiac cycle, explain the physiology of the pulse and conduct a pulse measurement

9. explain the factors that affect blood pressure

10. outline the relationships between blood volume, pressure and flow

11. describe the factors affecting resistance and their overall effect on blood flow and pressure

12. explain the factors contributing to venous blood return

13. outline the relationships between cardiac output and mean arterial pressure, and relate these to the effects of exercise on cardiovascular function.

KEY TERMS

Arteriole

Artery

Atrioventricular (AV) node

Atrioventricular valves

Atrium

Blood pressure (BP)

Blood vessel

Capillary

Cardiac conduction system

Cardiac cycle

Cardiac output (CO)

Circulatory system

Coronary arteries

Diastolic

Endocardium

Heart

Heart rate (HR)

Myocardium

Pericardium

Pulmonary circuit

Pulse

Resistance

Semilunar valves

Sinoatrial (SA) node

Systemic circuit

Systolic

Vasoconstriction

Vasodilation

Vein

Ventricle

Venule

ACTIVITY 16.1: STRUCTURE AND FUNCTION OF THE HEART

The chief organ of the cardiovascular system is the **heart**, which acts as a pump to distribute blood throughout the network of blood vessels (Fig. 16.1). The heart is a four-chambered muscular organ, weighing approximately 250–350 g. It contains specialised internal structures that assist its function as a pump and promote the flow of blood within its chambers – the **endocardium**, **atrioventricular valves** and **semilunar valves** – and structures that protect and nourish the heart externally – the **pericardium** and **coronary arteries** respectively.

This activity outlines the structure, function, and blood circulation through the heart.

1. Describe the location of the heart.

   _____

   _____

   _____

2. Identify each of the structures in Fig. 16.1A using the terms provided.

Left coro-nary artery/ cardiac vein	Left pulmonary veins	Pulmonary trunk	Conus arteriosus
Left ventricle	Apex	Auricle of right atrium	Arch of aorta
Right pulmonary veins	Auricle of left atrium	Brachioce-phalic trunk	Right coronary artery/ cardiac vein
Adipose tissue/ epicardium	Right ventricle	Left common carotid artery	Ligamentum arteriosum
Great car-diac vein	Superior vena cava	Ascending aorta	Left subclavian artery

   a. Structure A: _____

   b. Structure B: _____

   c. Structure C: _____

   d. Structure D: _____

   e. Structure E: _____

   f. Structure F: _____

   g. Structure G: _____

   h. Structure H: _____

   i. Structure I: _____

   j. Structure J: _____

   k. Structure K: _____

   l. Structure L: _____

   m. Structure M: _____

   n. Structure N: _____

   o. Structure O: _____

   p. Structure P: _____

   q. Structure Q: _____

   r. Structure R: _____

   s. Structure S: _____

   t. Structure T: _____

3. Consider the following questions, with reference to Fig. 16.1A:

   a. What is the function of structures B and Q?

      _____

      _____

      _____

   b. What is the function of structures C and N?

      _____

      _____

      _____

   c. What is the function of structure E?

      _____

      _____

      _____

   d. What is the function of structure M?

      _____

      _____

      _____

4. Identify each of the structures in Fig. 16.1B using the terms provided.

Right atrium	Papillary muscle	Brachioce-phalic trunk	Myocardium
Aorta	Inferior vena cava	Left pulmonary artery	Left pulmonary veins
Left ventricle	Arch of aorta	Right pulmonary veins	Pulmonary semilunar valve
Chordae tendineae	Tricuspid valve	Pulmonary artery trunk	Interventricular septum
Superior vena cava	Aortic semilunar valve	Left atrium	Left common carotid artery
Bicuspid (mitral) valve	Right ventricle	Left subclavian artery	Right pulmonary artery

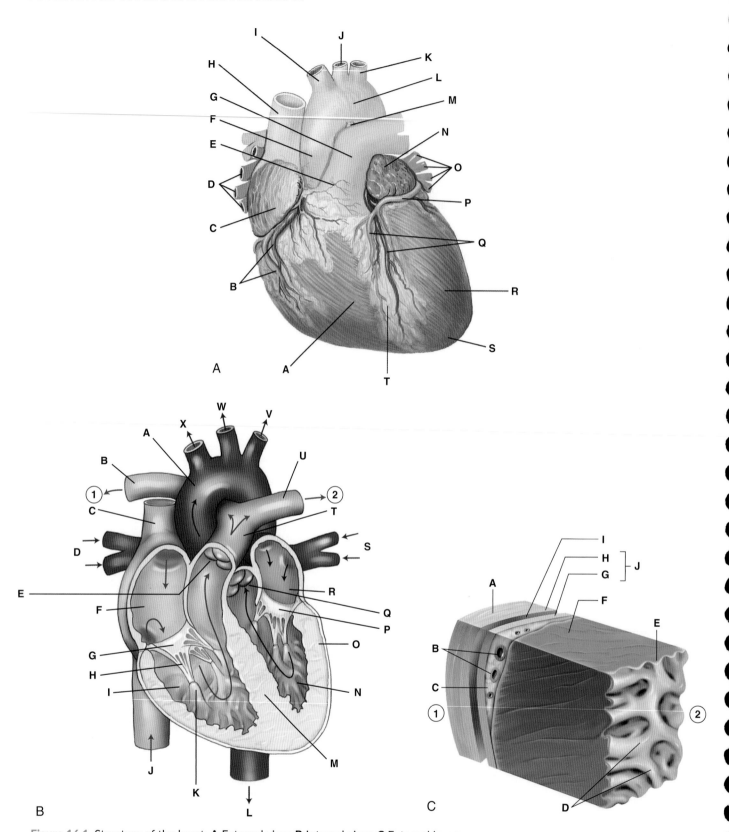

Figure 16.1 Structure of the heart. **A** External view. **B** Internal view. **C** External layers.
(*Source:* **A** *Rothrock, J. C. (2019). Alexander's care of the patient in surgery. Elsevier.* **B** *Shiland, B. J. (2018). Mastering healthcare terminology. Elsevier.* **C** *Patton, K. T., Thibodeau, G. A., & Hutton, A. (2016). Anatomy and physiology. Elsevier.*)

a. Structure A: _____

b. Structure B: _____

c. Structure C: _____

d. Structure D: _____

e. Structure E: _____

f. Structure F: _____

g. Structure G: _____

h. Structure H: _____

i. Structure I: _____

j. Structure J: _____

k. Structure K: _____

l. Structure L: _____

m. Structure M: _____

n. Structure N: _____

o. Structure O: _____

p. Structure P: _____

q. Structure Q: _____

r. Structure R: _____

s. Structure S: _____

t. Structure T: _____

u. Structure U: _____

v. Structure V: _____

w. Structure W: _____

x. Structure X: _____

5. Consider the following questions, with reference to Fig. 16.1B:

a. What is the destination of the blood in structure 1?

_____

b. From which structure did the blood in structure 1 arise?

_____

c. What is the destination of the blood in structure 2?

_____

d. From which structure did the blood in structure 2 arise?

_____

e. In order, list the structures of the right side of the heart through which blood flows.

_____

_____

_____

f. In order, the structures of the left side of the heart through which blood flows.

_____

_____

_____

g. What is the source of the blood in structure C?

_____

h. What is the destination of the blood in structures D and S?

_____

i. What is the function of structures E, G, P and Q?

_____

_____

_____

j. Which blood circuit would be affected if structure G failed to operate effectively? Suggest a reason based on the structure of G.

_____

_____

_____

k. Which blood circuit would be affected if structure P failed to operate effectively? Suggest a reason based on the structure of P.

_____

_____

_____

l. What is the function of structures F and R?

_____

_____

_____

m. What is the function of structure H?

_____

_____

_____

n. What is the function of structures I and N?

_____

_____

_____

o. What is the source of the blood in structure J?

_____

p. What is the function of structure K?

_____

_____

_____

q. What is the destination of the blood in structure L?

_____

r. What is the function of structure M?

_____

_____

_____

s. What is the destination of the blood in structure T?

_____

t. Where are the base and apex of the heart located?

_____

_____

_____

6. Identify each of the structures in Fig. 16.1C using the terms provided.

Epicardium	Pericardial space	Trabeculae carneae	Parietal layer
Serous pericardium	Adipose tissue	Endocardium	Coronary vessels
	Myocardium	Fibrous pericardium	

a. Structure A: _____

b. Structure B: _____

c. Structure C: _____

d. Structure D: _____

e. Structure E: _____

f. Structure F: _____

g. Structure G: _____

h. Structure H: _____

i. Structure I: _____

j. Structure J: _____

7. Consider the following questions with reference to Fig. 16.1C:

a. The surface at number 1 faces which body structures?

_____

b. The surface at number 2 faces which body structures?

_____

c. What is the function of structure A?

_____

_____

d. What is the function of structure B?

_____

_____

e. What is the function of structure C?

_____

_____

f. What is the function of structure D?

_____

_____

g. What is the function of structure E?

_____

_____

h. What is the function of structure F?

_____

_____

i. What is the composition and arrangement of structure F within the heart?

_____

_____

_____

j. What is the function of structure G?

_____

_____

k. What is the function of structure H

_____

_____

l. What is found within structure I and what is its function?

_____

_____

_____

m. What is the function of structure J?

_____

_____

Apply the Concepts

1. Is there any mixing of blood in the heart? Suggest a reason for this.

_____

_____

_____

2. What is pericarditis and how does it occur?

_____

_____

_____

3. Is there a distinction between coronary artery disease and coronary heart disease? Explain.

_____

_____

_____

4. What is rheumatic heart disease and how does it occur?

_____

_____

_____

5. What is myocardial infarction (MI) and how does it occur?

_____

_____

_____

6. How is myocardial infarction diagnosed chemically?

_____

_____

_____

Additional Activities

For additional activities visit Activity 16A: Blood Circuits and Circulation on Evolve˙.

For additional activities visit Activity 16B: Examination of Heart Structure (Heart Dissection) on Evolve˙.

ACTIVITY 16.2: STRUCTURE AND FUNCTION OF THE BLOOD VESSELS

The blood vessels form a closed blood delivery system (Fig. 16.2). Vessels that diverge from the heart are **arteries** and **arterioles**, and vessels that converge towards the heart are **venules** and **veins**. These vessels distribute and collect blood, but do not directly serve the requirements of the tissue cells. **Capillaries** have an intimate association with the tissue cells, forming beds within organs to increase the surface area for diffusion and exchange of substances (Fig. 16.3). All blood vessels are composed of concentric tissue layers, or tunics, of varying composition and thickness related to the functions of the vessel.

This activity outlines the structure and function of the blood vessels.

1. Identify each of the blood vessels, their functions, and the associated numbered structures in Fig. 16.2:

   a. Vessel A: _____

      i. Function: _____

      ii. Structure 1: _____

      iii. Structure 2: _____

      iv. Structure 3: _____

   b. Vessel B: _____

      i. Function: _____

      ii. Structure 1: _____

   iii. Structure 2: _____

   iv. Structure 3: _____

   c. Vessel C: _____

      i. Function: _____

      ii. Structure 1: _____

      iii. Structure 2: _____

   d. Vessel D: _____

      i. Function: _____

      ii. Structure 1: _____

      iii. Structure 2: _____

      iv. Structure 3: _____

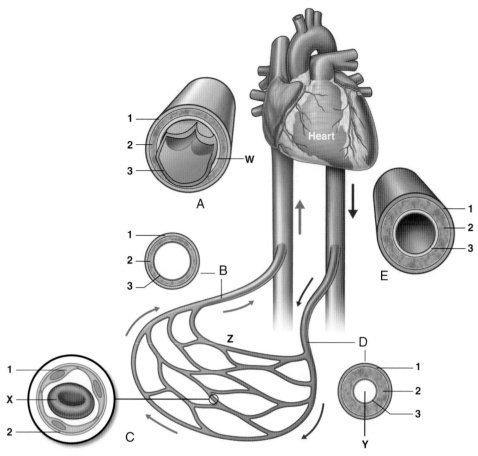

Figure 16.2 Structure of the blood vessels.
(Source: Waugh, A., & Grant, A. (2014). Ross & Wilson anatomy and physiology in health and illness. Elsevier.)

e. Vessel E: _____

   i. Function: _____

   ii. Structure 1: _____

   iii. Structure 2: _____

   iv. Structure 3: _____

2. Consider the following questions, with reference to Fig. 16.2:

  a. Starting from the heart, trace the flow of blood through the vessels that form the vascular system.

  _____

  _____

  _____

b. What is the function of structure 1 in vessels A, B, D and E?

  _____

  _____

  _____

c. What is the composition of structure 1 in vessels A, B, D and E?

  _____

  _____

d. What is the function of structure 2 in vessels A, B, D and E?

  _____

  _____

  _____

e. What is the composition of structure 2 in vessels A, B, D and E?

_____

_____

_____

f. Increased sympathetic stimulation of structure 2 in vessels A, B, D and E will have what effect?

_____

_____

_____

g. Decreased sympathetic stimulation of structure 2 in vessels A, B, D and E will have what effect?

_____

_____

_____

h. What is the function of structure 3 in vessels A, B, D and E?

_____

_____

_____

i. What is the composition of structure 3 in vessels A, B, D and E?

_____

_____

j. Vessels A and E contain structures referred to as the nervi vasorum. What are these structures, in which layer are they located, and what is their function?

_____

_____

_____

k. Vessels A and E contain structures referred to as the vasa vasorum. What are these structures, in which layer are they located, and what is their function?

_____

_____

_____

l. Vessel C is composed of two layers. Explain how this aids the function of this vessel but can also impede haemostasis.

_____

_____

_____

m. What is structure W and what is the function of this structure?

_____

_____

_____

n. Why is structure W found in this type of blood vessel?

_____

_____

_____

o. What is structure X? What does the comparative size of structure X indicate about the diameter of vessel C?

_____

_____

_____

p. What is structure Y and what is contained there?

_____

_____

_____

q. What is structure Z? Which blood vessels form this structure and what is its function?

_____

_____

_____

r. Explain how blood leaking from structure Z is recaptured by the circulation.

_____

_____

_____

s. Why are veins referred to as capacitance vessels?

_____

_____

_____

3. Identify each of the capillary types, their structure, their function, and their location in Fig. 16.3:

  a. Capillary A: _____

    i. Structure: _____

    ii. Function: _____

    iii. Location: _____

  b. Capillary B: _____

    i. Structure: _____

    ii. Function: _____

    iii. Location: _____

  c. Capillary C: _____

    i. Structure: _____

    ii. Function: _____

    iii. Location: _____

4. Consider the following questions, with reference to Fig. 16.3:

  a. What is structure A and what is its function?

    _____

    _____

    _____

b. What is structure B and what is its function?

    _____

    _____

    _____

c. What is structure C and what is its function?

    _____

    _____

    _____

d. What is structure D and what is its function?

    _____

    _____

    _____

e. What is structure E and what is its function?

    _____

    _____

    _____

f. What is structure F and what is its function?

    _____

    _____

    _____

g. How do luminal cells of capillaries and blood vessels receive nutrition?

    _____

    _____

    _____

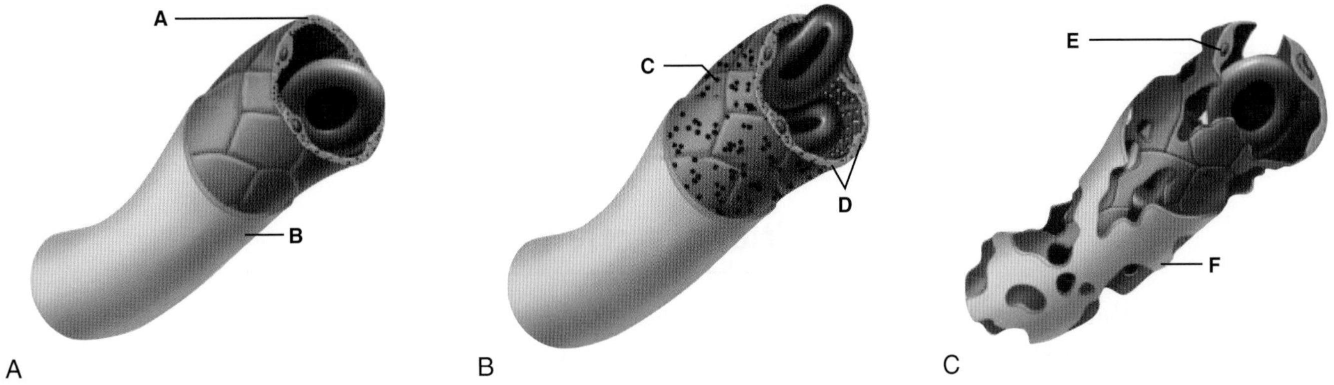

Figure 16.3 Types of capillaries.
(Source: Craft, J., Gordon, C., Huether, S. E., McCance, K. L., & Brashers, V. L. (2019). Understanding pathophysiology – ANZ adaptation. Elsevier Australia.)

h. A capillary bed is also referred to by which other term?

_____

_____

_____

i. Which types of capillary form beds within tissues and organs?

_____

_____

_____

j. How is blood flow through a capillary bed regulated by arterioles?

_____

_____

_____

k. Which tissues do not have a capillary supply?

_____

_____

_____

Apply the Concepts

1. How many types of arteries exist and how do they differ in their structure and function?

_____

_____

_____

2. How many types of veins exist and how do they differ in their structure and function?

_____

_____

_____

3. What is perfusion and how is this process achieved within capillary beds?

_____

_____

_____

4. What is ischaemia and how does it occur?

_____

_____

_____

Additional Activities

For additional activities visit Activity 16C: Identification of Heart and Blood Vessel Structures on Evolve®.

For additional activities visit Activity 16D: Microscopic Examination of the Heart and Blood Vessels on Evolve®.

For additional activities visit Activity 16E: Cardiac Conduction System and the Electrocardiogram (ECG) on Evolve®.

ACTIVITY 16.3: THE CARDIAC CYCLE AND PULSE

The cardiac cycle involves the continuous cycling of blood through the heart. This is accompanied by pressure and volume changes as the atria and ventricles empty and fill with blood and involves the contraction and relaxation of the heart myocardium. In addition, the actions of the atrioventricular valves and semilunar valves, which can be heard as the heart sounds, ensure that blood flows through the heart in one direction, preventing backflow.

This activity provides an overview of the cardiac cycle and demonstrates the heart sounds, heart rate, and palpating, observing and measuring pulse.

Part 1: The Cardiac Cycle

The pressure changes accompanying the emptying and filling of the atria and ventricles signify the **systolic** and **diastolic** phases of the cardiac cycle (Fig. 16.4) by which blood is pumped through the circulatory system. The blood exerts force against blood vessel walls which can be monitored and measured as **blood pressure (BP).**

1. What is the cardiac cycle?

   _____

   _____

   _____

2. To what does the term systole refer?

   _____

   _____

   _____

3. To what does the term diastole refer?

   _____

   _____

   _____

4. Identify each of the stages of the cardiac cycle in Fig. 16.4 and outline the events occurring in each stage in relation to the opening or closing of the heart valves, blood flow and pressure within the heart, and heart activity based on contraction and relaxation.

   a. Stage 1: _____

      i. Valves: _____

      ii. Blood flow: _____

      iii. Pressure: _____

      iv. Heart activity: _____

   b. Stage 2: _____

      i. Valves: _____

      ii. Blood flow: _____

      iii. Pressure: _____

      iv. Heart activity: _____

   c. Stage 3: _____

      i. Valves: _____

      ii. Blood flow: _____

      iii. Pressure: _____

      iv. Heart activity: _____

   d. Stage 4: _____

      i. Valves: _____

      ii. Blood flow: _____

      iii. Pressure: _____

      iv. Heart activity: _____

   e. Stage 5: _____

      i. Valves: _____

      ii. Blood flow: _____

      iii. Pressure: _____

      iv. Heart activity: _____

5. Consider the following questions, with reference to Fig. 16.4:

   a. What do the arrows at stage 1 indicate?

      _____

      _____

371

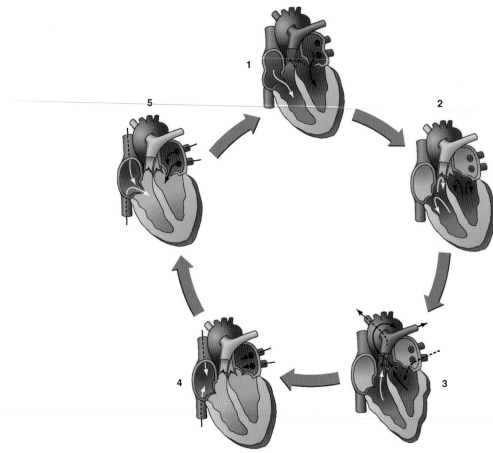

Figure 16.4 The cardiac cycle.
(Source: Hazinski, M. F. (2013). Nursing care of the critically ill child. Elsevier.)

b. What do the arrows at stage 2 indicate?

_____

_____

c. Stage 2 is also referred to as isovolumetric contraction. Explain this process further.

_____

_____

_____

d. What do the arrows at stage 3 indicate?

_____

_____

_____

e. What do the arrows at stage 4 indicate?

_____

_____

_____

f. Stage 4 is also referred to as isovolumetric relaxation. Explain this process further.

_____

_____

_____

g. Explain the absence of arrows in the ventricles in stage 4.

_____

_____

h. What do the arrows at stage 5 indicate?

_____

_____

_____

Part 2: Auscultating Heart Sounds and Determining Heart Rate

The sounds that accompany the cardiac cycle, often described as lub-dub sounds, can be auscultated or heard externally over various regions of the thorax, relating to the locations of the atrioventricular valves and semilunar valves (Fig. 16.5). The timing of these sounds provides an indication of the duration of the various phases of the cardiac cycle, and allows determination of the **heart rate**, or the number of heart beats per minute.

1. This activity is best conducted in pairs.

2. Obtain a human subject, a stethoscope, some alcohol swabs and a stopwatch.

3. Heart sounds are best auscultated if the subject's outer clothing is removed, so a male subject may be preferable.

4. Clean the earpieces of the stethoscope with the alcohol swabs.

5. Place the earpieces into your ears. Note that the earpieces are angled. For comfort, the earpieces should be angled in a forward direction when placed in the ears.

6. Place the diaphragm of the stethoscope on the subject's thorax, just medial to the left nipple at the fifth intercostal space.

   a. What is located in this region?

   _____

7. Listen carefully for heart sounds.

8. Once located, count the number of pulse beats for 15 seconds.

9. Multiply the number of beats in 15 seconds by 4. This gives the heart rate in beats per minute.

10. Record your observations in the table provided.

11. Continue auscultating heart sounds, calculating the heart rate based on the different areas of the thorax auscultated as indicated in Fig. 16.5, and recording your observations in the table provided.

Area of auscultation	Number of beats (15 seconds)	Heart rate (bpm)
Tricuspid valve		
Aortic valve		
Pulmonary valve		
Mitral valve		

12. Consider the following questions:

    a. In which area of auscultation were heart sounds most audible?

    _____

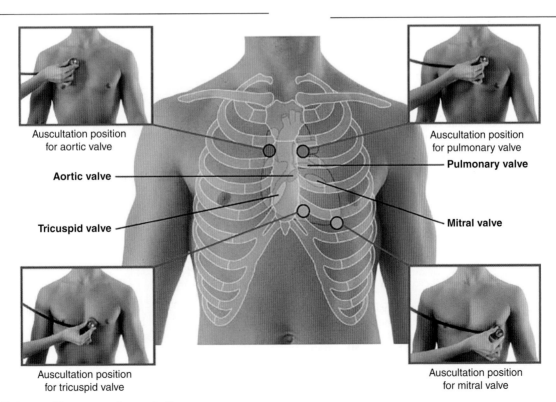

Auscultation position for aortic valve

Aortic valve

Tricuspid valve

Auscultation position for tricuspid valve

Auscultation position for pulmonary valve

Pulmonary valve

Mitral valve

Auscultation position for mitral valve

Figure 16.5 Areas of heart sound auscultation.
(*Source: Piano, M. R., & Law, W. R. (2008). Cardiac nursing: A companion to Braunwald's heart disease. Elsevier.*)

b. Was the heart rate the same in all locations?

_____

_____

c. What causes the heart sounds?

_____

_____

d. How are the heart sounds typically described?

_____

_____

e. Do the heart sounds sound the same?

_____

_____

f. How can the heart sounds be distinguished?

_____

_____

_____

g. The heart sounds are also referred to as S1 and S2 sounds. To what do these sounds relate?

_____

_____

h. What function do the heart valves serve?

_____

_____

i. Are the atrioventricular valves able to invert into the atria? Explain.

_____

_____

_____

Part 3: Palpating the Pulse

The **pulse** occurs as a result of the expansion and recoil of the arteries due to the beating of the heart. The pulse may be felt easily on any artery close to the body surface when the artery is compressed over a bone or other firm tissue (Fig. 16.6).

1. This activity is best conducted in pairs, but can also be conducted on yourself.

2. Obtain a human subject, a chair and a stopwatch.

3. Ask the subject to sit in the chair without moving.

4. Select a body site for palpating a regional artery from Fig. 16.6.

5. To palpate the pulse, place the fingertips of the first two fingers of one hand over the artery until throbbing can be felt (you should never use the thumb when measuring an individual's pulse as the thumb has a faint pulse of its own).

6. Count the pulse for 15 seconds and record your result in the table provided.

7. Calculate the pulse rate in beats per minute by multiplying the pulse by 4 and record your result in the table provided.

8. Assess the force of the pulse and record this in the table provided.

9. Repeat this procedure for each of the body sites indicated in Fig. 16.6, recording your results in the table provided.

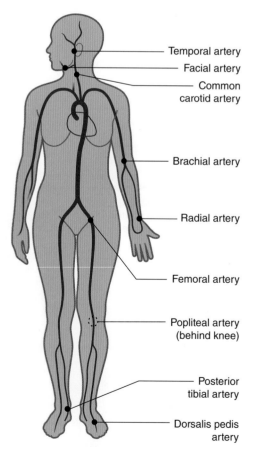

Figure 16.6 Body sites for palpating the pulse.
(*Source: Waugh, A., & Grant, A. (2014). Ross & Wilson anatomy and physiology in health and illness. Elsevier.*)

Artery palpated	Force strength (1 = weak; 5 = strong)	Number of pulses (30 seconds)	Pulse rate (bpm)
Temporal artery			
Facial artery			
Carotid artery			
Brachial artery			
Radial artery			
Femoral artery			
Popliteal artery			
Posterior tibial artery			
Dorsalis pedis artery			

10. Consider the following questions:

a. Which pulse point had the greatest force?

_____

b. Which pulse point had the least force?

_____

c. What is the explanation for this?

_____

_____

d. What do the results indicate about the blood vessels used for taking pulse?

_____

_____

_____

e. What is pulse?

_____

f. Is heart rate the same as pulse rate? Explain.

_____

_____

_____

g. Suggest a reason for discrepancies in pulse rate determined by palpation and heart rate determined by ECG.

_____

_____

_____

h. What is the typical heart rate for adults?

_____

i. How is heart rate regulated?

_____

_____

_____

Part 4: Observing and Measuring Pulse

In many cases, the pulse that occurs as a result of the expansion and recoil of the arteries due to the beating of the heart can be observed visually in peripheral blood vessels. This allows for the pulse to be measured through simple observation.

1. This activity is best conducted in pairs, but can also be conducted on yourself.

2. Obtain a human subject, a small ball of plasticine, a toothpick, stopwatch, electronic blood pressure monitor and an exercise bike.

3. Flatten the ball of plasticine and stand the toothpick in the middle of the ball.

4. To observe the pulse at rest in the seated position, relax the subject's arm and rest their hand on the table.

5. Balance the plasticine ball on the inside of the subject's wrist where the pulse can be felt and note your observations.

a. Are you able to see the toothpick move?

_____

6. Count how many times the toothpick moves in 15 seconds with the stopwatch and record your observations in the table provided.

7. Multiply this reading by 4 to obtain beats per minute and record your observations in the table provided.

8. Take the subject's pulse rate with the electronic blood pressure monitor and record your observations in the table provided.

9. Repeat the process this time asking the subject to stand up and observe the pulse with the same wrist facing upward, recording your observations in the table provided.

10. Repeat the process this time asking the subject to complete 2 minutes of exercise on the exercise bike.

11. Once the 2 minutes have elapsed, observe the pulse with the same wrist facing upward, recording your observations in the table provided.

Pulse taken	Manual pulses (15 seconds)	Manual pulse rate (bpm)	Electronic pulse rate (bpm)
Seated			
Standing			
Exercise			

12. Consider the following questions:

a. Explain why the toothpick could be seen moving.

_____

_____

b. Were any differences observed in the pulse rate between the seated, standing and exercise conditions?

_____

c. Provide a possible explanation for any differences noted between conditions.

_____

_____

_____

d. Did the electronic pulse rate match the manual pulse rate? Explain.

_____

_____

_____

Apply the Concepts

1. What are S3 and S4 heart sounds or gallops, and how do they occur?

_____

_____

_____

2. What is tachycardia and how does it occur?

_____

_____

_____

3. What is bradycardia and how does it occur?

_____

_____

_____

4. What is a heart murmur and how does it occur?

_____

_____

_____

5. What is asystole?

_____

_____

_____

Additional Activities

For additional activities visit Activity 16F: Factors Affecting Blood Pressure on Evolve˙.

For additional activities visit Activity 16G: Volume, Pressure, and Flow Relationships on Evolve˙.

ACTIVITY 16.4: FACTORS AFFECTING RESISTANCE

Blood flow (mL/min) through vessels is related to the driving pressure (mmHg) and the resistive factors affecting flow (mmHg/mL/min). The pressure gradient assists flow, whereas resistance opposes flow. The main factors contributing to resistance within the cardiovascular system are blood viscosity, vascular diameter and vascular length. These factors have implications for blood circulation, principally in the veins returning blood to the heart under decreased blood pressure and against gravity.

This activity demonstrates the factors affecting resistance associated with blood circulation.

Part 1: Blood Viscosity

The viscosity or thickness of the blood is affected by the concentrations of cellular elements, plasma proteins and water. The viscosity of the blood determines how easily the blood's components can move past each other, affecting blood flow. As viscosity increases, resistance increases and blood flow decreases. The opposite occurs as blood viscosity decreases.

1. These activities are best conducted in pairs or groups of four.

2. Obtain three 100 mL measuring cylinders, one 250 mL beaker, deionised water, glycerine (or corn syrup), red food colouring, stirrer, three 5-cent coins (or marbles, metal bolts), glass marker and a stopwatch.

3. Label the measuring cylinders 1 to 3 with the glass marker.

4. Pour 100 mL deionised water into the beaker, add 4 drops of food colouring, and ensure that the solution is well mixed with the stirrer.

5. Pour this solution into the measuring cylinder labelled 1. This is solution 1.

6. Pour 50 mL deionised water and 50 mL glycerine into the beaker.

   Add 4 drops of food colouring, and ensure that the solution is well mixed with the stirrer.

7. Pour this solution into the measuring cylinder labelled 2. This is solution 2.

8. Pour 100 mL glycerine into the beaker, add 4 drops food colouring, and ensure that the solution is well mixed with the stirrer.

9. Pour this solution into the measuring cylinder labelled 3. This is solution 3.

10. Drop one coin into each cylinder, using the stopwatch to record the time taken for each coin to fall to the bottom of the cylinder.

11. Note your results below:

    a. Time taken in solution 1 (100% water):

    _____

    b. Time taken in solution 2 (50% water and 50% glycerine):

    _____

    c. Time taken in solution 3 (100% glycerine):

    _____

12. Retain the solutions for the experiments that follow.

13. Consider the following questions:

    a. Compare the times taken for the coins to fall between solutions.

    _____

    b. Is viscosity related to density? Explain.

    _____

    _____

    _____

    c. How does blood viscosity affect resistance?

    _____

    _____

    d. What factors affect blood viscosity?

    _____

    _____

    e. How does blood viscosity affect blood flow?

    _____

    _____

    f. How does blood viscosity affect blood pressure?

    _____

    _____

    g. Is blood flow through the vascular lumen slower in the centre of the vessel or towards the vascular walls? Explain.

    _____

    _____

Part 2: Vascular Diameter

Vascular diameter is affected by a number of factors including the actions of adrenaline, noradrenaline, antidiuretic hormone, and angiotensin II. These act on smooth muscle of the vascular tunica media, and can cause **vasodilation**, widening of the vessel, or **vasoconstriction**, narrowing of the vessel. As the diameter of the blood vessel increases, the blood encounters less of the internal vascular surface, resistance decreases and blood flow increases. The opposite occurs as vessel diameter decreases.

1. Obtain solution 2 from Part 1, a retort stand, a boss head clamp, 50 mL burette, 1 mL disposable pipette, 3 mL disposable pipette, metric ruler (mm), scissors, 250 mL beaker and a stopwatch.

2. Attach the clamp to the retort stand and place the burette into the clamp, securing the burette end approximately 12 cm from the retort stand base.

3. Ensure that the tap at the bottom of the burette is in the closed position.

4. Place the funnel into the top of the burette and pour 50 mL of solution 2 into the funnel, allowing it to settle in the burette.

5. Cut both disposable pipettes 3.5 cm from the tip with the scissors.

6. Attach the 1 mL pipette (diameter 1) to the burette tip and place the beaker underneath, ensuring that the pipette is situated above the beaker.

7. Dispense 10 mL of solution into the beaker, recording the time taken for the volume of fluid to empty into the beaker.

8. Repeat this process with the 3 mL pipette (diameter 2).

9. Note your results below:

    a. Time taken for diameter 1: _____

    b. Time taken for diameter 2: _____

10. Retain this set-up for the experiment that follows.

11. Consider the following questions:

    a. Compare the times taken for the fluid to drain through the different tube diameters.

    _____

    _____

    b. How does vascular diameter affect resistance?

    _____

    _____

c. What factors affect vascular diameter?

_____

_____

_____

d. How does vascular diameter affect blood flow?

_____

_____

e. How does vascular diameter affect blood pressure?

_____

_____

Part 3: Vascular Length

Vascular length is affected mainly by the size of an individual, as this will determine the length of the vessels required to distribute blood throughout the body. For example, children have a smaller body size and require shorter blood vessels to supply that size, so a child's vascular resistance is likely to be less than that of an adult. As the length of a blood vessel increases, resistance increases because blood encounters greater internal vascular surface area, and blood flow decreases. The opposite occurs as vessel length decreases.

1. Retain the set-up and materials from Part 2 and obtain 3 plastic (or silicone) drinking straws (0.5 cm diameter).

2. Top up the fluid in the burette with solution 2 to 50 mL.

3. Cut the drinking straws to 6 cm, 12 cm, and 18 cm lengths with the scissors.

4. Attach the 6cm straw length (length 1) to the burette tip and place the beaker underneath, ensuring that the straw is situated above the beaker.

5. Dispense 10 mL of solution into the beaker, recording the time taken for the fluid to empty into the beaker.

6. Repeat this process with the 12 cm (length 2) and 18 cm (length 3) lengths.

7. Note your results below:

   a. Time taken for Length 1 (6 cm): _____

   b. Time taken for Length 2 (12 cm): _____

   c. Time taken for Length 3 (18 cm): _____

8. Consider the following questions:

   a. Compare the times taken for the fluid to drain through the different lengths of tube.

   _____

   _____

   b. How does vascular length affect resistance?

   _____

   c. What factors affect vascular length?

   _____

   d. How does vascular length affect blood flow?

   _____

   _____

   e. How does vascular length affect blood pressure?

   _____

   _____

Part 4: Blood Viscosity, Flow, and Gravity

Increasing blood viscosity causes an increase in resistance, reducing the flow of blood through blood vessels. This presents a special problem in the venous system, which carries blood at reduced pressure due to resistance already encountered in the arteries, arterioles and capillaries. During extended periods of sitting or standing, in particular, blood of low pressure and flow must return to the heart against gravity. Reducing blood viscosity, amongst other measures, can assist with venous return.

1. Obtain a dimple tile, deionised water, glycerine, red food colouring, 2 disposable pipettes, toothpicks, pencil, metric ruler (mm), thin layer chromatography plate (5 cm × 8 cm), 3 microhaematocrit tubes, a jar or container with lid, chromatography mobile phase fluid and paper towels.

2. Pour approximately 0.5 cm of chromatography fluid into the container and close the lid.

3. Place the dimple tile on a paper towel.

4. Place 5 drops of glycerine into each of three separate dimples on the tile.

5. Add 1 drop of food colouring to each pool of glycerine.

6. To dimple 1, add 8 drops of water. This is sample 1.

7. To dimple 2, add 4 drops of water. This is sample 2.

8. To dimple 3, do not add water. This is sample 3.

9. Gently stir each sample in the dimples with a separate toothpick until well mixed.

10. Place the thin layer chromatography (TLC) plate on a paper towel, so that the plate is aligned in portrait mode.

11. Gently rule a line 1 cm from the bottom of the plate with the pencil, and mark three evenly distributed points across the line, leaving a margin of approximately 0.5 cm from the edges of the plate. Number these points 1, 2 and 3.

12. Using a microhaematocrit tube, dab enough of sample 1 onto the TLC plate at point 1 so that a circle of approximately 0.5 cm diameter is formed.

13. Repeat the process with samples 2 and 3 at points 2 and 3, using new microhaematocrit tubes to prevent contamination.

14. Place the TLC plate into the chamber with the fluid so that base of the plate where the samples are located is sitting in the fluid (the fluid should not be touching the sample circles).

15. Close the lid to prevent evaporation and wait approximately 10–15 minutes, or until the samples have progressed halfway up the plate.

16. Once the time has elapsed, remove the plate from the fluid to a paper towel.

17. Consider the following questions:

   a. Which sample travelled more completely up the TLC plate?

   _____

   b. Suggest a reason for this observation.

   _____

   _____

c. Imagine the samples represent blood. Which sample would be most likely to represent a state of dehydration?

   _____

d. Imagine the samples represent blood. Which samples would be most likely to experience greater resistance against the walls of a blood vessel?

   _____

e. Imagine the TLC plate represents a vein returning blood from the feet to the heart. What implications do the results have in terms of venous blood return?

   _____

   _____

   _____

f. What implications do the results have in terms of cardiac function?

   _____

   _____

g. Excluding dehydration, what type of medication may be prescribed for an individual with blood similar to sample 3?

   _____

h. How is blood flow intrinsically and extrinsically controlled?

   _____

   _____

   _____

Apply the Concepts

1. What is laminar flow and how does it affect blood flow within blood vessels?

_____

_____

_____

2. What is preload and afterload?

_____

_____

_____

3. What is cor pulmonale and how does it occur?

_____

_____

_____

4. Is there a distinction between right-sided and left-sided heart failure? Explain.

_____

_____

_____

ACTIVITY 16.5: VENOUS BLOOD RETURN

A number of physiological factors aid the return of venous blood to the heart. In the absence of these factors, venous blood, which has experienced a greater amount of resistance, has a low pressure and often flows against gravity, would remain within the veins for longer as flow is reduced. This would increase the likelihood of blood clot (thrombus) formation, slow venous return and the potential obstruction of blood flow completely.

This activity demonstrates the actions of skeletal muscle and venous valves on venous blood return against gravity.

Part 1: Skeletal Muscle and Venous Blood Return Against Gravity

Deep veins located in the lower limbs are situated between skeletal muscles and cannot be observed externally, as can superficial veins. Since blood within veins experiences low pressure and is often returned to the heart against gravity, the actions of skeletal muscle contraction during walking and other movements presses on the embedded veins, assisting venous return.

1. This activity is best conducted individually or in pairs.

2. Obtain a plastic (or silicone) drinking straw (0.5 cm diameter), metric ruler (mm), scissors, plasticine, 3 small foldback clips, 50% glycerine solution coloured red and 1 mL disposable pipette.

3. Cut the straw with the scissors so that it measures 18 cm.

4. Plug one end of the straw with plasticine so that the end is completely sealed.

5. Gently fill the straw with the glycerine solution using the disposable pipette until the straw is half-filled with solution.

6. Holding the straw in one hand, gently squeeze the solution up the straw with your fingers, from the bottom of the straw.

7. Once you have moved the solution up the straw by approximately 2 cm, quickly attach a foldback clip to the straw in that location while your fingers are still squeezing the straw.

8. Release the straw with your fingers and note the action of the solution within the straw.

9. Repeat this process two more times, noting the action of the solution within the straw.

10. Consider the following questions:

   a. The solution in the straw represents which cardiovascular structure?

   _____

   b. The straw represents which cardiovascular structure?

   _____

   c. The foldback clips represent which vascular structures?

   _____

   d. The squeezing action of your fingers on the straw represents which physiological process?

   _____

   e. Was solution present in the spaces between the foldback clips and how does this relate to blood within veins?

   _____

   _____

   _____

   f. Based on your observations, are the actions of venous valves and skeletal muscle contraction sufficient to propel blood through the veins against gravity? Suggest an additional mechanism that assists venous return within the body.

   _____

   _____

   _____

Part 2: Venous Valves and Venous Blood Return Against Gravity

Venous valves, much like the atrioventricular valves and semilunar valves of the heart, enforce a one-way flow of blood through the venous system. They are formed as folds originating from the tunica intima and project into the venous lumen. They are most abundant in the veins of the lower limbs, where blood experiencing small pressure gradients is returned towards the heart against gravity. Venous valves are assisted in their function by the actions of skeletal muscles.

1. This activity is best conducted in pairs.

2. Obtain a human subject and a stopwatch.

3. Allow the subject's dominant arm to hang to the side of their body.

4. Wait for 60 seconds or until the blood vessels on the dorsal aspect of the hand distend with blood.

5. Place two fingers against one of the distended veins while the arm is still hanging to the side of the body.

6. Press firmly upwards along the vein towards the wrist, keeping your fingers in place.

   a. What effect did this have on the vein?

   _____

   b. Relate your observations to the effect of gravity on blood flow in the vein.

   _____

7. Remove your fingers from the vein.

   a. What effect did this have on the vein?

   _____

   b. From where did this blood flow?

   _____

   c. In which direction did the blood flow?

   _____

   d. What do the results indicate about how blood is assisted to flow against gravity?

   _____

8. Consider the following questions:

   a. Identify and explain three factors that aid venous return to the heart.

   _____

   _____

   _____

   _____

   _____

   _____

   b. Identify two locations within the body where venous valves are absent and suggest a reason why.

   _____

   _____

   _____

Apply the Concepts

1. What are varicose veins and how do they occur?

   _____

   _____

   _____

2. What are haemorrhoids and how do they occur?

   _____

   _____

   _____

3. What is deep vein thrombosis (DVT) and how does it occur?

   _____

   _____

   _____

4. What is phlebotomy?

   _____

   _____

   _____

5. What is phlebitis and how does it occur?

   _____

   _____

   _____

Additional Activities

For additional activities visit Activity 16H: Cardiac Output, Mean Arterial Pressure, and Cardiovascular Response to Exercise on Evolve®.

Additional Resources

Atlas of Human Cardiac Anatomy

The Atlas of Human Cardiac Anatomy is a resource providing access to virtual models and information relating to heart anatomy and physiology, including 3-D models and plastinates, as well as tutorials relating to cardiac anatomy, physiology, MRIs and ECGs.

www.vhlab.umn.edu/atlas/index.shtml

Cardiovascular Physiology Concepts

This Cardiovascular Physiology Concepts site provides materials related to the physiology of the cardiovascular system that serve as the basis for cardiovascular disease, and has been specifically designed for students, physicians, allied health professionals and educators.

www.cvphysiology.com/Intro

ECG and Echo Learning

The ECG and Echo Learning resource provides access to a number of resources related to electrocardiography and echocardiography and contains options for registration, ebooks, test interpretation, progress tracking and results.

ecgwaves.com/

GetBodySmart: Circulatory System

GetBodySmart presents fully animated, illustrated and interactive eBooks about human anatomy and physiology body systems.

www.getbodysmart.com/circulatory-system

Gizmos: Circulatory System

An interactive simulation with lesson materials where users trace the flow of blood through a beating heart, observe the network of blood vessels, and analyse blood samples from different blood vessels for metabolic substances.

gizmos.explorelearning.com/index.cfm?method5cResource.dspDetail&resourceID5662

Histology Guide Virtual Microscopy Laboratory: Cardiovascular System

Histology Guide is an online resource providing a virtual microscopy laboratory experience, by allowing users to view microscope slides from professional collections for the purpose of interpreting cellular and tissue structures as seen through a microscope.

https://histologyguide.com/slidebox/09-cardiovascular-system.html

Innerbody Research: Cardiovascular System

Innerbody Research provides objective, science-based advice to help readers make more informed choices about home health products and services with most up-to-date reviews, guides and research, including information about the cardiovascular system.

www.innerbody.com/image/cardov.html

Osmosis – Cardiovascular System

The Cardiovascular System module of Osmosis provides videos, notes, quiz questions, and links to further resources related to the anatomy, physiology, and conditions of the cardiovascular system.

www.osmosis.org/library/md/organ-systems/cardiovascular-system/physiology/electrocardiography/introduction-to-electrocardiography

The Histology Guide: Circulatory System

The Histology Guide is a virtual experience of using a microscope with zoom features divided into topics and offering histological slides with labels and quizzes for each topic, such as the circulatory system. It is provided by the University of Leeds.

www.histology.leeds.ac.uk/circulatory/index.php

Visible Body: Circulatory System

Visible Body provides interactive and highly accurate visualisations and apps for learning and teaching anatomy and physiology for students and healthcare professionals, including body systems such as the circulatory system.

www.visiblebody.com/learn/circulatory

CHAPTER 17
The Respiratory System

The function of the respiratory system is to exchange the gases required and produced by tissue cells as a result of cell metabolism and ATP production. (Refer to Chapter 6: Cells and Metabolism, for further information on cell function and ATP production.) The respiratory system consists of a series of passageways of the conducting zone which filter, humidify and warm inhaled air before it enters the respiratory zone for gas exchange within the lungs. Breathing, or inspiration and expiration, is maintained through the coordinated contraction of the diaphragm and intercostal muscles, achieved via the nervous system, which adjusts thoracic volume and intrapulmonary pressures, causing the flow of respiratory gases. In addition, respiratory gases transported within the blood are detected by the nervous system which adjusts respiratory rate based on their concentration (Refer to Chapter 12: The Nervous System, for further information on nervous tissue and the brain.)

The respiratory gases, oxygen and carbon dioxide, are exchanged at the alveoli within the lungs before and after being transported within the blood. (Refer to Chapter 15: Blood, for further information on oxygen transport and haemoglobin structure.) The respiratory system also shares a unique relationship with the cardiovascular system, which acts to transport gas-containing blood throughout the body. (Refer to Chapter 16: The Cardiovascular System, for further information on heart and blood vessels functions.) Conditions affecting the respiratory system may result from infection, trauma or structural alterations, and can be detected through spirometry, radiography and physical assessment.

LEARNING OUTCOMES

On completion of these activities, the student should be able to:

1. describe the structure and function of the upper respiratory system
2. outline the structure and function of mucus
3. describe the structure and function of the lower respiratory system
4. conduct a radiographic examination of the lung structures
5. identify, describe, and examine the microscopic structures of the respiratory system
6. describe the mechanics of breathing and observe the actions of the model lung

LEARNING OUTCOMES—cont'd

7. outline the gas laws influencing breathing and respiration

8. outline respiratory volumes and capacities with reference to spirometry

9. describe the processes of respiration and gas exchange

10. outline the pH and buffering of carbon dioxide within the circulation

11. describe the factors affecting respiratory rate and relate this to the diving reflex

12. conduct a basic physical respiratory assessment.

KEY TERMS

Acidosis

Alkalosis

Alveolar surfactant

Alveoli

Breathing

Bronchi

Bronchioles

Buffer

Cilia

Conducting zone

Diaphragm

Epiglottis

Expiration

Hyperventilation

Hypoventilation

Inspiration

Intercostal muscles

Larynx

Lungs

Mucus

Nasal cavity

Paranasal sinuses

Pharynx

Pleura

Respiratory zone

Thorax

Trachea

Ventilation

ACTIVITY 17.1: STRUCTURE AND FUNCTION OF THE UPPER RESPIRATORY SYSTEM

The upper respiratory system consists of a series of tracts responsible for conducting air towards the respiratory organs contained within the **thorax**, where gas exchange occurs (Fig. 17.1). Incoming air is humidified, warmed to body temperature, and filtered of debris by the unique epithelium which lines the tract. Since the **trachea** and oesophagus run parallel to each other, the **epiglottis** prevents swallowed food from entering the **lungs** by sealing off the opening to the trachea and directing food into the oesophagus (Fig. 17.2). In addition, the **larynx** contains the vocal cords, which form the voice as air rushes through its inlet, vibrating the cords.

This activity outlines the structure and function of the upper respiratory organs.

1. Identify each of the structures in Fig. 17.1 using the terms provided.

Thyroid cartilage	Palatine tonsil	Oral cavity
Larynx	Cribriform plate	True vocal cord
Epiglottis	Pharyngeal tonsil (adenoids)	Laryngopharynx
Nasal conchae	Tongue	Frontal sinus
Oesophagus	Hard palate	Vocal cords
Cricoid cartilage	Oropharynx	Hyoid bone
Vestibule	Uvula	Thyroid gland
False vocal cord	Soft palate	Glottis
Sphenoid sinus	Lingual tonsil	Trachea
Nasopharynx		Nasal cavities

a. Structure A: _____

b. Structure B: _____

c. Structure C: _____

d. Structure D: _____

e. Structure E: _____

f. Structure F: _____

g. Structure G: _____

h. Structure H: _____

i. Structure I: _____

j. Structure J: _____

k. Structure K: _____

l. Structure L: _____

m. Structure M: _____

n. Structure N: _____

o. Structure O: _____

p. Structure P: _____

q. Structure Q: _____

r. Structure R: _____

s. Structure S: _____

t. Structure T: _____

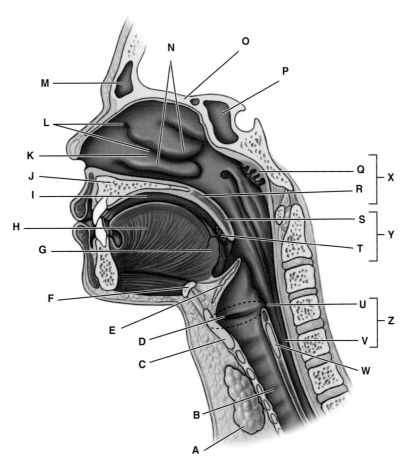

Figure 17.1 Upper respiratory structures.
(Source: Herlihy, B. (2018). The human body in health and illness. Elsevier.)

u. Structure U: _____

v. Structure V: _____

w. Structure W: _____

x. Structure X: _____

y. Structure Y: _____

z. Structure Z: _____

2. Consider the following questions, with reference to Fig. 17.1:

a. What is the function of structure B?

_____

_____

b. What is the function of structure C?

_____

_____

c. What is the function of structure E and of what type of tissue is it composed?

_____

_____

d. What is the function of structure J?

_____

e. What is the function of structures M and P?

_____

f. What is the function of structure N?

_____

_____

g. What is the function of structure R?

_____

_____

h. What is the function of structure S?

_____

_____

i. What is the function of structure U?

_____

_____

j. Relate the names of structures X, Y, and Z to their locations.

_____

_____

k. What is the pharynx and what is its function?

_____

_____

3. Identify each of the structures in Fig. 17.2 using the terms provided.

Trachea	Cartilage	Elastic fibres
Epithelium	Epiglottis	True vocal cord
False vocal cord	Mucosa	Lamina propria
Submucosa	Trachealis muscle	Adventitia
Seromucous glands	Lumen	Glottis

a. Structure A: _____

b. Structure B: _____

c. Structure C: _____

d. Structure D: _____

e. Structure E: _____

f. Structure F: _____

g. Structure G: _____

h. Structure H: _____

i. Structure I: _____

j. Structure J: _____

k. Structure K: _____

l. Structure L: _____

m. Structure M: _____

n. Structure N: _____

o. Structure O: _____

p. Structure P: _____

q. Structure Q: _____

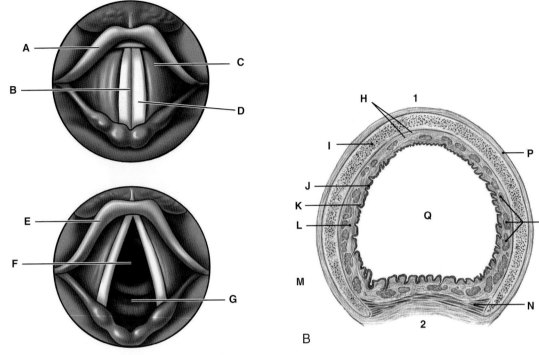

Figure 17.2 Structures of the pharynx. **A** Larynx. **B** Trachea.
*(Source: **A** Herlihy, B. (2018). The human body in health and illness. Elsevier. **B** Paulsen, F., & Waschke, J. (2018). Sobotta atlas of human anatomy: Head, neck and neuroanatomy. Elsevier.)*

4. Consider the following questions with reference to Fig. 17.2:

   a. In Fig. 17.2B, number 1 faces which structures?

   _____

   b. In Fig. 17.2B, number 2 faces which structures?

   _____

   c. What is the function of structures B and F?

   _____

   _____

   d. What is the function of structure C and of what tissue is it composed?

   _____

   _____

   e. What is the function of structure D and of what tissue is it composed?

   _____

   _____

   f. Note that structure I is incomplete posteriorly. Suggest a reason for this arrangement.

   _____

   _____

   g. Of what tissue is structure I composed?

   _____

   h. Structure J is composed of which type of tissue? Relate this to its function.

   _____

   _____

   i. What is the function of structure N?

   _____

   _____

   j. What is the function of structure O?

   _____

   _____

Apply the Concepts

1. What is sinusitis and how does it occur?

_____

_____

_____

2. What are nasal polyps and how do they occur?

_____

_____

_____

3. What is epistaxis and how does it occur?

_____

_____

_____

4. What is allergic rhinitis and how does it occur?

_____

_____

_____

5. Is there a distinction between laryngitis and pharyngitis? Explain.

_____

_____

_____

6. What occurs during the Valsalva manoeuvre and how is this beneficial functionally?

_____

_____

_____

7. How does choking occur?

_____

_____

_____

ACTIVITY 17.2: STRUCTURE AND FUNCTION OF MUCUS

Mucus is a thick, sticky fluid that is secreted by mucous glands and goblet cells which are embedded within the epithelial tissue lining the respiratory tract. Mucus keeps the respiratory membrane surfaces moist and acts to moisten and humidify incoming air, while trapping inhaled debris for subsequent propulsion by the **cilia** towards the **pharynx** and **nasal cavity** for expulsion. The **paranasal sinuses** are the chief region of the upper respiratory tract where mucus is secreted.

This activity demonstrates the structure and function of mucus within the respiratory system.

 To conduct this activity, it is important to ensure the following safety precautions:

- *Exercise care when handling and pouring boiling water into glassware to avoid skin scalding.*

- *Avoid directly touching the sides of hot glassware to minimise risk of skin injury.*

1. This activity is best conducted in pairs.

2. Obtain a 100 mL beaker, electric kettle, deionised water, two teaspoons, gelatine powder, 25 mL measuring cylinder, glycerine, two watch glasses, talcum powder, small paintbrush, cotton swab, compound microscope, microscope slides, coverslips and a stopwatch.

3. Boil the deionised water in the kettle and pour 20 mL boiling water into the beaker.

4. Gently sprinkle 1 teaspoon of gelatine over the water and stir so that the gelatine dissolves.

5. Measure 10 mL glycerine with the measuring cylinder and pour this into the beaker, stirring well to incorporate.

6. Place 1 teaspoon of gelatine mixture onto one of the watch glasses.

7. Allow the mixture in the beaker and the watch glass to stand for 20 minutes.

8. After 20 minutes, gently stir the mixture in the beaker, noting the consistency.

9. Note the consistency of the mixture in the watch glass.

   a. Which process contributed to the change in consistency of the mixture?

   _____

   b. Relate this to the processes occurring in the respiratory tract.

   _____

   _____

   _____

10. Gently sweep over the mixture in the watch glass with the paintbrush attempting to move the mixture from one side of the watch glass to the other, noting the behaviour of the mixture.

    a. How did the mixture behave in response to the actions of the paint brush?

    _____

    _____

    b. What does the action of the paintbrush represent in relation to respiratory function?

    _____

11. Add 1 teaspoon of the gelatine mixture in the beaker to the other watch glass, spreading it thinly around the surface.

12. Gently tilt the watch glass and observe the behaviour of the mixture.

13. Gently sprinkle a very small amount of talcum powder onto the mixture on the second watch glass, and tilt the watch glass in different directions, observing the result.

    a. What effect was observed in the talcum powder?

    _____

    _____

14. Gently stir the talcum powder into the mixture on the second watch glass with the cotton swab, observing the result.

    a. What effect was observed in the mixture?

    _____

    _____

    b. What does the talcum powder represent in relation to respiratory function?

    _____

    _____

15. Working quickly, smear a small amount of this mixture onto a microscope slide with the cotton swab and place a coverslip over the top, pressing gently onto the coverslip to spread the mixture thinly onto the slide.

16. Observe the mixture with the compound microscope under low power.

17. Draw a diagram of what you can see in the circle below.

Magnification of diagram: × _____

    a. What are the small particles that are observed in the mixture?

    _____

    b. Explain the behaviour of these particles within the mixture.

    _____

    _____

    c. What do these particles and the surrounding medium represent in relation to respiratory function?

    _____

    _____

18. Consider the following:

    a. Explain how the composition of this mixture represents the composition of real mucus.

    _____

    _____

    b. Explain how the consistency of this mixture represents the consistency of real mucus.

    _____

    _____

    _____

    c. What is the role of mucus in the respiratory system?

    _____

    _____

    d. What is the role of cilia in the respiratory system?

    _____

    _____

    e. What is mucociliary clearance and how does it aid immune function?

    _____

    _____

    _____

Apply the Concepts

1. Explain the relationship between cigarette smoking and the function of cilia.

   _____

   _____

   _____

2. What is sputum? Relate the presence of sputum to respiratory health.

   _____

   _____

   _____

3. Relate the following sputum colours to respiratory pathology:

   a. Clear sputum: _____

   b. Brown sputum: _____

   c. Yellow sputum: _____

   d. Green sputum: _____

   e. White sputum: _____

   f. Red sputum: _____

   g. Black sputum: _____

4. What is cystic fibrosis and how does it occur?

   _____

   _____

   _____

5. What is diphtheria and how does it affect respiratory function?

   _____

   _____

   _____

6. What is bronchitis and how does it occur?

   _____

   _____

   _____

ACTIVITY 17.3: STRUCTURE AND FUNCTION OF THE LOWER RESPIRATORY SYSTEM

The lower respiratory system consists of structures extending from the **conducting zone**, such as the **bronchi** and **bronchioles**, to structures forming the **respiratory zone** (Fig. 17.3). Structures of the respiratory zone, particularly the **alveoli**, are actively engaged in gas exchange and are located within the lungs. The lungs are housed within the thorax, which provides physical protection, and are surrounded by **intercostal muscles** that drive **ventilation**. In addition, the **pleurae** provide a protective moist environment around each lung, reducing friction against the thoracic cage caused by **breathing** movements (Fig. 17.4).

This activity outlines the structure and function of the lower respiratory organs.

1. Identify each of the structures in Fig. 17.3 using the terms provided.

Cartilaginous rings	Hilus	Superior lobe
Superior lobe	Bronchiole	Primary bronchi
Inferior lobe	Pulmonary venule	Terminal bronchiole
Trachea	Smooth muscle	Alveolar pore
Alveolar duct	Carina	Lung base
Lung apex	Middle lobe	Secondary bronchi
Cardiac impression	Thyroid cartilage	Pulmonary arteriole
Alveolar sacs	Tertiary bronchi	Capillaries
	Alveoli	

a. Structure A: _____

b. Structure B: _____

c. Structure C: _____

d. Structure D: _____

e. Structure E: _____

f. Structure F: _____

g. Structure G: _____

h. Structure H: _____

i. Structure I: _____

j. Structure J: _____

k. Structure K: _____

l. Structure L: _____

m. Structure M: _____

n. Structure N: _____

o. Structure O: _____

p. Structure P: _____

q. Structure Q: _____

r. Structure R: _____

s. Structure S: _____

t. Structure T: _____

u. Structure U: _____

v. Structure V: _____

w. Structure W: _____

x. Structure X: _____

y. Structure Y: _____

z. Structure Z: _____

2. Consider the following questions with reference to Fig. 17.3:

a. What is the function of structure B?

_____

_____

b. Structure B is composed of which type of tissue?

_____

_____

c. What is the function of structure J?

_____

_____

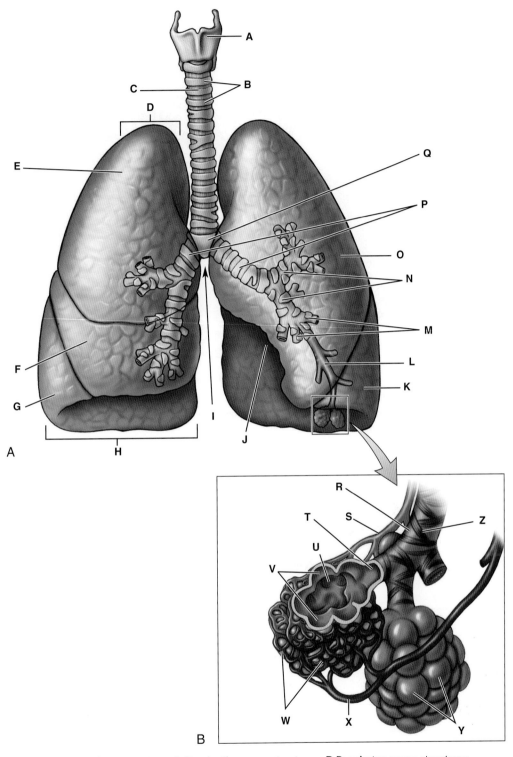

Figure 17.3 Structures of the respiratory system. **A** Conducting zone structures. **B** Respiratory zone structures.
(Source: Herlihy, B. (2018). The human body in health and illness. Elsevier.)

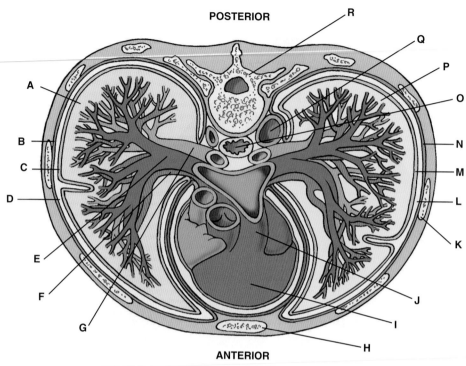

Figure 17.4 The pleurae and associated structures.
(Source: Heuer, A., & Rodriguez, N. E. (2021). Egan's fundamentals of respiratory care. Elsevier.)

d. What type of blood is contained in structure S and what is the source of this blood?

_____

_____

e. What type of blood is contained in structure X and what is the destination of this blood?

_____

_____

f. Structures N, P, and R form part of which respiratory structure?

_____

_____

g. What is the function of structure U?

_____

_____

h. Which cell types are found in structure V and what are their functions?

_____

_____

i. What is the function of structure W?

_____

_____

j. Structure Y is surrounded by elastic fibres. Suggest a reason for this arrangement.

_____

_____

k. What is the function of structure Z?

_____

_____

l. Compare the number of lobes present in each lung and suggest a reason for any differences.

_____

_____

_____

m. What are the bronchopulmonary segments of the lungs and what is their functional significance?

_____

_____

_____

3. Identify each of the structures in Fig. 17.4 using the terms provided.

Sternum	Heart	Right lung
Primary bronchus	Pulmonary trunk	Rib
Left lung	Intrapleural space	Oesophagus
Parietal pleura	Aorta	Vertebra
Pulmonary artery	Visceral pleura	Pulmonary vein

a. Structure A: _____

b. Structure B: _____

c. Structure C: _____

d. Structure D: _____

e. Structure E: _____

f. Structure F: _____

g. Structure G: _____

h. Structure H: _____

i. Structure I: _____

j. Structure J: _____

k. Structure K: _____

l. Structure L: _____

m. Structure M: _____

n. Structure N: _____

o. Structure O: _____

p. Structure P: _____

q. Structure Q: _____

r. Structure R: _____

4. Consider the following questions with reference to Fig. 17.4:

a. What is the function of structure B?

_____

_____

b. What is the function of structure C?

_____

_____

c. What is contained within structure D and what is its function?

_____

_____

_____

d. What is the function of the pleural membranes and serous fluid?

_____

_____

e. How do the pleurae facilitate breathing?

_____

_____

Apply the Concepts

1. What is pleurisy and how does it occur?

_____

_____

_____

2. What is pleural thickening and how does it occur?

_____

_____

_____

3. What is pleural effusion and how does it occur?

_____

_____

_____

4. What is respiratory distress syndrome and why are premature infants at risk?

_____

_____

_____

5. Is there a distinction between influenza and the common cold? Explain.

_____

_____

_____

6. What is COVID-19 and how does it affect respiratory function?

_____

_____

_____

Additional Activities

For additional activities visit Activity 17A: Radiographic Examination of Lung Structures on Evolve˙.

For additional activities visit Activity 17B: Identification of Respiratory Structures on Evolve˙.

For additional activities visit Activity 17C: Microscopic Examination of Respiratory Structures on Evolve˙.

ACTIVITY 17.4: MECHANICS OF BREATHING AND THE MODEL LUNG

Breathing, or **inspiration** and **expiration**, incorporates the repeated and rhythmic events of the respiratory organs such as the lungs and structures of the thorax such as the diaphragm and intercostal muscles of the rib cage (Fig. 17.5). These events are carefully coordinated by the nervous system in response to the concentrations and pressure gradients of carbon dioxide and oxygen in the blood.

This activity outlines the mechanics of breathing and demonstrates the processes of breathing using a model lung apparatus.

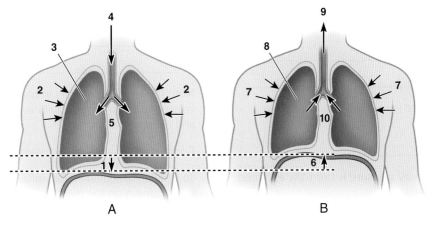

Figure 17.5 Mechanics of breathing.
(Source: Klieger, D. M. (2009). Saunders essentials of medical assisting. Elsevier.)

Part 1: Mechanics of Breathing

Inspiration and expiration involve the rhythmic contraction and relaxation of the diaphragm and the external intercostal muscles. These change the volume of the thoracic cage, which has an inverse effect on the air pressure within the lungs. Air flows into and out of the lungs in response to these changes, relying on the natural recoil of lung tissue.

1. Examine Fig. 17.5, and identify each of the breathing stages and the events occurring in each stage:

   a. Stage A: _____

      i. Event 1: _____

      ii. Event 2: _____

      iii. Event 3: _____

      iv. Event 4: _____

      v. Event 5: _____

   b. Stage B: _____

      i. Event 6: _____

      ii. Event 7: _____

      iii. Event 8: _____

      iv. Event 9: _____

      v. Event 10: _____

2. Consider the following questions:

   a. What type of tissue comprises the diaphragm?

      _____

   b. Is control of the diaphragm voluntary, involuntary, or both? Explain.

      _____

      _____

      _____

   c. During event A, do the external intercostal muscles and diaphragm contract or relax?

      _____

   d. During event A, does thoracic volume increase or decrease?

      _____

   e. Which factors contributed to this increase or decrease in thoracic volume?

      _____

      _____

   f. During event B, do the external intercostal muscles and diaphragm contract or relax?

      _____

   g. During event B, does thoracic volume increase or decrease?

      _____

h. Which factors contributed to this increase or decrease in thoracic volume?

_____

_____

i. Atmospheric pressure is normally assumed to be what value?

_____

j. At rest, intrapulmonary pressure is normally assumed to be what value?

_____

k. Does air flow into the lungs as a result of increased or decreased intrapulmonary pressure?

_____

l. Does air flow out of the lungs as a result of increased or decreased intrapulmonary pressure?

_____

m. How is intrapulmonary pressure decreased?

_____

n. How is intrapulmonary pressure increased?

_____

o. What would occur if the intrapulmonary and atmospheric pressures were equalised?

_____

Part 2: The Model Lung

A model lung demonstrates the principle involved in gas flow into and out of the lungs. It is a simple apparatus consisting of a bell jar, bottle or dome which represents the thorax, a rubber membrane which represents the diaphragm, and a pair of balloons which represent the lungs.

1. This activity is best conducted in pairs.

2. Obtain a model lung apparatus.

3. Operate the model lung by moving the rubber diaphragm up and down.

   a. Do the balloons fully inflate and deflate?

   _____

b. Suggest a reason for this observation.

_____

_____

4. Note the relative changes in balloon (lung) size as the volume of the thoracic cavity is alternately increased and decreased.

5. Complete the table below, based on your observations.

6. To simulate pneumothorax, inflate the balloon lungs by pulling down on the diaphragm.

7. Allow air to enter into the bell jar thorax by loosening the rubber stopper.

   a. What occurs to the balloon lungs when pneumothorax is simulated?

   _____

	Diaphragm pushed up		Diaphragm pulled down	
Change in:	Increased	Decreased	Increased	Decreased
Internal volume of bell jar (thoracic cage)				
Internal pressure of bell jar (thoracic cage)				
Size of balloons (lungs)				
	Into/out of lungs	Into/out of lungs	Into/out of lungs	Into/out of lungs
Direction of air flow				

b. How does the structural relationship between the balloon-lungs and the jar-thorax differ from that seen in the human lungs and thorax?

_____

_____

_____

c. Under what internal conditions does air tend to flow into the lungs?

_____

_____

d. Under what internal conditions does air tend to flow out of the lungs?

_____

_____

e. Is breathing under voluntary or involuntary control?

_____

f. Is breathing under sympathetic or parasympathetic control?

_____

Apply the Concepts

1. Explain whether inhalation and exhalation can be monitored by the use of external cues.

_____

_____

_____

2. What is pneumothorax and how does it occur?

_____

_____

_____

3. What is respiratory arrest?

_____

_____

_____

Additional Activities

For additional activities visit Activity 17D: Gas Laws Influencing Breathing and Respiration on Evolve˙.

For additional activities visit Activity 17E: Respiratory Volumes and Capacities - The Spirogram on Evolve˙.

For additional activities visit Activity 17F: Respiratory Volumes and Capacities - Wet and Dry Spirometry on Evolve˙.

ACTIVITY 17.5: RESPIRATION AND GAS EXCHANGE

The exchange of respiratory gases – oxygen and carbon dioxide – occurs at the alveoli, which are in direct contact with the pulmonary capillaries, together forming the respiratory membrane (Fig. 17.6). The respiratory membrane offers a large surface area and is extremely thin and moist, which contributes to fast gas diffusion and exchange. The membrane is kept moist by the secretion of **alveolar surfactant** by alveolar type II cells. The alveolar surfactant acts to prevent the alveoli from collapsing, keeps the alveolar membrane tight, and provides a moist medium within which respiratory gases can be exchanged (Fig. 17.7).

This activity demonstrates the processes associated with respiration and gas exchange.

1. For the four processes of respiration provided, outline the process occurring in each:

   a. Pulmonary ventilation: _____

   _____

   b. External respiration: _____

   _____

   c. Transport of respiratory gases: _____

   _____

   d. Internal respiration: _____

   _____

2. Examine Fig. 17.6, and identify the structures indicated:

   a. Structure A: _____

   b. Structure B: _____

   c. Structure C: _____

   d. Structure D: _____

   e. Structure E: _____

   f. Structure F: _____

   g. Structure G: _____

   h. Structure H: _____

   i. Structure I: _____

   j. Structure J: _____

   k. Structure K: _____

   l. Structure L: _____

   m. Structure M: _____

   n. Structure N: _____

3. Consider the following questions:

   a. Identify four characteristics of the alveoli that make them ideal sites for gas diffusion.

   _____

   _____

   _____

   _____

   b. Which structures comprise the respiratory membrane?

   _____

   _____

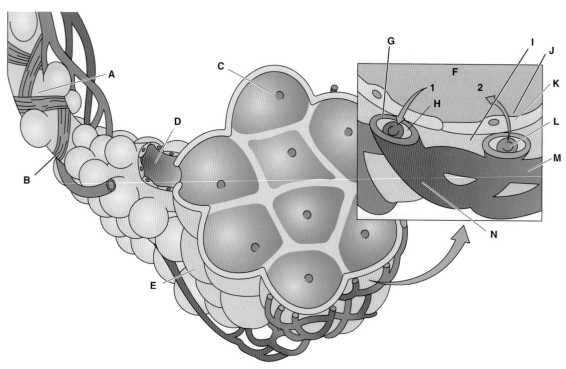

Figure 17.6 The respiratory membrane and gas exchange.
(Source: Gartner, L. P. (2020). Textbook of histology. Elsevier.)

c. What might occur if structure B were to constrict?

_____

_____

d. Structure E is composed of what type of cells?

_____

e. What is found within structure I and what is its function?

_____

_____

f. What substance is found lining structure J, and which structures secrete this substance?

_____

_____

g. What is the function of alveolar surfactant?

_____

_____

h. Which cells located within the alveoli have an immune function?

_____

i. Which process drives the transport of gases across the respiratory membrane?

_____

j. What type of blood is being transported at structure M and what is its source?

_____

k. What type of blood is being transported at structure N and what is its destination?

_____

l. Which gas is being exchanged at number 1?

_____

m. Which gas is being exchanged at number 2?

_____

4. Consider the following questions with reference to Fig. 17.7:

a. In Fig. 17.7A, why does oxygen move from the systemic capillary wall into the body tissue?

_____

_____

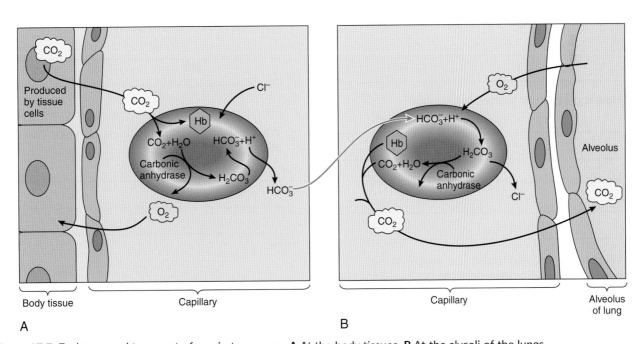

Figure 17.7 Exchange and transport of respiratory gases. **A** At the body tissues. **B** At the alveoli of the lungs.
(Source: Gartner, L. P. (2020). Textbook of histology. Elsevier.)

b. What is the source and destination of this oxygen?

_____

_____

c. In Fig. 17.7A, why does carbon dioxide move from the body tissue into the systemic capillary wall?

_____

_____

d. What is the source and destination of this carbon dioxide?

_____

_____

e. In Fig. 17.7B, why does oxygen move from the alveoli into the pulmonary capillary wall?

_____

_____

f. What is the destination of this oxygen and why?

_____

_____

g. In Fig. 17.7B, why does carbon dioxide move from the pulmonary capillary wall into the alveoli?

_____

_____

h. What is the source of this carbon dioxide and why?

_____

_____

i. How is oxygen transported in the blood?

_____

_____

j. How is carbon dioxide transported in the blood?

_____

_____

k. What terms are used to describe oxygen-loaded haemoglobin and oxygen-depleted haemoglobin?

_____

l. Provide the equations for the binding of oxygen and carbon dioxide to haemoglobin.

_____

_____

m. Provide the equation for the reaction between carbon dioxide and water within the blood.

_____

_____

n. The method of carbon dioxide transportation within the blood is known as which system?

_____

o. What is a buffer?

_____

_____

p. Why is carbonic acid (H_2CO_3) an ideal method of transport for carbon dioxide in the blood?

_____

_____

q. What is carbonic anhydrase and what is its function?

_____

_____

_____

r. Explain the presence of chloride ions (Cl^-) in Fig. 17.7, relating this to chloride shift.

_____

_____

_____

s. What is ventilation–perfusion coupling and how is this regulated?

_____

_____

_____

Apply the Concepts

1. Is there a distinction between buffering and neutralisation? Explain.

_____

_____

_____

2. What is the phosphate buffer system and how does it operate?

_____

_____

_____

3. What is the protein buffer system and how does it operate?

_____

_____

_____

Additional Activities

For additional activities visit Activity 17G: pH and Buffering of Carbon Dioxide on Evolve˙.

ACTIVITY 17.6: RESPIRATORY HOMEOSTASIS AND FACTORS AFFECTING RESPIRATORY RATE

The processes associated with breathing are carefully coordinated by mechanisms that involve a number of body systems and structures. The variable most strongly influencing the maintenance of respiratory homeostasis is carbon dioxide (Fig. 17.8). When the metabolic demands of the tissue cells increase, as during exercise, the production of carbon dioxide increases. This in turn, affects respiratory rate.

This activity outlines the factors associated with respiratory homeostasis and respiratory rate.

Part 1: Respiratory Homeostasis

Respiratory rate is largely regulated by the concentration of respiratory gases within the blood. For example, during exercise the metabolic requirements of the tissue cells increase, increasing the demand for oxygen and increasing the output of carbon dioxide. The increase in circulating carbon dioxide reduces plasma pH, which is detected by chemoreceptors located centrally (in the brain stem) and peripherally (in the carotid and aortic bodies). These send afferent impulses to the medullary respiratory centres (clusters of neurons associated with the pons and glossopharyngeal nerve) which regulate the respiratory muscles via efferent pathways to increase respiratory rate, thereby causing excess carbon dioxide to be exhaled. As carbon dioxide accumulates in the blood, carbonic acid levels increase, causing a further drop in plasma pH and further stimulating the activity of chemoreceptors.

1. Examine Fig. 17.8, and identify each of the stages forming the respiratory feedback loop:

   a. Stage A: _____

   b. Stage B: _____

   c. Stage C: _____

   d. Stage D: _____

   e. Stage E: _____

2. Examine Fig. 17.8, and identify each of the structures and events occurring within the respiratory feedback loop:

   a. Event 1: _____

   b. Structures 2: _____

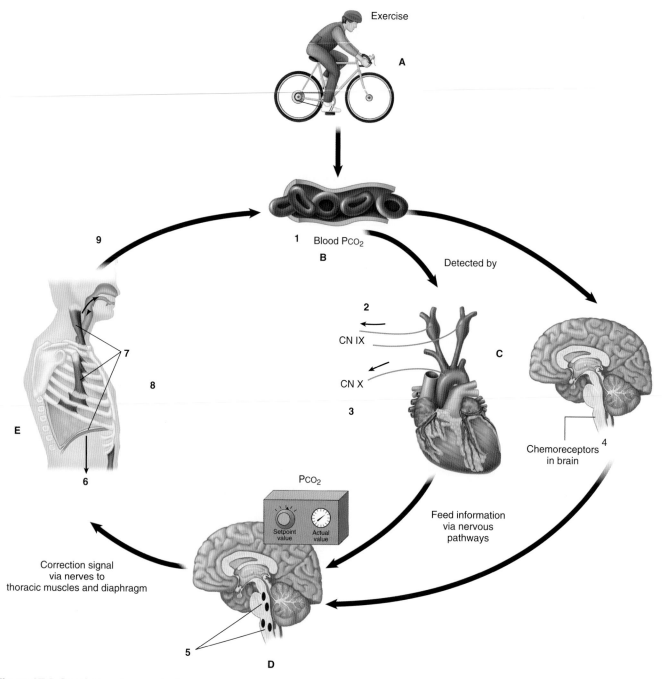

Figure 17.8 Respiratory homeostasis.
(Thibodeau, G. A., & Patton, K. T. (2017). The human body in health and disease, 7th ed. Elsevier Mosby.)

c. Structure 3: _____

d. Structure 4: _____

e. Structure 5: _____

f. Event 6: _____

g. Event 7: _____

h. Event 8: _____

i. Event 9: _____

3. Consider the following questions with reference to Fig. 17.8:

a. Which variable is responsible for initiating respiratory homeostasis?

_____

b. CN IX represents which structure? What is its function in respiration?

_____

_____

c. CN X represents which structure? What is its function in respiration?

_____

_____

d. Structures 2 and 3 represent which type of receptors?

_____

e. Structure 4 represents which type of receptor?

_____

f. Where are the neural control centres of respiratory rhythm located?

_____

g. Which nerves are responsible for communication between structures 5 and 6?

_____

_____

Part 2: Alterations in Respiratory Rate

Respiratory rate, although coordinated via the autonomic nervous system, is largely influenced by the concentration of carbon dioxide in the blood. Similarly, hyperventilation and hypoventilation will affect the rate at which carbon dioxide is removed from the blood.

⚠ To conduct this activity, it is important to ensure the following safety precautions:

- *Individuals with respiratory conditions may wish to avoid this activity.*

1. This activity is best conducted in pairs.

2. Obtain a human subject, a large paper bag and a stopwatch.

3. Ask the subject to open the paper bag fully, and swirl it through the air to ensure that the bag is full of air.

4. Have the subject gather the top of the bag in both hands, leaving a small opening in the centre large enough to surround their nose and mouth.

5. Ask the subject to breath into the bag as normally as possible for 4 minutes, or as long as they are able while they are standing.

6. Record the time with the stopwatch.

7. Note any changes in respiratory rate (the number of breaths per minute) and respiratory depth (the amount of air inhaled with each breath).

8. This can be observed either by noting changes in the rise and fall of the chest or by observing how the creases in the bag change with each breath.

9. Repeat the activity with another subject, timing the process and comparing respiratory rate and respiratory depth between subjects.

10. Consider the following questions:

a. What is considered a normal respiratory rate for adults?

_____

b. What is considered a normal time ratio of inspiration to expiration (I:E) for adults?

_____

c. How did the composition of the gases in the bag change during the activity?

_____

_____

d. How did respiratory rate change as the subject continued to breathe into the bag?

_____

e. Suggest a reason for the alteration in respiratory rate over time.

_____

_____

_____

f. Is this an example of negative or positive feedback?

_____

g. Which structures in the nervous system are responsible for adjusting respiratory rate and depth?

_____

h. What are these structures collectively called, with reference to their role in respiration?

_____

i. Suggest one possible outcome if respiratory rate did not change throughout this activity.

_____

_____

_____

Apply the Concepts

1. What is hypercapnia and how does it occur?

_____

_____

_____

2. What is hypocapnia and how does it occur?

_____

_____

_____

3. What is aspiration and how might this present challenges clinically?

_____

_____

_____

4. What is sudden infant death syndrome (SIDS) and how does it occur?

_____

_____

_____

Additional Activities

For additional activities visit Activity 17H: The Diving Reflex on Evolve°.

ACTIVITY 17.7: PHYSICAL RESPIRATORY ASSESSMENT

The physical examination of an individual with a respiratory condition is a structured approach, as with any physical examination, and generally consists of the following processes in order of assessment – inspection, palpation, percussion and auscultation. This is often conducted using the landmarks of the chest (Fig. 17.9). Although physical examination of respiratory function can assist with the diagnosis and monitoring of an underlying respiratory condition, it also provides the basis for understanding the normal and abnormal functions of the respiratory system.

This activity demonstrates the application of percussion and auscultation in the assessment of respiratory function.

Part 1: Respiratory Percussion

Percussion is a technique that is used to determine the presence of solid and hollow structures beneath the surface of the body. The middle finger, or occasionally the middle finger and adjoining finger of one hand, is placed over the area that is being assessed. The middle finger of the other hand is used to tap on the middle finger of the placed hand, with a flick of the wrist. Percussion should be conducted by working across the chest from side to side, so that the right and left sides of the body can be compared. Practise by percussing and listening to solid and hollow objects first. Solid objects sound dull, whereas hollow objects sound resonant.

1. This activity is best conducted in pairs.

2. Obtain a human subject.

3. Respiratory percussion is best performed if the subject's outer clothing is removed, so a male subject may be preferable.

4. Start at the front of the chest, and moving downwards from side to side, percuss the locations in the table provided using Fig. 17.9 to assist.

5. Listen for the following percussion sounds in each of the indicated locations:

   - Flat – an extremely dull sound (presence of fluid).

   - Dull – a moderate thud-like sound (presence of solid mass or bone).

   - Resonant – loud, low-pitched, hollow sound (presence of normal lung tissue).

   - Hyper-resonant – a light sound of reduced density (presence of air).

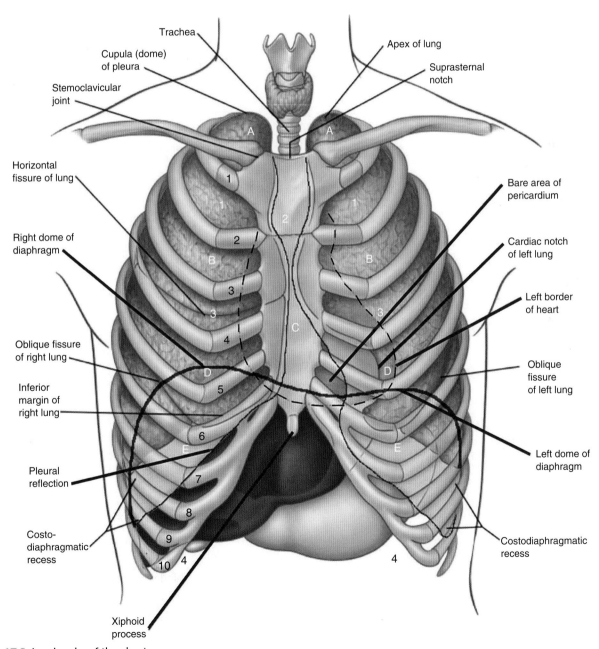

Figure 17.9 Landmarks of the chest.

(*Source: Smith, S. E., & Darling, G. E. (2011). Surface anatomy and surface landmarks for thoracic surgery: Part II. Thoracic Surgery Clinics, 21(2), 139–155.*)

6. Repeat the process at the back of the chest, moving downwards from side to side following the locations in Fig. 17.9 to assist.

7. Note the expansion of the chest with breathing and any asymmetry that may be present.

8. Record your observations in the table provided.

Percussion location	Description	Underlying structures	Sound
Front			
Location A	Above clavicles		
Location B	Between 2nd and 3rd ribs		
Location C	Sternum		
Location D	Between 4th and 5th ribs		
Location E	Between 6th and 7th ribs		
Back			
Location 1	Scapula		
Location 2	Spinus process		
Location 3	Between 3rd and 4th ribs		
Location 4	Below 10th ribs		

Part 2: Respiratory Auscultation

Auscultation is a technique that allows the respiratory sounds to be heard through the use of a stethoscope. During auscultation, the minimum number of locations to auscultate is normally four areas on each side of the chest, a total of eight areas. This would be repeated on the back of the chest. Conditions affecting the respiratory system, such as those associated with obstruction or restriction, can often be diagnosed using this technique.

1. This activity is best conducted in pairs.

2. Ask a third person to be a subject. Obtain a stethoscope and some alcohol swabs.

3. Respiratory auscultation is best performed if the subject's outer clothing is removed, so a male subject may be preferable.

4. Clean the earpieces of the stethoscope with the alcohol swabs.

5. Place the earpieces into your ears. Note that the earpieces are angled. For comfort, the earpieces should be angled in a forward direction when placed in the ears.

6. Place the diaphragm of the stethoscope on the subject's throat just below the larynx.

   a. This area forms which region of the respiratory system?

   _____

7. Listen for bronchial sounds on inspiration and expiration.

   a. Which of the respiratory sounds are heard primarily during inspiration?

   _____

   b. Which of the respiratory sounds are heard primarily during expiration?

   _____

   c. Bronchial sounds are produced by which structure during normal breathing?

   _____

   d. How are bronchial sounds heard in the presence of a respiratory condition?

   _____

   e. Suggest a condition that may affect bronchial sounds.

   _____

8. Move the stethoscope down toward the region of the bronchi until you can no longer hear the sounds of inspiration and expiration.

   a. This area forms which region of the respiratory system?

   _____

9. Place the stethoscope over the following chest areas and listen for breathing sounds, heard primarily during inspiration, using Fig. 17.9 to assist.

   • Under the clavicle.

   • At various intercostal spaces.

   • Triangle of auscultation (on the back just under the scapula).

10. Listen for breathing sounds on inspiration and expiration, taking note of any additional sounds that may be present, such as:

   • *crackles* – an intermittent crackling sound, usually during inhalation.

- *wheezing* – a high-pitched sound, usually during exhalation.
- *rhonchi* – a low-pitched rattling sound, usually during exhalation.
- *stridor* – a loud high-pitched sound, usually during inhalation.
- *rales* – a clicking sound, usually during inhalation.
- *crepitation* – a crackling sound, usually during inhalation.
- *pleural rub* – a raspy sound usually, during inhalation and exhalation.

a. Describe the breathing sounds during inspiration and expiration.

_____

_____

b. What term is used to describe the regular sounds associated with breathing?

_____

c. Suggest a condition that may increase the volume of respiratory sounds.

_____

_____

d. Suggest a condition that may reduce the volume of respiratory sounds.

_____

Apply the Concepts

1. Suggest a possible cause of crackles.

_____

2. Suggest a possible cause of wheezing.

_____

3. Suggest a possible cause of rhonchi.

_____

4. Suggest a possible cause of stridor.

_____

5. What is barrel chest and how does it occur?

_____

_____

6. What is pigeon chest and how does it occur?

_____

_____

7. What is funnel chest and how does it occur?

_____

_____

Additional Resources

GetBodySmart: Respiratory System and Spirometry

GetBodySmart presents fully animated, illustrated, and interactive eBooks about human anatomy and physiology body systems.

www.getbodysmart.com/respiratory-system
www.getbodysmart.com/spirometry/pulmonary-function-tests

Histology Guide Virtual Microscopy Laboratory: Respiratory System

Histology Guide is an online resource providing a virtual microscopy laboratory experience, by allowing users to view microscope slides from professional collections for the purpose of interpreting cellular and tissue structures as seen through a microscope.

histologyguide.com/slidebox/17-respiratory-system.html

Innerbody Research: Respiratory System

Innerbody Research provides objective, science-based advice to help readers make more informed choices about home health products and services with most up-to-date reviews, guides and research, including information about the respiratory system.

www.innerbody.com/anatomy/respiratory

JavaLab: Boyle's Law

An online animation that allows users to interact with the interface and adjust the factors that affect the behaviour of gases associated with Boyle's law.

javalab.org/en/boyles_law_en/

Osmosis – Respiratory System

The Respiratory System module of Osmosis provides videos, notes, quiz questions and links to further resources related to the respiratory system.

www.osmosis.org/library/md/foundational-sciences/physiology#respiratory_system

The Histology Guide: Respiratory System

The Histology Guide is a virtual experience of using a microscope with zoom features divided into topics and offering histological slides with labels and quizzes for each topic, such as the respiratory system. It is provided by the University of Leeds.

www.histology.leeds.ac.uk/respiratory/index.php

The McGill Physiology Virtual Lab: Respiration Laboratory

A series of interactive tutorials on a variety of physiology topics created for students enrolled in introductory physiology courses at McGill University.

www.medicine.mcgill.ca/physio/vlab/Other_exps/resp/vlabmenuresp.htm

Visible Body: Respiratory System

Visible Body provides interactive and highly accurate visualisations and apps for learning and teaching anatomy and physiology for students and healthcare professionals. It includes body systems such as the respiratory system.

www.visiblebody.com/learn/respiratory

CHAPTER 18
The Lymphatic System

Lymph, (from the Latin *lympha*, meaning clear liquid), is a fluid that is drained from interstitial spaces everywhere in the body and returned to the blood vascular system via lymphatic vessels. The lymphatic system comprises an extensive network of lymphatic vessels, lymphatic tissue and lymph nodes.

In a blood capillary bed, the blood's hydrostatic pressure forces fluid out of the blood at the arterial end and colloid osmotic pressures force most of it to return to the blood at the venous end. The fluid that remains behind forms the interstitial fluid and this must eventually be returned to the blood to ensure that blood volume is maintained. (Refer to Chapter 21: The Urinary System and Electrolyte Balance, for further information on fluid and electrolyte balance.) A major role of the lymphatic system is to drain the body's tissues of this excess fluid and return it to the blood. Once interstitial fluid enters a lymphatic vessel it is known as lymph.

The lymph nodes of the lymphatic system are also part of a system of lymphoid organs and tissues, which provide the structural basis of the immune system and include the spleen, tonsils, thymus and other lymphoid tissues. (Refer to Chapter 19: Immunity and Infection, for information on immunity and infection control.)

LEARNING OUTCOMES

On completion of these activities, the student should be able to:

1. discuss the general structure and the roles of the lymphatic system
2. describe the arrangements and morphology of lymphatic vessels and lymph nodes
3. describe the general nature of lymphoid tissues and their arrangement in lymphoid organs
4. characterise the cells of the immune system and identify the sites of their production and storage
5. distinguish between the dual roles of the spleen in the immune and cardiovascular systems
6. clarify the dual roles of the thymus in the immune and endocrine systems
7. discuss the nature and role of mucosa-associated lymphoid tissue
8. compare the structures and functions of the various lymphoid organs and tissues.

KEY TERMS

Appendix
Hilum
Lingual tonsil
Lymph
Lymph lacteal
Lymph node
Lymph sinus
Lymph vessel
Lymphatic capillary
Lymphatic duct

Lymphatic trunk
Lymphatic valve
Lymphocytes
Lymphoid cells
Lymphoid follicle
Lymphoid organ
Lymphoid tissue
Macrophage
Mucosa-associated lymphoid tissue (MALT)

Palatine tonsil
Peyer's patches
Pharyngeal tonsil
Red pulp
Spleen
Thymic lobule
Thymus gland
Trabecula
Tubal tonsil
White pulp

ACTIVITY 18.1: LYMPH AND LYMPHATIC VESSELS

The lymphatic system is composed of a number of structures that assist in the circulation and filtration of **lymph**, which is drained into **lymphatic ducts** and **lymphatic vessels**, and then **lymphatic trunks** (Fig. 18.1). **Lymph vessels**, similar in structure to veins, form an extensive network throughout the body, but are structurally different in that they contain **lymphatic valves** that prevent fluid backflow, and eventually branch to form **lymphatic capillaries** or **lymph lacteals**. Lymph vessels and their associated **lymph nodes** perform several important functions.

This activity examines the nature and role of lymph and the lymphatic system.

1. Identify each of the labelled structures shown in Fig. 18.1, by matching the number of each structure with its correct term.

   a. Axillary lymph node: _____

   b. Bone marrow: _____

   c. Cervical lymph node: _____

   d. Cisterna chyli: _____

   e. Cubital lymph node: _____

   f. Inguinal lymph node: _____

   g. Peyer patches: _____

   h. Right lymphatic duct: _____

   i. Spleen: _____

   j. Submandibular lymph nodes: _____

   k. Thoracic duct: _____

   l. Thymus: _____

   m. Tonsils: _____

2. Identify the lymphatic vessel that drains:

   a. The upper right side of the body

   _____

   b. The lower half and left side of the body

   _____

3. What is the function of the cisterna chyli?

   _____

   _____

4. Explain why, unlike the blood vascular system, the lymphatic system carries fluid in one direction only.

   _____

   _____

   _____

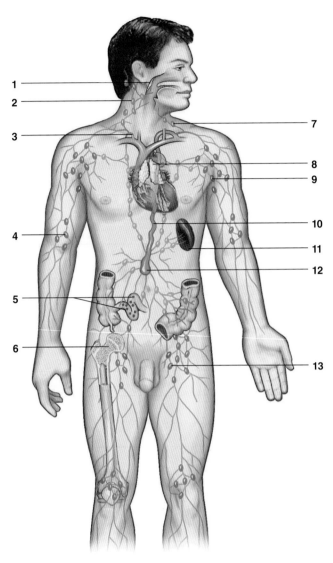

Figure 18.1 Structures of the lymphatic system.
(Source: Walker, S., Wood, M., & Nicol, J. (2021). Mastering medical terminology: Australia and New Zealand, 3rd edn. Elsevier.)

5. How many lymphatic trunks are there and which regions of the body do they drain?

_____

_____

_____

6. Consider the following questions:

a. Identify three ways in which lymphatic capillaries differ from blood capillaries.

_____

_____

_____

b. Where are lymph lacteals found and what is their function?

_____

_____

_____

c. What blood vessels do lymphatic vessels most closely resemble?

_____

d. How is unidirectional flow in lymphatic vessels achieved?

_____

7. Since the lymphatic system does not have a pumping organ to maintain lymph flow, what mechanisms drive the movement of lymph through lymphatic vessels?

_____

_____

_____

8. Complete the following sentences by filling in the blanks with the terms provided.

Capillaries	Subclavian
Ducts	Thoracic duct
Internal jugular	Trunks
Right lymphatic duct	

a. Lymph enters the lymphatic system in the lymphatic

_____ and flows through collecting vessels

to lymphatic _____, which drain large

parts of the body.

b. These drain into one of two large _____

called the _____ and the _____.

c. These in turn drain into the venous circulation at the

junction of the _____ and

_____ on each side of the body.

9. Which important component of blood is not found in lymph?

_____

Apply the Concepts

1. a. What is elephantiasis and how does it occur?

_____

_____

   b. Explain why the swelling associated with elephantiasis is significant and lasts so long without treatment.

_____

_____

_____

2. What is lymphoma and how does it occur?

_____

_____

3. What is lymphangiomatosis and how does it occur?

_____

_____

4. What is lymphadenopathy and how does it occur?

_____

_____

ACTIVITY 18.2: LYMPH NODES

Lymph nodes are the principal lymphoid organs of the body and are found in their hundreds along lymphatic vessels (Fig. 18.2). They are the only lymphoid organs that have both afferent and efferent lymph vessels. Other lymphoid organs and lymphoid tissues have only efferent lymphatics. Lymph is filtered within the node by circulating through the **lymph sinuses**, which are separated by connective tissue in the form of **trabeculae**.

This activity examines the structure and function of lymph nodes.

1. Examine Fig. 18.2, and match the number of each labelled structure with its correct term.

   a. Afferent lymphatic vessels _____

   b. Capsule _____

   c. Efferent lymphatic vessel _____

   d. Germinal centre _____

   e. Hilum _____

   f. Lymph nodules _____

   g. Medullary cords _____

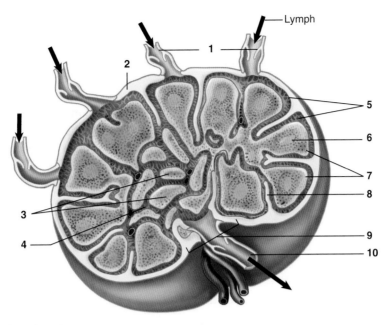

Figure 18.2 Section of a lymph node.
(Source: Turgeon, M. L. (2022). Immunology and serology in laboratory medicine. Elsevier.)

h. Medullary sinus _____

i. Subcapsular sinuses _____

j. Trabecula _____

2. What are the two main functions of lymph nodes?

_____

_____

3. Match the following lymph node structures with the function or description provided:

Afferent lymphatic vessels	Hilum
Capsule	Lymph nodules
Cortex	Lymph sinuses
Efferent lymphatic vessels	Medulla
Germinal centres	Trabeculae

a. Carry the lymph into the lymph node

_____

b. The outermost region, containing densely packed follicles

_____

c. Large lymph capillaries with criss-crossing reticular fibres

_____

d. Strands of connective tissue dividing the node into compartments

_____

e. Layer of fibrous tissue encasing the lymph node

_____

f. Carry the lymph away from the lymph node

_____

g. Indented region on the efferent side of the lymph node

_____

h. Irregular compartments within the cortex

_____

i. Parts of the cortex where proliferating B cells abound

_____

j. The region containing most large blood vessels

_____

4. Consider the following questions:

a. Through approximately how many lymph nodes does lymph pass before entering the bloodstream?

_____

b. Why does lymph need to pass through more than one lymph node?

_____

_____

c. What structural features of a lymph node ensure that lymph flows slowly through it?

_____

_____

d. Why is this beneficial?

_____

_____

e. What are macrophages?

_____

_____

f. What is their function in the lymph nodes?

_____

_____

g. Lymph nodes are distributed unevenly throughout the body, being most concentrated in three regions. What are these regions?

_____

_____

Apply the Concepts

1. A person with an infected throat often experiences swollen glands in the neck. What are these glands and why are they swollen?

_____

_____

2. Individuals who have undergone a radical mastectomy (surgical removal of a breast and axillary lymph nodes) often experience painful swelling of the arm on that side.

   a. What causes this swelling?

   _____

   _____

   b. The swelling often reduces with time and the arm returns to normal. What allows this to happen?

   _____

   _____

3. Bubonic plague is thought to have killed up to half the population of Europe in the 14th century. It is caused by bacteria transmitted in the bites of fleas, and still results in hundreds of deaths around the world each year. An infected individual develops painful buboes in the area close to the flea bite.

   a. What are buboes?

   _____

   _____

   b. How are plague bacteria conducted to the sites of the buboes?

   _____

   _____

ACTIVITY 18.3: MICROSCOPIC EXAMINATION OF LYMPHATIC STRUCTURES

The primary function of lymph nodes is to filter lymph before returning it to the lymphatic circulation (Fig. 18.4). In order to filter lymph, the lymph nodes must receive lymph via lymph vessels, which unlike blood vessels, contain lymphatic valves to aid their function (Fig. 18.3).

This activity examines the microscopic structure of lymph vessels and lymph nodes.

Lymph Vessel (LS)

1. Examine the prepared slide of a lymph vessel LS (H&E) under low power. Refer to Fig. 18.3 to assist with identification of the structures examined.

2. Locate a lymphatic valve in the lymph vessel.

3. In the space to the right, sketch a portion of the examined lymph vessel containing a valve.

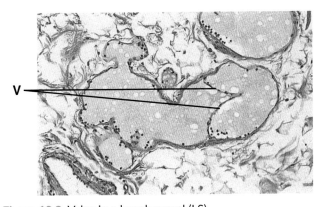

Figure 18.3 Valve in a lymph vessel (LS).
(Source: Burkitt, H. G., Young, B., Wheater, P. R., & Heath, J. W. (2006). Wheater's functional histology: A text and colour atlas. Elsevier.)

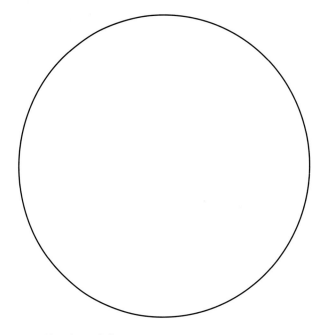

Magnification of diagram: × _____

a. From observing the structure of the valve, is it possible to identify the direction of lymph flow through the vessel?

_____

b. Indicate flow direction with an arrow on your diagram.

4. Lymphatic vessels are sometimes said to be similar to veins, but there are important differences.

a. What differences are visible in the specimen?

_____

_____

Lymph Node (TS)

1. Examine the prepared slide of a lymph node TS (H&E) under low power. Refer to Fig. 18.4 to assist with identification of the structures examined.

2. Identify the *cortex* containing *lymph follicles* with their *germinal centres* and the inner *medulla*. Note the *fibrous capsule* surrounding the gland and the *lymph vessels* running through it.

419

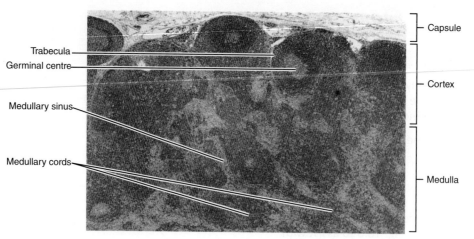

Figure 18.4 Lymph node (TS).
(Source: Shankar, N. D., & Vaz, M. (2022). Textbook of applied anatomy and applied physiology for nurses. Elsevier.)

3. Draw an outline sketch showing as many of these features as you can see in the space below and label your diagram.

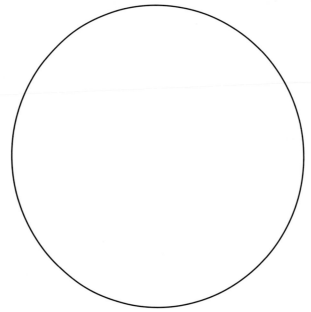

Magnification of diagram: × _____

Apply the Concepts

1. What is lymphoedema and how does it occur?

   _____

   _____

2. Distinguish between Hodgkin lymphoma and non-Hodgkin lymphoma.

   _____

   _____

   _____

ACTIVITY 18.4: LYMPHOID CELLS AND TISSUES

Lymphoid cells are cells of the immune system found in **lymphoid tissues**, and include supporting cells within those tissues. The major active cells of the immune system are the **lymphocytes**, which are manufactured in bone marrow and then mature into T lymphocytes (T cells) or B lymphocytes (B cells), which protect the body from foreign antigens. Lymphoid tissue is found in all **lymphoid organs** and serves the purposes of storing and increasing the numbers of lymphocytes, and of providing surveillance points for both lymphocytes and **macrophages**. A loose connective tissue, called reticular connective tissue, dominates most lymphoid organs and includes solid structures called **lymphoid follicles**, often containing germinal centres where B lymphocytes proliferate.

This activity examines the cells and tissues of the immune system and their roles in immunity.

1. Define the following terms:

   a. Antigen _____

   _____

   b. Antibody _____

   _____

2. Lymphoid tissue is the dominant tissue in all but one of the lymphoid organs. Which organ is the exception?

   _____

3. Complete the following sentences by filling in the blanks.

   a. Lymphoid tissue consists mainly of _____

   tissue which includes _____ lymphoid

   tissue, found in almost all body organs.

   b. Another type of lymphoid tissue comprising solid,

   spherical bodies and _____ fibres are the

   lymphoid _____.

   c. These often have lighter-staining centres called

   _____ , which contain proliferating

   _____ cells.

   d. Aggregations of these structures in the intestinal

   walls are called _____.

4. Consider the following questions:

   a. In which lymphoid organ are B lymphocytes produced?

   _____

   b. In which lymphoid organ are T lymphocytes produced?

   _____

   c. Due to their role in producing lymphocytes, what general name is given to these two organs?

   _____

Apply the Concepts

1. What is Castleman disease and how does it occur?

   _____

   _____

2. What is lymphatic filariasis and how does it occur?

   _____

   _____

ACTIVITY 18.5: OTHER LYMPHOID ORGANS – THE SPLEEN

The **spleen** is a secondary lymphoid organ and the largest of all the organs of the immune system (Fig. 18.5). Splenic tissue provides a site for lymphocytes to proliferate and maintain a surveillance for pathogens (Fig. 18.6). It is composed of **red pulp**, consisting of blood-filled venous sinuses, and **white pulp**, consisting of lymphoid tissue. In addition to its role in the immune system, the spleen has important functions in the cardiovascular system.

This activity examines the structure of the spleen and its dual physiological roles.

1. Obtain a model or chart of the human torso and locate the spleen.

   _____

2. Identify each of the labelled structures shown in Fig. 18.5, by matching the number of each structure with its correct term.

   a. Capsule _____

   b. Hilum _____

   c. Red pulp _____

   d. Splenic artery _____

   e. Splenic vein _____

   f. Trabecula _____

   g. Venous sinuses _____

   h. White pulp _____

3. Unlike lymph nodes, the spleen has a rich blood supply. What are the functions of the spleen in the blood vascular system?

   _____

   _____

   _____

   _____

4. Consider the following questions:

   a. What structures are responsible for the immune functions of the spleen?

   _____

   b. What types of cells mostly make up these structures?

   _____

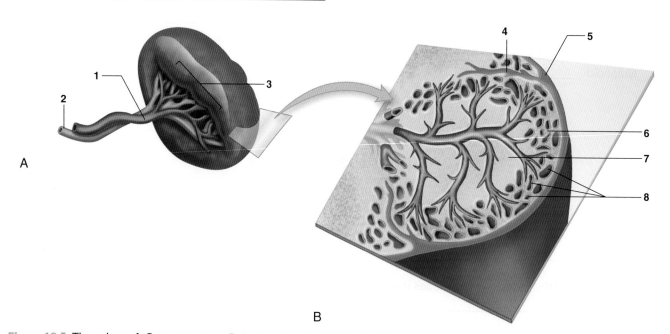

Figure 18.5 The spleen. **A** Gross structure. **B** Section showing histological features.
(*Source: Patton, K. T., Bell, F. B., Matusiak, D. J. et al. (2021). Anatomy and physiology laboratory manual. Elsevier.*)

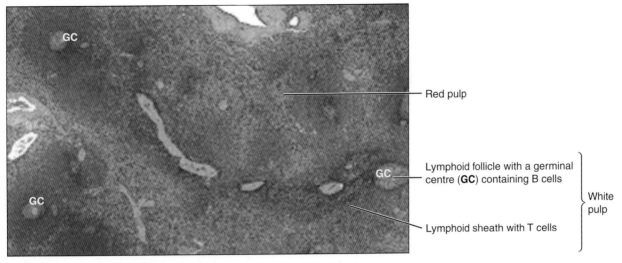

Figure 18.6 Photomicrograph of spleen tissue.
(Source: Davis, K., & Guerra, A. (2021). Mosby's pharmacy technician: Principles and practice. Elsevier.)

c. Explain the function of the splenic cords.

_____

_____

_____

d. The splenic cords are composed of which tissue?

_____

5. Obtain a prepared slide of spleen tissue TS (H&E) and examine it under the low power of a compound microscope. Refer to Fig. 18.6 to assist with identification of the structures examined.

a. Describe the arrangement of white pulp and red pulp in spleen tissue.

_____

_____

_____

b. Which structure(s) are also found in lymph nodes?

_____

6. Draw an outline sketch showing the capsule, white pulp and red pulp in the space below, and label your diagram.

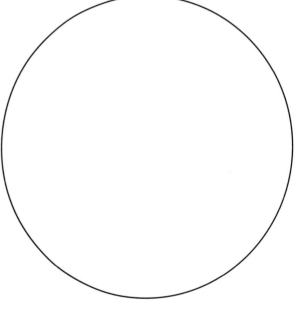

Magnification of diagram: ✕ _____

a. What roles does the spleen have in relation to blood filtration?

_____

_____

b. In which area of the splenic tissue does this process occur?

_____

Apply the Concepts

1. What is splenomegaly and how does it occur?

   _____

   _____

2. What is hypersplenism and how does it occur?

   _____

   _____

3. What is splenic rupture and how does it occur?

   _____

   _____

4. What is a splenectomy and what is the result systemically?

   _____

   _____

ACTIVITY 18.6: OTHER LYMPHOID ORGANS – THE THYMUS

The bilobed **thymus gland** has roles in both the endocrine and lymphatic systems (Fig. 18.7). It extends from the lower neck to the upper thorax and partly overlies the heart. It is divided into the left and right lobes, which are composed of **thymic lobules**, each containing regions of medulla and cortex. The thymus gland is prominent in babies and is active until puberty, when it starts to atrophy and to produce immunocompetent cells at a declining rate.

This activity examines the functions and structure of the thymus gland.

1. Obtain a model or chart of the human torso and locate the thymus.

   a. Which organs lie close or adjacent to the thymus?

   _____

   _____

2. Consider the endocrine role of the thymus and identify the:

   a. Hormones secreted _____

   _____

   b. Role(s) of the hormones _____

   _____

3. What type of lymphoid cells are produced in the thymus?

   _____

4. Examine Fig. 18.7, showing the structure of the thymus gland. Note that it is lobular and that each lobule is separated from the others by inward extensions called trabeculae. The cortex of each lobule is more densely stained than the medulla and within the medulla thymic corpuscles can sometimes be seen.

   a. What cell types are densely packed in the cortical regions?

   _____

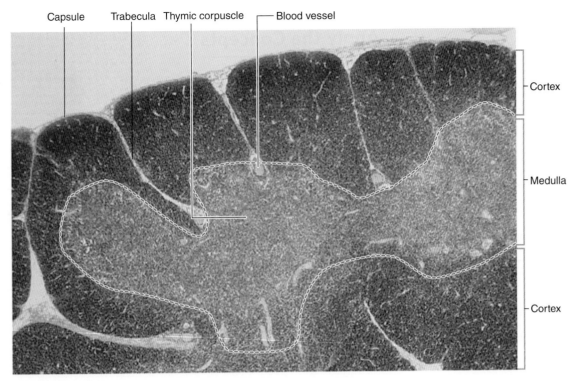

Capsule   Trabecula   Thymic corpuscle   — Blood vessel

Cortex

Medulla

Cortex

Figure 18.7 Structure of the thymus gland.
(Source: VanMeter, K. C., & Hubert, R. J. (2022). Pathophysiology for the health professions. Elsevier.)

b. What is considered to be the function of the thymic corpuscles?

_____

_____

c. What structures, found in other lymphoid organs, are absent from the thymus gland?

_____

5. Obtain a prepared slide of thymus tissue TS (H&E) and examine it under the low and high powers of a compound microscope. Refer to Fig. 18.7 to assist with identification of the structures examined.

6. In the space to the right, make a low-power sketch of thymus tissue, labelling any structures you can identify.

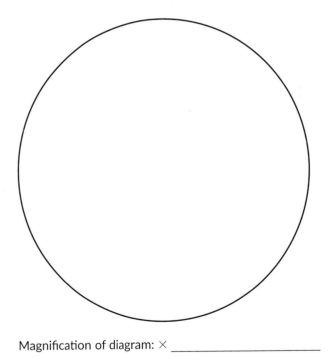

Magnification of diagram: ✕ _____

Apply the Concepts

1. What is myasthaenia gravis (MG) and how does it occur?

_____

_____

2. What is pure red cell aplasia (PRCA) and how does it occur?

_____

_____

3. What is hypogammaglobulinaemia and how does it occur?

_____

_____

4. What is thymoma and how does it occur?

_____

_____

ACTIVITY 18.7: MUCOSA-ASSOCIATED LYMPHOID TISSUE (MALT)

Mucosa-associated lymphoid tissue (MALT) constitutes about 50 per cent of all lymphoid tissue and is found in mucous membranes throughout the body. The role of MALT is to initiate immune responses to specific antigens encountered along all mucosal surfaces. The largest aggregations of MALT occur in the tonsils (**palatine tonsils, pharyngeal tonsils, lingual tonsils, tubal tonsils**), **Peyer's patches** and the **appendix**. The palatine tonsils are most commonly referred to simply as the tonsils (Fig. 18.8).

This activity examines the structure of the palatine tonsil in comparison with other lymphoid organs.

1. Obtain appropriate charts or diagrams and describe the exact locations of each type of tonsil in the table provided.

Tonsil	Location
Palatine	
Lingual	
Pharyngeal	
Tubal	

2. Why are the tonsils found in those parts of the body?

_____

_____

3. Pharyngeal tonsils are also known by which common name?

_____

4. Examine Fig. 18.8, showing the microscopic structure of a palatine tonsil.

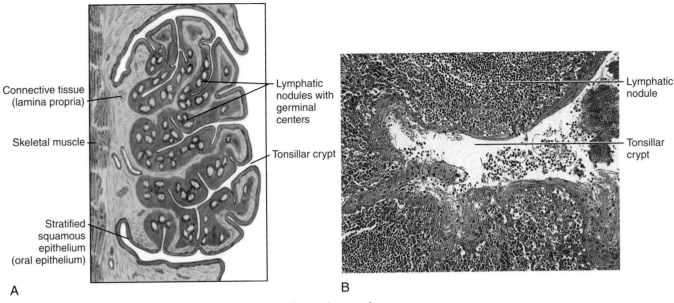

Figure 18.8 A palatine tonsil. **A** Schematic diagram. **B** Photomicrograph.
(Source: Fehrenbach, M. J., & Popowics, T. (2016). Illustrated dental embryology, histology, and anatomy. Elsevier.)

5. Palatine tonsils are the largest tonsils and are the only tonsils that are paired. Notice the follicles containing germinal centres and the tonsillar crypts arising from invaginations of the epithelium.

   a. Which structures in the palatine tonsil are absent from the thymus gland?

   _____

   b. What is the function of the tonsillar crypts?

   _____

6. Obtain a prepared slide of a section of palatine tonsil TS (H&E) and examine under the low and high powers of a compound microscope. Refer to Fig. 18.8 to assist with identification of the structure examined.

7. In the space below, make a low-power sketch of tonsil tissue, labelling any structures you can identify.

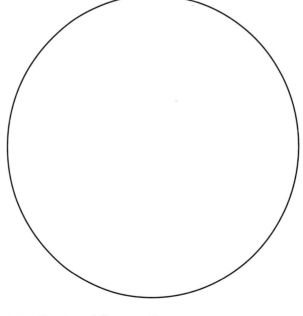

Magnification of diagram: × _____

8. The following table lists a number of properties of lymph nodes and lymphoid organs. Decide which organ fits each property by placing a tick in the column of that organ.

(Note: More than one organ may be ticked for each property.)

Property	Lymph node	Spleen	Thymus gland	Palatine tonsil
Has an endocrine function				
Located in the pharynx				
Atrophies in old age				
Contains lymphatic follicles				

Property	Lymph node	Spleen	Thymus gland	Palatine tonsil
Has afferent lymphatic vessels				
Found all over the body				
Has a rich blood supply				
Filters lymph				
A type of MALT				
Contains white and red pulp				
Has a bilobed structure				
Destroys cell fragments				

Apply the Concepts

1. What is tonsillitis and how does it occur?

_____

_____

2. Tonsillectomy (surgical removal of the tonsils) used to be commonly performed on children, but is now rare.

   a. Why is this procedure no longer routinely practised?

   _____

   _____

3. What are tonsilloliths and how do they occur?

_____

_____

4. What is a MALT lymphoma and where does it occur?

_____

_____

Additional Resources

Innerbody Research: Immune and Lymphatic Systems

Innerbody Research provides objective, science-based advice to help readers make more informed choices about home health products and services with most up-to-date reviews, guides and research, including information about the immune and lymphatic systems.

www.innerbody.com/image/lympov.html

Lumen Learning: Lymphatic System Structure and Function

Lumen Learning provides a number of online courses and modules related to the anatomy and physiology of a variety of body systems, including the lymphatic system.

courses.lumenlearning.com/boundless-ap/chapter/lymphatic-system-structure-and-function/

NursesLabs: Lymphatic System Anatomy and Physiology

NursesLabs is an educational resource for student nurses and covers care plans, exams, test banks and study notes on a variety of health-related topics.

nurseslabs.com/lymphatic-system-anatomy-physiology/

Osmosis – Lymphatic System Anatomy and Physiology

The Lymphatic System module of Osmosis provides videos, notes, quiz questions and links to further resources related to the lymphatic system.

www.osmosis.org/learn/Lymphatic_system_anatomy_and_physiology?from=/md/foundational-sciences/physiology/cardiovascular-system/anatomy-and-physiology

Physiopedia: Lymphatic System

Physiopedia is a free knowledge resource relating to physiotherapy, but also provides information on a number of body systems, such as the lymphatic system.

www.physio-pedia.com/Lymphatic_System

Teach Me Anatomy: The Lymphatic System and Tonsils

Teach Me Anatomy provides basic information on anatomical subjects and systems, with reference to the clinical relevance of the system being reviewed.

teachmeanatomy.info/the-basics/ultrastructure/lymphatic-system/
teachmeanatomy.info/neck/misc/tonsils-and-adenoids/

Visible Body: Lymphatic System

Visible Body provides interactive and highly accurate visualisations and apps for learning and teaching anatomy and physiology for students and healthcare professionals, including body systems such as the lymphatic system.

www.visiblebody.com/learn/lymphatic

CHAPTER 19
Immunity and Infection

In a world where all living things are under constant attack from a host of competitors, bacteria, viruses, parasites and noxious chemicals, animals have survived only by developing sophisticated defence mechanisms. The capacity of the human body to resist organisms, disease vectors and toxins that tend to damage tissues and organs is called immunity. Much of this resistance is provided by a special immune system that forms antibodies and activated lymphocytes which target specific invading organisms and toxins. (Refer to Chapter 18: The Lymphatic System, for further information on lymphatic tissue and the immune response.) This type of immunity is called acquired immunity and develops in response to the invasion of foreign agents, a time-consuming process. The other type is innate immunity, a defence system that provides constant, ready-made barricades to invasion. (Refer to Chapter 9: The Integumentary System, for further information on skin function.) Skin and mucosal linings prevent the entry of many invaders, stomach acid destroys pathogens in food, and the blood and tissues contain cells and chemicals which are prepared to break down invaders.

The immune system is best considered a functional system rather than a discrete anatomical system. Previously, the term immune system was only used in reference to acquired immunity, but it is now understood that acquired immunity and innate immunity are closely connected, and the mechanisms they develop to combat infection are interdependent.

LEARNING OUTCOMES

On completion of these activities, the student should be able to:

1. distinguish between innate and acquired immunity
2. describe the body's protective mechanisms against the entry of pathogens
3. describe the body's non-specific internal mechanisms for destroying pathogens
4. outline the sequence of events in the inflammatory response
5. distinguish between B and T lymphocytes in terms of their origins and functions
6. discuss the roles of antibodies in humoral immunity
7. describe the nature of cell-mediated immunity and the role of T lymphocytes
8. identify the mechanisms by which microorganisms can be transmitted between people.

KEY TERMS

Acquired immunity
Antibody
Antibody-mediated immunity
Antigen
B lymphocyte
Cell-mediated immunity
External innate defences
Fever
First line of defence

Humoral immunity
Immunoglobulins
Infection
Inflammation
Inflammatory response
Innate immunity
Internal innate defences
Monocyte
Non-specific immunity

Pathogen
Phagocytosis
Plasma cells
Second line of defence
Specific immunity
T lymphocyte
Third line of defence

ACTIVITY 19.1: EXTERNAL INNATE DEFENCES

The body's **innate immune** defences against attack are divided into two groups: those defences which prevent the entry of **pathogens** into the body (physical barriers) and those which deal with pathogens that gain entry, such as through cuts and scratches. These form the body's **external innate defences**, and are considered the body's **first line of defence**.

This activity examines the main features of external innate immunity.

1. Complete the following sentences by filling in the blanks.

    a. The outer layer of the skin, called the

       _____ forms the main physical barrier to

       the entry of micro-organisms.

    b. It contains high concentrations of the protein

       _____, which is resistant to weak acids and

       bases, and to bacterial enzymes and toxins.

    c. In addition, bacterial growth on the skin is inhibited

       by the _____ pH of the skin.

    d. Body cavities that open to the exterior, such as the

       _____, _____, _____,

       and _____ are lined with a type of tissue

       called _____ tissue, which also protects the

       body from invasion.

2. Consider the arrangements of the cells in the skin epidermis and in mucosal membranes.

    a. What do they have in common?

       _____

b. What is the importance of this arrangement?

   _____

   _____

3. List the defensive secretions produced by mucous membranes.

   _____

4. Bacteria that reach the stomach can be destroyed by stomach acid, but those that reach the lungs find conditions more conducive to growth and reproduction.

    a. Describe two protective mechanisms found in the respiratory system which prevent bacteria from reaching the lungs.

       _____

       _____

       _____

       _____

       _____

       _____

5. Which enzyme is found in lachrymal fluid and helps to protect the eyes from invading pathogens?

_____

6. Explain what is meant by the body's 'acid mantle'.

_____

_____

_____

ACTIVITY 19.2: INTERNAL INNATE DEFENCES

When microorganisms penetrate the external defences and enter the deeper tissues, the body's **internal innate defences** are triggered. These comprise **non-specific immunity**, which involves agents that react quickly to destroy foreign objects, such as in the process of **phagocytosis** (Fig. 19.1). This is considered the body's **second line of defence**.

This activity considers the mechanisms involved in the internal innate defences.

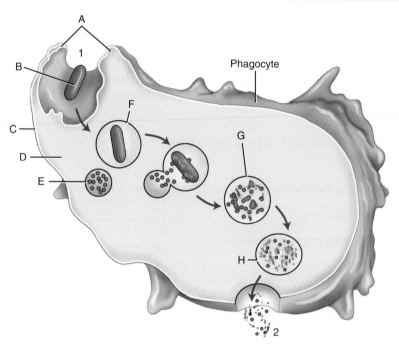

Figure 19.1 Phagocytosis.
(Source: Herlihy, B., Kirov, E. (2022). The human body in health and illness. Elsevier.)

1. Define the following terms:

   a. Phagocyte _____

   _____

   b. Macrophage _____

   _____

   c. Chemotaxis _____

   _____

2. Which leukocytes give rise to macrophages?

   _____

3. Which other leukocytes can become phagocytic?

   _____

4. Identify the locations in the body where the following can be found:

   a. Fixed macrophages

   _____

   b. Free macrophages

   _____

5. Examine Fig. 19.1 and match the letter of each labelled structure with its correct term or the event occurring.

   a. Cytoplasm _____

   b. Lysosome _____

   c. Pathogen _____

   d. Phagolysosome _____

   e. Phagosome _____

   f. Plasma membrane _____

   g. Pseudopodia _____

   h. Residual body _____

6. Consider the following questions, with reference to Fig. 19.1:

   a. What is contained in structure E?

   _____

   b. What is released from structure H?

   _____

c. Identify the process occurring:

   i. At event 1

   _____

   ii. At event 2

   _____

   iii. In structure G

   _____

7. If a phagocyte is unable to destroy a pathogen by enzyme action alone, it may introduce bactericidal chemicals into the phagocytic vesicle.

   a. Identify some of these chemical agents.

   _____

   _____

8. What name is given to the small group of large granular leukocytes which circulate in blood and lymph and kill cancer cells and virus-infected cells before acquired immunity is activated?

   _____

ACTIVITY 19.3: THE INFLAMMATORY RESPONSE

When tissue injury occurs from any cause, the injured tissues release multiple substances that cause secondary changes in those tissues. This suite of tissue changes is called the **inflammatory response**, and includes local vasodilatation, leakage of fluid from capillaries into interstitial spaces, clot formation in interstitial fluid, and migration of leukocytes into interstitial spaces (Fig. 19.2). The **second line of defence** against invading organisms involves cells which invade the injured area in large numbers from the blood. When the **inflammation** is severe, concentrations of these cells in the blood can increase five-fold. The **third line of defence** can take several days to develop and is mediated by **monocytes**, which are normally in low concentrations in the blood. If an **infection** develops, a **fever** occurs.

This activity explores the mechanisms and consequences of the inflammatory response.

1. One of the first effects of inflammation is that the area of injury is 'walled off' from surrounding tissues.

   a. Explain how this occurs.

   _____

   _____

   b. Why is this important?

   _____

   _____

2. The process of inflammation begins with the release of many chemicals into the tissue surrounding the injury.

   a. Identify some of these chemicals.

   _____

   _____

   b. Describe three important roles these chemicals play in the inflammatory response.

   _____

   _____

   _____

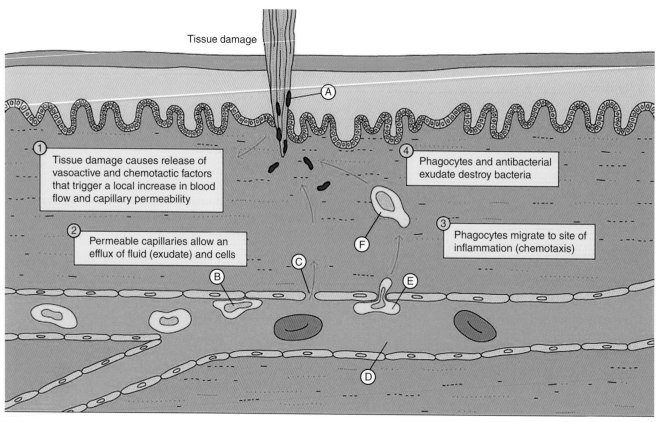

Figure 19.2 Initial response to injury.
(Source: Kumari, R., Inflammation – process, factors and anti-inflammatory agents. Microbiology notes, 2021. https://microbiologynotes.org/inflammation-process-factors-and-anti-inflammatory-agents/)

3. What are the five cardinal signs of inflammation?

_____

_____

_____

4. When the body's cells are damaged or exposed to foreign substances, many release chemicals to elevate body temperature, resulting in fever.

a. What are these chemicals called?

_____

b. How do they act to elevate body temperature?

_____

_____

c. Why might this be advantageous?

_____

_____

_____

5. What is the first line of defence?

_____

_____

a. Which type of tissue provides the first line of defence?

_____

b. Give the locations of some of these tissues.

_____

_____

6. What is the second line of defence?

_____

_____

a. What type of cells provide the second line of defence?

_____

b. What are the names of these cells?

_____

c. What body tissue is the source of these new cells?

_____

d. What is the name of the process whereby these cells squeeze through spaces that form between epithelial cells in capillary walls to enter the injured tissue?

_____

7. What is the third line of defence?

_____

_____

_____

a. In which tissue is the storage pool of monocytes found?

_____

b. When monocytes arrive at the injured tissue they are immature cells which take 8 hours or more to differentiate into what type of phagocytic cells?

_____

8. Examine Fig. 19.2 and match the structures or processes with the terms provided.

Bacteria   Diapedesis
Capillary   Margination
Capillary exudate   Neutrophil

a. A: _____

b. B: _____

c. C: _____

d. D: _____

e. E: _____

f. F: _____

9. Since viruses are not living organisms, explain how they are able to replicate.

_____

_____

_____

10. Some infected cells can produce interferons.

a. What are interferons and how do they help protect cells from viral infections?

_____

_____

_____

Apply the Concepts

1. In severely infected areas, a creamy-yellow pus may form in a wound.

   a. Describe the composition of pus.

   _____

   _____

2. If the inflammatory response fails to clear a wound of debris, collagen fibres may be laid down to wall off the sac of pus.

   a. What structure is formed by this mechanism?

   _____

   b. What procedure may need to be performed on this structure?

   _____

3. As part of the inflammatory response, capillary permeability increases to the point that plasma proteins leak into the interstitial fluid.

   a. Why is this desirable?

   _____

   _____

4. Explain why steroids are often prescribed for inflammation.

   _____

   _____

ACTIVITY 19.4: THE ROLE OF LYMPHOCYTES IN ACQUIRED IMMUNITY

In addition to innate immunity, the body has mechanisms to develop **specific immunity** against particular invading agents such as bacteria, viruses, toxins or transplanted foreign cells and tissues. This is called **acquired immunity** and has two components. The first is **humoral immunity**, also called **antibody-mediated immunity**, and the second is **cell-mediated immunity**.

This activity explores the nature of humoral immunity.

1. B and T lymphocytes are both involved in acquired immunity, but have different sources and functions. Tick the appropriate box on each line of the table provided based on their characteristics.

Characteristic	B Lymphocytes	T Lymphocytes
Originate in bone marrow		
Mature in the thymus		
Mature in the bone marrow		
Responsible for humoral immunity		
Responsible for cell-mediated immunity		
Produce antibodies		

2. Distinguish between an antigen and an antibody.

   _____

   _____

   _____

3. Complete the following sentences by filling in the blanks with the terms provided.

   Antigen   Proliferate
   Clonal selection   Receptors
   Effector   Secondary
   Immunocompetence   Self-tolerance
   Memory

   a. During maturation, lymphocytes must become

   capable of recognising one specific _____

   and binding to it. This ability is called _____.

   b. Lymphocytes bind to foreign antigens by means of

   _____ on their cell membranes, but must

   be unresponsive to the antigens of the body's own

   cells, a property called _____.

c. After differentiation, B and T cells travel to _____ lymphoid organs, the bone marrow and thymus.

d. When a foreign antigen binds to the surface receptors of B and T cells, the lymphocytes _____ rapidly, forming a clone of similar cells, a process called _____.

e. These cells then specialise into _____ cells and _____ cells, increasing the speed of the response when exposed to further antigens.

Apply the Concepts

1. What is a hapten?

   _____

   _____

2. How do haptens and antigens differ?

   _____

   _____

ACTIVITY 19.5: HUMORAL IMMUNITY

Humoral immunity, mediated by **B lymphocytes**, involves the production of **antibodies** in the body's humors (fluids such as blood and lymph). These antibodies bind mainly to **antigens** or invading agents such as bacteria, viruses and toxins (Fig. 19.3).

This activity explores the nature of humoral immunity.

1. B lymphocytes differentiate to form which two effector cells of the humoral response?

   _____

2. Identify the functions of the following B cells:

   a. Memory cells _____

   _____

   b. Plasma cells _____

   _____

3. Consider the following questions with reference to Fig. 19.3:

   a. Is the secondary immune response to antigen A less than, similar to, or greater than the primary immune response?

   _____

   b. Is the primary immune response to antigen B less than, similar to, or greater than the primary response to antigen A?

   _____

   c. How long is the delay between the first exposure to antigen A and the response to it?

   _____

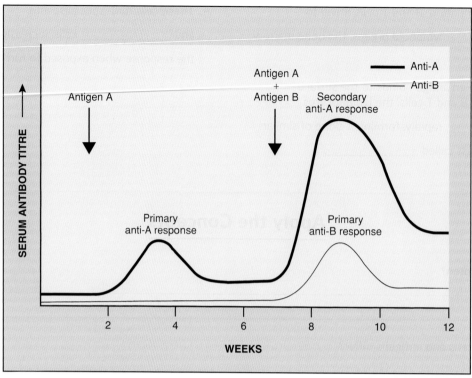

Figure 19.3 Primary and secondary immune responses to two antigens.
(Source: Gould, B. E., & Dyer, R. (2011). Pathophysiology for the health professions. Elsevier.)

d. What causes this delay?

_____

_____

e. How long is the delay between the second exposure to antigen A and the response to it?

_____

f. Why is the delay different from that in the first exposure?

_____

g. What cells mediate the secondary response?

_____

h. Why is the secondary response so much greater than the primary response?

_____

_____

i. Why is the response to antigen B so much smaller than the secondary response to antigen A?

_____

_____

4. The events shown in Fig. 19.3 are examples of active humoral immunity.

a. What is passive humoral immunity?

_____

_____

_____

b. Provide an example of:

i. Natural passive immunity _____

_____

ii. Artificial passive immunity _____

_____

Apply the Concepts

1. What is an allergen and how does it cause an allergic response?

   _____

   _____

   _____

2. Explain the meaning of self-tolerance.

   _____

   _____

3. Is there a distinction between vaccination and immunisation? Explain.

   _____

   _____

   _____

4. What is serology testing?

   _____

   _____

ACTIVITY 19.6: ANTIBODIES

Antibodies are gamma globulin proteins, collectively called **immunoglobulins**, secreted by effector B lymphocytes called **plasma cells** (Fig. 19.4).

This activity explores the nature and functions of antibodies.

1. Consider the following questions, with reference to Fig. 19.4:

   a. How many classes of antibodies are found in the human body?

   _____

   b. Provide the function of each of the following human antibodies:

      i. IgA _____

      ii. IgD _____

      iii. IgE _____

      iv. IgG _____

      v. IgM _____

   c. How many peptide chains are found in the IgG antibody?

   _____

   d. Which labelled part(s) of the antibody are antigen binding site(s)?

   _____

   e. What name is given to the region labelled B?

   _____

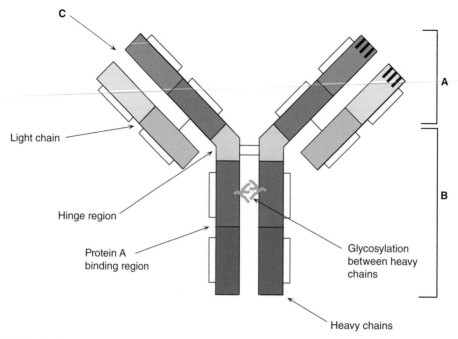

Figure 19.4 IgG antibody structure.
(Source: Hermanson, G. T. (2013). Bioconjugate techniques. Academic Press.)

f. Which parts of the antibody are variable?

_____

g. Why would you expect antibodies such as IgG to have variable parts?

_____

2. In which two ways do antibodies act to protect the body from invaders?

_____

_____

3. Define the following terms:

a. Precipitation _____

_____

b. Lysis _____

_____

c. Agglutination _____

_____

d. Neutralisation _____

_____

Apply the Concepts

1. Active humoral immunity may be artificially acquired when a person receives a vaccine. Most vaccines contain infecting agents that are either dead or severely weakened, or some components of those agents.

a. What components of a pathogen must be present in a vaccine in order to confer immunity?

_____

_____

b. How does a vaccine protect a person from a pathogen such as a virus?

_____

_____

c. Some vaccines require a follow-up booster shot. What is the purpose of these?

_____

_____

d. Would a booster shot have the same effect on the immune system as the initial injection? Explain why.

_____

_____

2. Is there a distinction between immunodeficiency and autoimmune disease? Explain.

_____

_____

_____

3. Is there a distinction between HIV and AIDS? Explain.

_____

_____

_____

ACTIVITY 19.7: CELL-MEDIATED IMMUNITY

Cell-mediated immunity, or **T lymphocyte immunity**, is best suited to respond to invading cells and is achieved through the formation of activated lymphocytes. T cells are more complex and diverse than B cells and do not produce antibodies.

This activity explores the diversity and roles of T cells in cell-mediated immunity.

1. Where are immature lymphocytes formed?

_____

2. Where do immature lymphocytes mature and differentiate?

_____

3. Identify the function of each type of lymphocyte:

a. Helper T cells _____

_____

b. Cytotoxic T cells _____

_____

c. Regulatory T cells _____

_____

4. Why is it necessary to have regulatory T cells?

_____

_____

_____

5. How could regulatory T cells be useful in tissue transplant procedures?

_____

_____

_____

6. What are cytokines?

_____

_____

_____

a. What effect do cytokines have on T cells?

_____

_____

7. Complete the following sentences by filling in the blanks with the terms provided.

Antigens	Cytotoxic
Apoptosis	Killer
Bacteria	Perforins
Cancer	Viruses
Cell membrane	

a. Cytotoxic T cells, also known as _____ T cells, roam the body in search of cells displaying _____ that the T cells recognise.

b. Their main targets are cells containing _____ but they also attack cells infected by _____ as well as the body's own _____ cells.

c. After binding to a target cell, the cytotoxic T cells secrete hole-forming proteins called _____ which punch holes in the _____ of the attacked cell.

d. The T cells then inject _____ substances, leading to the death of the target cell.

e. Cytotoxic T cells may also stimulate a target cell to kill itself, a process called _____.

8. Natural killer cells and cytotoxic T cells use similar mechanisms to kill their target cells.

a. How do they differ in the way they identify target cells?

_____

_____

_____

Apply the Concepts

1. When the immune system loses its ability to distinguish foreign cells from the body's own cells it may start to destroy its own tissues.

a. What name is given to this condition?

_____

b. Give examples of diseases that are caused by this condition.

_____

_____

c. How can this condition be treated?

_____

_____

2. A person suffers a bee sting and 20 minutes later the area stung is red, swollen, and painful.

   a. What type of agent has been injected by the bee?

   _____

   b. What type of immune response has been elicited?

   _____

   c. If the sting produces an allergic reaction, what drug may be administered to reduce the allergic response?

   _____

3. Explain why immunosuppressive therapy is often prescribed following transplant surgery.

   _____

   _____

4. What is systemic lupus erythematosus (SLE) and what are its consequences?

   _____

   _____

   _____

   _____

ACTIVITY 19.8: MICROORGANISMS AND INFECTION

Infection occurs when a microorganism or virus enters the body and causes harm. Infections can be transmitted from one person to another by inhaling airborne microorganisms, the transfer of body fluids, ingesting liquids or solids, or touching an object that an infected person has touched.

This activity will demonstrate the ease with which infections can be transferred between individuals.

Part 1: Simulation of Infection Transmission

1. This activity is best conducted in groups of four.

2. Assign each person in the group a number from 1 to 4.

3. Have person 1 dispense a small amount of Glitterbug potion onto their right hand and rub in well.

4. Examine the right hand of person 1 under UV light.

5. Have person 1 firmly shake hands with person 2.

6. Have person 2 firmly shake hands with person 3.

7. Have person 3 firmly shake hands with person 4.

8. Examine each person's right hand under the UV light.

9. All members of the group should wash their hands before proceeding further.

10. Consider the following questions:

   a. Which group member had the most potion on their hand?

   _____

   b. What do the results indicate about the ease with which microorganisms can be transmitted?

   _____

   _____

   _____

c. What factors contribute to the ease of transmission of microorganisms?

_____

_____

_____

_____

Part 2: Hand Hygiene

1. Have all members in the group dispense a small amount of Glitterbug potion onto their hands and rub in well.

2. Allow to air dry.

3. Have all group members wash their hands well with soap and water, following the handwashing technique displayed in the laboratory.

4. Gently pat dry with paper towels.

5. All members of the group should now examine their hands under UV light.

6. Consider the following questions:

a. Which areas of the hands were not cleaned?

_____

b. What could you have done to improve your handwashing technique?

_____

c. What does the result indicate about the importance of correct handwashing technique?

_____

_____

Additional Resources

BioInteractive: The Immune System
BioInteractive provides tools, resources, and professional learning materials that reflect current knowledge and evidence-based strategies on topics such as the immune system.

www.biointeractive.org/classroom-resources/immune-system

Histology Guide Virtual Microscopy Laboratory: Lymphoid System
Histology Guide is an online resource providing a virtual microscopy laboratory experience, by allowing users to view microscope slides from professional collections for the purpose of interpreting cellular and tissue structures as seen through a microscope.

histologyguide.com/slidebox/10-lymphoid-system.html

Innerbody Research: Immune and Lymphatic Systems
Innerbody Research provides objective, science-based advice to help readers make more informed choices about home health products and services with most up-to-date reviews, guides and research, including information about the immune and lymphatic systems.

www.innerbody.com/image/lympov.html

Osmosis – Immune System
The Immune System module of Osmosis provides videos, notes, quiz questions, and links to further resources related to the immune system.

www.osmosis.org/library/md/foundational-sciences/physiology#immune_system

Physiopedia: Immune System
Physiopedia provides a knowledge and resource base for physiotherapists and on a range of topics including the immune system and complement system.

www.physio-pedia.com/Immune_System
www.physio-pedia.com/Complement_System

The Histology Guide: Lymphoid Tissue
The Histology Guide is a virtual experience of using a microscope with zoom features. It is divided into topics and offers histological slides with labels and quizzes for each topic, such as lymphoid tissue. It is provided by the University of Leeds.

www.histology.leeds.ac.uk/lymphoid/index.php

The McGill Physiology Virtual Lab: Immunology Laboratory
A series of interactive tutorials on a variety of physiology topics created for students enrolled in introductory physiology courses at McGill University.

www.medicine.mcgill.ca/physio/vlab/immun/vlabmenuimmun.htm

The Vaccine Makers Project
The Vaccine Makers Project provides scientifically supported content and a variety of resources to educate about how the immune system works and how vaccines work to prevent disease.

vaccinemakers.org/resources/videos/innate-immune-system-animation

CHAPTER 20
The Digestive System

The digestive system acts as a deconstruction line that processes food, absorbs nutrients and supplies molecules obtained from the nutrient pool to the tissues and cells of the body. This helps to build, repair and replace biological structures. The digestive system consists of the gastrointestinal tract, also referred to as the alimentary canal, which extends from the mouth or oral cavity to the rectum, and terminates at the anus. Accessory digestive organs consisting of the salivary glands, liver, gall bladder and pancreas produce secretions outside the gastrointestinal tract that are subsequently emptied into the tract. These secretions aid the digestive process and include bile which emulsifies fats, digestive enzymes which hydrolyse macromolecules, and mucus which assists the passage of food through the gastrointestinal tract. (Refer to Chapter 4: Biological Chemistry, for further information on enzyme function and macromolecule structure.)

The digestive system carries out six main processes. These are: ingestion, which involves eating; propulsion, which involves the movement of food through the gastrointestinal tract and includes peristalsis; mechanical digestion, which involves physically reducing the size of food particles and includes chewing, stomach churning and segmentation; chemical digestion, which involves breaking molecular bonds via the actions of digestive enzymes; absorption, which extracts nutrients from the digestive tract and releases them into the blood circulation; and defecation, which eliminates food residue and indigestible remains from the body.

LEARNING OUTCOMES

On completion of these activities, the student should be able to:

1. outline the structure and function of the digestive system
2. explain the activities associated with the digestive process
3. describe the macroscopic and microscopic structure, and function of the gastrointestinal wall
4. outline the structure and function of the upper digestive structures
5. describe the process of deglutition
6. outline the structure and function of the stomach and its digestive processes
7. outline the structure and function of the intestines and relate this to intestinal absorption

LEARNING OUTCOMES—cont'd

8. identify the location of the digestive organs within the abdomen
9. outline the structure and function of the accessory digestive organs
10. explain the functions of accessory digestive organ secretions on the digestive process
11. describe the location of the secretion and functions of digestive system enzymes
12. describe the emulsification of fats.

KEY TERMS

Absorption
Accessory digestive organs
Bile
Bolus
Chemical digestion
Chyme
Defecation
Deglutition
Digestion
Duodenum
Elimination

Emulsification
Epiglottis
Gall bladder
Gastrointestinal tract
Ingestion
Large intestine
Liver
Mechanical digestion
Oesophagus
Oral cavity
Pancreas

Peristalsis
Propulsion
Rugae
Saliva
Salivary glands
Segmentation
Small intestine
Sphincter
Stomach
Tongue
Villi

ACTIVITY 20.1: STRUCTURE AND FUNCTION OF THE DIGESTIVE SYSTEM

The digestive system consists of the **gastrointestinal tract**, or alimentary canal, and the **accessory digestive organs**, which aid the gastrointestinal tract in its processes of **digestion** (Fig. 20.1). Food is mechanically and chemically broken down in the gastrointestinal tract, which secretes a variety of digestive substances and enzymes. Additional digestive enzymes are produced by the accessory digestive organs and secreted into the gastrointestinal tract at various locations along the digestive pathway to further assist **chemical digestion** (Fig. 20.2).

This activity provides an overview of the structure and function of the digestive system and the pathway of food through the digestive tract.

1. Identify the structures of the digestive system in Fig. 20.1:

   a. Structure A: _____

   b. Structure B: _____

   c. Structure C: _____

   d. Structure D: _____

   e. Structure E: _____

   f. Structure F: _____

   g. Structure G: _____

   h. Structure H: _____

   i. Structure I: _____

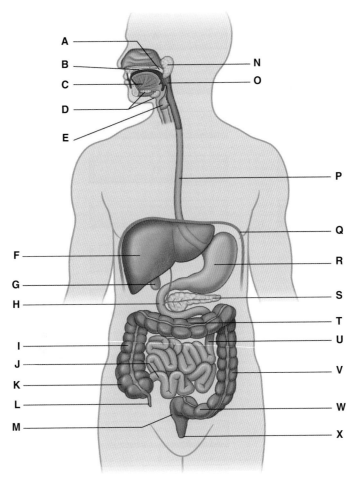

Figure 20.1 Structures of the digestive system.
(Source: Waugh, A., & Grant, A. (2014). Ross & Wilson anatomy and physiology in health and illness. Elsevier.)

j. Structure J: _____

k. Structure K: _____

l. Structure L: _____

m. Structure M: _____

n. Structure N: _____

o. Structure O: _____

p. Structure P: _____

q. Structure Q: _____

r. Structure R: _____

s. Structure S: _____

t. Structure T: _____

u. Structure U: _____

v. Structure V: _____

w. Structure W: _____

x. Structure X: _____

2. Consider the following questions with reference to Fig. 20.1:

   a. Structures A, B, and C form which part of the digestive system?

   _____

   b. Structures H, J, and U form which part of the digestive system?

   _____

   c. Structures I, K, L, T, V and W form which part of the digestive system?

   _____

   d. Structures D, F, G, N and S form which part of the digestive system?

   _____

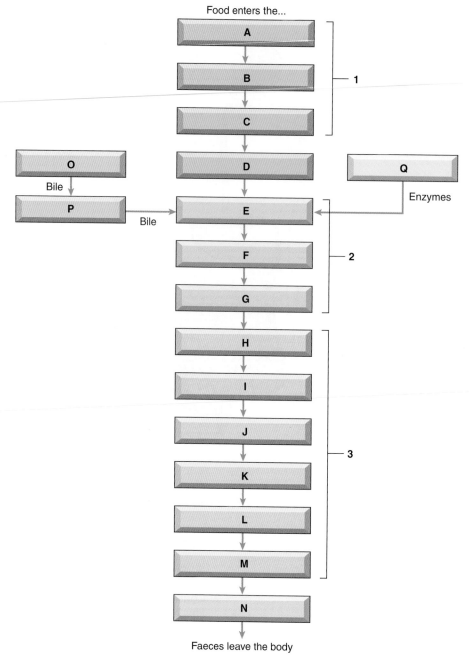

Food enters the...

Figure 20.2 Pathway of food through the digestive tract.
(Source: Chabner, D. E. (2020). The language of medicine. Elsevier.)

3. Briefly state the digestive function of each of the structures below:

a. Mouth: _____

_____

b. Teeth: _____

c. Tongue: _____

_____

d. Salivary glands: _____

_____

e. Pharynx: _____

_____

f. Oesophagus: _____

_____

g. Stomach: _____

_____

h. Liver: _____

_____

i. Gall bladder: _____

_____

j. Pancreas: _____

_____

k. Duodenum _____

_____

l. Small intestine _____

_____

m. Large intestine: _____

_____

n. Rectum: _____

_____

o. Anus: _____

_____

4. The gastrointestinal tract is also referred to by which other term?

_____

5. Identify the structures associated with the pathway of food through the digestive tract in Fig. 20.2:

a. Structure A: _____

b. Structure B: _____

c. Structure C: _____

d. Structure D: _____

e. Structure E: _____

f. Structure F: _____

g. Structure G: _____

h. Structure H: _____

i. Structure I: _____

j. Structure J: _____

k. Structure K: _____

l. Structure L: _____

m. Structure M: _____

n. Structure N: _____

o. Structure O: _____

p. Structure P: _____

q. Structure Q: _____

6. Identify the six main digestive processes and, based on Fig. 20.2, list the structures involved in the table below.

Digestive process	Structures involved

7. Which region of the digestive system is indicated by the following colours:

a. Green: _____

b. Orange: _____

c. Purple: _____

d. Yellow: _____

8. Are peristalsis and segmentation voluntary or involuntary processes? Explain.

_____

_____

9. Compare the processes of peristalsis and segmentation in the table provided.

	Peristalsis	Segmentation
Digestive process		
Purpose		
Location		
Direction of movement		
Description of process		

ACTIVITY 20.2: STRUCTURE AND FUNCTION OF THE GASTROINTESTINAL WALL

The wall of the gastrointestinal tract consists of four layers, each with its own structural arrangement (Fig. 20.3). The thickness and characteristics of each layer changes throughout the tract, based on the functions of that particular region. For example, the **oesophagus** is lined with stratified squamous epithelium to allow for abrasion caused by swallowing food, whereas the **small intestine** is lined with simple columnar epithelium to allow for **absorption** of nutrients. In addition, mucus is produced throughout most of the gastrointestinal tract for the purpose of lubrication and protection, while the movement of food through the gastrointestinal tract via **peristalsis** is an involuntary process which requires the coordinated contraction of smooth muscle within the intestinal wall.

This activity examines the structure and function of the gastrointestinal wall.

1. Identify the layers of the gastrointestinal wall and their associated structures based on Fig. 20.3:

   a. Layer A: _____

      i. Structure 1: _____

      ii. Structure 2: _____

   b. Layer B: _____

      i. Structure 3: _____

      ii. Structure 4: _____

   c. Layer C: _____

      i. Structure 5: _____

      ii. Structure 6: _____

      iii. Structure 7: _____

   d. Layer D: _____

      i. Structure 8: _____

      ii. Structure 9: _____

2. Consider the following questions:

   a. What is the purpose of the lymphatic tissue?

      _____

      _____

   b. Which tissue comprises the mesenteries and what is their function?

      _____

      _____

      _____

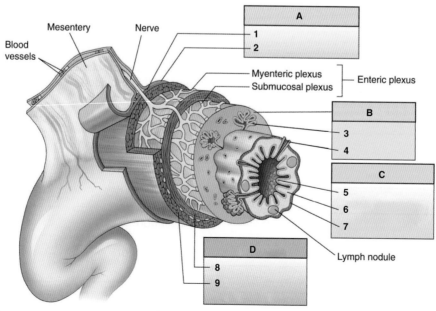

Figure 20.3 Wall of the gastrointestinal tract.
(Source: McCance, K. L., & Huether, S. E. (2019). Pathophysiology: The biologic basis for disease in adults and children. Elsevier.)

c. Which tissue comprises the omenta and what is the function of the omenta?

_____

_____

_____

d. Which tissue comprises the mucosa and what is the function of the mucosa?

_____

_____

_____

e. Which tissue comprises the serosa and what is the function of the serosa?

_____

_____

_____

f. Which tissue comprises the muscularis and what is the function of the muscularis?

_____

_____

_____

g. What is the function of the blood vessels present within the submucosa?

_____

_____

h. What is the function of the nerves present within the muscularis?

_____

_____

Apply the Concepts

1. What is a hernia and how does it occur?

_____

_____

_____

2. What is Crohn's disease and how does it occur?

_____

_____

_____

3. What is ulcerative colitis and how does it occur?

_____

_____

_____

Additional Activities

For additional activities visit Activity 20A: Microscopic Examination of the Gastrointestinal Tract on Evolve˙.

For additional activities visit Activity 20B: Structure and Function of the Upper Digestive Structures on Evolve˙.

ACTIVITY 20.3: PROCESS AND MECHANICS OF DEGLUTITION

Deglutition, or swallowing, occurs once food has been ingested, mechanically broken down, lubricated with **saliva**, and a **bolus** has been formed.

This activity outlines the process and mechanics of deglutition.

Part 1: Process of Deglutition

The process of swallowing occurs in three phases, and requires the coordinated activity of the upper digestive structures, particularly the **epiglottis** (Fig. 20.4).

1. Identify and explain the process occurring in each phase of deglutition in Fig. 20.4:

   a. Phase 1: _____

      i. Process: _____

      _____

   b. Phase 2: _____

      i. Process: _____

      _____

   c. Phase 3: _____

      i. Process: _____

      _____

2. Consider the following questions with reference to Fig. 20.4:

   a. What is a bolus?

   _____

   _____

b. Which stages of deglutition are under voluntary control?

   _____

   _____

c. Which stages of deglutition are under involuntary control?

   _____

   _____

d. Which process propels food through the oesophagus and how is this achieved?

   _____

   _____

e. Explain how the bolus is conveyed into the oesophagus once it reaches the entrance of the oesophagus.

   _____

   _____

   _____

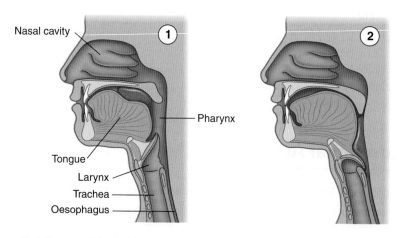
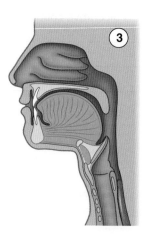

Figure 20.4 Stages of deglutition.
(Source: Waugh, A., & Grant, A. (2014). Ross & Wilson Anatomy and physiology in health and illness. Elsevier.)

f. With reference to pharyngeal structures, explain how choking occurs.

_____

_____

_____

Part 2: Mechanics of Deglutition

The goal of deglutition is **propulsion**, where the bolus is pushed into the oesophagus for delivery to the **stomach** for further chemical digestion and the formation of **chyme**.

1. This activity is best conducted in pairs.

2. Obtain two disposable cups, potable water, stethoscope, alcohol wipes and a stopwatch.

3. Fill both cups with water for each subject.

4. Swallow a mouthful of water, consciously noting the movement of your tongue.

   a. What was noted regarding the movement of the tongue?

   _____

5. One subject should repeat the swallowing process, while the other subject watches.

6. Notice the movement of the larynx, which is visible externally (this movement is more obvious in males).

   a. What was noticeable regarding the movement of the larynx?

   _____

7. Obtain a stethoscope and clean the earpieces with the alcohol wipes before use.

8. Place the bell of the stethoscope over the subject's abdominal wall approximately 2 cm below the xiphoid process and slightly to the left.

9. Listen for sounds as the subject takes two or three swallows of water. There should be two audible sounds.

10. Determine the time interval between these two sounds.

    a. Number of seconds: _____

11. Consider the following questions:

    a. What does the movement of the larynx accomplish?

    _____

    _____

    b. What does the first audible sound indicate?

    _____

    _____

    c. What does the second audible sound indicate?

    _____

    _____

    d. What is the composition of the gastroesophageal (cardiac) sphincter?

    _____

    _____

    e. What is the function of the gastroesophageal (cardiac) sphincter?

    _____

    _____

Apply the Concepts

1. What is heartburn and how does it occur?

_____

_____

_____

2. What is gastroesophageal reflux disease (GORD) and how does it occur?

_____

_____

_____

3. What is achalasia and how does it occur?

_____

_____

_____

ACTIVITY 20.4: STRUCTURE AND FUNCTION OF THE STOMACH

The stomach is a temporary storage tank for partially digested food. It is highly motile due to having three specialised muscular layers, which are able to contract the stomach wall in multiple directions to facilitate mechanical digestion (Fig. 20.5). The stomach is bound by two muscular **sphincters**, one at the junction of the oesophagus and stomach entrance (gastroesophageal sphincter), the other at the junction of the stomach exit and the entrance to the small intestine (pyloric sphincter). In addition, the stomach contains internal folds of tissue called **rugae**, which serve to increase the internal volume of the stomach as it fills and the lining stretches. The stomach receives mechanically digested food which has been physically broken down and conveyed from the oral cavity via the oesophagus in the form of a bolus. Once in the stomach, the food is mixed with gastric juice and chemically digested by enzymes to form chyme.

This activity examines the structure and function of the stomach.

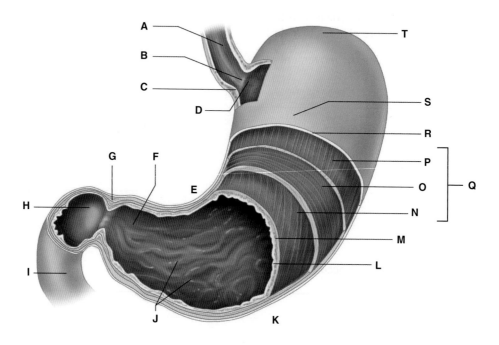

Figure 20.5 Structure of the stomach.
(Source: Thibodeau, G. A., and T Patton, K. (2012). Anthony's textbook of anatomy and physiology. Mosby, Elsevier.)

1. Identify the structures of the stomach in Fig. 20.5:

    a. Structure A: _____

    b. Structure B: _____

    c. Structure C: _____

    d. Structure D: _____

    e. Structure E: _____

    f. Structure F: _____

    g. Structure G: _____

    h. Structure H: _____

    i. Structure I: _____

    j. Structure J: _____

    k. Structure K: _____

    l. Structure L: _____

    m. Structure M: _____

    n. Structure N: _____

    o. Structure O: _____

    p. Structure P: _____

    q. Structure Q: _____

    r. Structure R: _____

    s. Structure S: _____

    t. Structure T: _____

2. Consider the following questions:

    a. Identify the three main functions of the stomach.

    _____

    _____

    b. What are the rugae and what is their function?

    _____

    _____

c. What is the composition of gastric juice and how is it formed?

_____

_____

_____

d. What is food in the stomach called and what is its composition?

_____

_____

e. Does the chemical breakdown of food commence in the stomach? Explain.

_____

_____

_____

f. How is the muscularis externa of the stomach modified and why?

_____

_____

g. How long does food stay in the stomach before moving to the small intestine?

_____

_____

h. Where and how does normal stomach emptying occur?

_____

_____

_____

Apply the Concepts

1. What is gastritis and how does it occur?

_____

_____

_____

2. How does the process of emesis (vomiting) occur?

_____

_____

_____

3. Why does the blood become alkaline once emesis (vomiting) has occurred?

_____

_____

_____

Additional Activities

For additional activities visit Activity 20C: Paramecium - A Model of Ingestion and Digestion on Evolve˙.

ACTIVITY 20.5: THE STOMACH LINING AND MEDICATION pH

The gastric mucosa secretes a thick mucus-based lining which acts to protect the stomach wall from digestion by resident enzymes and gastric juice, the major component of which is hydrochloric acid. Occasionally, the mucosa may thin in certain areas of the stomach due to a number of factors, including stress, which compromises the integrity of the mucosa and exposes the stomach wall to erosion by gastric juice. In addition certain medications, by virtue of their pH, can similarly affect the integrity of the gastric mucosa.

This activity demonstrates the pH of some common medications and their effects on the stomach.

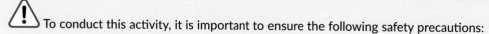 To conduct this activity, it is important to ensure the following safety precautions:

- *Wear disposable gloves at all times during the activity.*

- *Additional precautions, including safe disposal of medicinal compounds, may be required by your demonstrator.*

1. This activity is best conducted in pairs.

2. Obtain ten 100 mL beakers, a selection of medicinal compounds as indicated, mortar and pestle, deionised water, universal indicator with colour indicator chart, disposable pipettes, spatula and disposable gloves.

3. Fill each beaker with 50 mL deionised water.

4. Add 5 drops of universal indicator to each beaker.

5. Note the colour and pH based on the universal indicator chart provided. This is the initial pH.

6. Using a spatula add 1 tablet or 5 g of each substance listed in the table to each of the beakers, agitating gently to mix. It may be necessary to crush medications in tablet form with the mortar and pestle prior to adding.

7. Note the colour change and pH change based on the universal indicator chart provided. This is the final pH.

8. Record your results in the table provided, calculating the change in pH between the initial and final pH readings.

9. Dispose of materials as indicated by your demonstrator.

Sample	Medicinal compound	Colour change	Initial pH	Final pH	pH change
1	Alka Seltzer				
2	Aspirin				
3	Berocca				
4	Cough medicine				
5	ENO				
6	Gaviscon				
7	Ibuprofen				
8	Mylanta				
9	Paracetamol				
10	Vitamin C				

10. Consider the following questions:

a. What is the pH of gastric juice?

   _____

b. How is the stomach mucosa protected from digestion by internal enzymes and gastric juice?

   _____

   _____

   _____

c. What is likely to occur if the protection of the stomach mucosa is breached?

   _____

   _____

d. What effect might medicinal compounds 2, 3, 4, 7, 9 and 10 have on the stomach lining?

   _____

   _____

e. What effect might medicinal compounds 6 and 8 have on the stomach lining?

   _____

   _____

f. What effect might medicinal compounds 1 and 5 have on the stomach lining?

   _____

   _____

Apply the Concepts

1. What is a peptic ulcer and how does it occur?

   _____

   _____

   _____

2. Explain why gastric ulcers may form with overuse of non-steroidal anti-inflammatory medications.

_____

_____

_____

3. What are enteric-coated tablets?

_____

_____

4. What is the function of the enteric coating?

_____

_____

_____

5. How and where do enteric coated tablets deliver their medication within the digestive system?

_____

_____

_____

6. What is first pass metabolism and how does this affect medication delivery and absorption?

_____

_____

_____

ACTIVITY 20.6: ENZYMES OF THE GASTROINTESTINAL TRACT

Once food is ingested, it is mechanically broken down through chewing by the teeth, mixing by the **tongue**, churning by the stomach, and **segmentation** by the small intestine. To fully digest the food, chemical digestion by enzymes is required. This process breaks down foods into their chemical building blocks so that they are small enough for absorption across the wall of the small intestine. Digestive enzymes are distributed throughout the gastrointestinal tract, but are concentrated in the stomach and small intestine. Enzymes act on specific nutrient classes to break chemical bonds and are affected by local conditions such as temperature and pH.

This activity demonstrates the action of digestive enzymes on various food items.

To conduct this activity, it is important to ensure the following safety precaution:

- *Ensure disposable gloves are worn at all times during the activity, as the solvents used may cause skin irritation.*

1. This activity is best conducted in pairs.

2. Obtain four wide-mouthed test tubes, glass marker, test tube rack, 0.5 cm × 0.5 cm food cubes (bread, apple, cheese, cooked egg white, cooked liver), 4% amylase solution, 4% pepsin in 0.5% HCl, 4% trypsin in

0.5% $NaHCO_3$, 4% pancreatin in 0.5% $NaHCO_3$, pH paper, 20 mL measuring cylinder, water bath, stopwatch, Multistix and disposable gloves.

3. Label the test tubes 1 to 4 with the glass marker and place in the test tube rack.

4. Place one cube of each food item into each test tube. Each test tube should contain five different cubes of food.

5. To test tube 1, add 15 mL amylase solution.

6. To test tube 2, add 15 mL pepsin solution.

7. To test tube 3, add 15 mL trypsin solution.

8. To test tube 4, add 15 mL pancreatin solution.

9. Test the initial pH of each test tube with the pH paper and record your observations in the table provided.

10. Place the test tube rack containing the test tubes in the water bath set at 37°C for 1–2 hours, gently agitating each test tube every 10 minutes (the test tubes can be kept in the water bath for up to 24 hours).

11. Remove the test tube rack from the water bath once the time has elapsed.

12. Test the final pH of each test tube with the pH paper and record your observations in the table provided.

13. Observe any changes in the food items tested, noting your observations in the table provided.

14. Test the solution in each test tube with a Multistix to determine the presence of organic molecules as indicated in the table.

15. Record your observations in the table provided, indicating whether each solution tested positive or negative for each organic molecule.

Enzyme tested	Initial pH	Final pH	Observations	Organic molecule		
				Glucose	Proteins	Ketones
Amylase						
Pepsin						
Trypsin						
Pancreatin						

16. Consider the following questions:

a. Why were the samples in each activity incubated at 37°C?

_____

_____

b. What does the initial pH of each test tube imply about the action of each enzyme within the gastrointestinal tract?

_____

_____

_____

c. Which enzyme tested is produced outside the gastrointestinal tract?

_____

_____

d. Pancreatin contains which enzymes?

_____

e. What is the function of protease and where is it produced?

_____

_____

f. Which physiological processes did agitation of the test tubes simulate and why?

_____

_____

_____

g. What do the results indicate about the action of amylase?

_____

_____

h. What do the results indicate about the action of pepsin?

_____

_____

i. What do the results indicate about the action of trypsin?

_____

_____

j. What do the results indicate about the action of pancreatin?

_____

_____

k. What must occur before fats can be digested by lipase?

_____

_____

l. Why are the enzymes of the digestive system referred to as hydrolases?

_____

_____

m. Explain why gastric juice is buffered prior to entering the small intestine.

_____

_____

17. Complete the table below based on the functions of the digestive enzymes.

Macromolecule	Enzyme(s) involved	Site of action	Product(s)	Pathway of absorption
Carbohydrates (starch)				
Proteins				
Fats (triglycerides)				

ACTIVITY 20.7: STRUCTURE AND FUNCTION OF THE INTESTINES

The two main divisions of the intestine are named for their diameter rather than length, as the small intestine is longer (6.0 metres) than the **large intestine** (1.5 metres). The small intestine consists of three regions – the duodenum, jejunum and ileum – which are modified internally by **villi** and microvilli to increase surface area for the purpose of nutrient digestion and absorption (Fig. 20.6A). The **duodenum** contains openings to the ducts that convey secretions of the accessory digestive organs into the small intestine. The large intestine consists of five regions – the caecum, appendix, colon, rectum and anal canal – which conduct the absorption of excess water and the **elimination** of faeces through the process of **defecation** (Fig. 20.6B). The appendix plays an important role in immunity within the large intestine.

This activity examines the structure and functions of the small and large intestines.

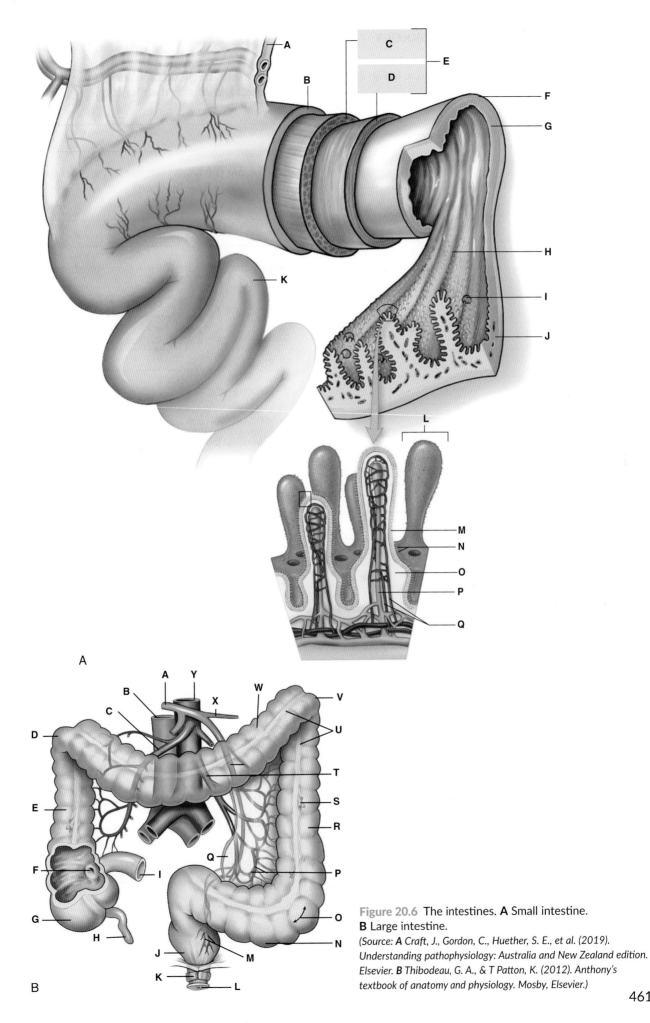

Figure 20.6 The intestines. **A** Small intestine.
B Large intestine.

*(Source: **A** Craft, J., Gordon, C., Huether, S. E., et al. (2019).
Understanding pathophysiology: Australia and New Zealand edition.
Elsevier. **B** Thibodeau, G. A., & T Patton, K. (2012). Anthony's
textbook of anatomy and physiology. Mosby, Elsevier.)*

1. Identify the structures of the small intestine in Fig. 20.6A:

   a. Structure A: _____

   b. Structure B: _____

   c. Structure C: _____

   d. Structure D: _____

   e. Structure E: _____

   f. Structure F: _____

   g. Structure G: _____

   h. Structure H: _____

   i. Structure I: _____

   j. Structure J: _____

   k. Structure K: _____

   l. Structure L: _____

   m. Structure M: _____

   n. Structure N: _____

   o. Structure O: _____

   p. Structure P: _____

   q. Structure Q: _____

2. Consider the following questions:

   a. Identify the three main functions of the small intestine.

   _____

   _____

   b. What is the function of the plicae circulares, villi and microvilli of the small intestine?

   _____

   _____

   c. Explain the location and structure of the brush border.

   _____

   _____

   _____

   d. Explain the functional benefit of the simple columnar epithelium located in the small intestine.

   _____

   _____

e. Where are the blood capillaries of the small intestine located and what is their function?

   _____

   _____

f. What are the lymph lacteals of the small intestine and what is their function?

   _____

   _____

3. Identify the structures of the large intestine in Fig. 20.6B:

   a. Structure A: _____

   b. Structure B: _____

   c. Structure C: _____

   d. Structure D: _____

   e. Structure E: _____

   f. Structure F: _____

   g. Structure G: _____

   h. Structure H: _____

   i. Structure I: _____

   j. Structure J: _____

   k. Structure K: _____

   l. Structure L: _____

   m. Structure M: _____

   n. Structure N: _____

   o. Structure O: _____

   p. Structure P: _____

   q. Structure Q: _____

   r. Structure R: _____

   s. Structure S: _____

   t. Structure T: _____

   u. Structure U: _____

   v. Structure V: _____

   w. Structure W: _____

   x. Structure X: _____

   y. Structure Y: _____

4. Consider the following questions:

a. Identify the three main functions of the large intestine.

_____

_____

b. Why are the hepatic and splenic flexures so-named?

_____

_____

c. To what do the terms ascending, transverse, descending and sigmoid refer, with reference to the colon?

_____

_____

_____

d. Is there a difference between the colon and the large intestine? Explain.

_____

_____

e. How are the haustra formed and what is their function?

_____

_____

_____

f. Explain the structure and function of the epiploic appendages.

_____

_____

_____

g. What is the function of the vermiform appendix and why is it so-named?

_____

_____

_____

h. Outline the relationship between the ileum, caecum, and the ileocaecal valve.

_____

_____

_____

i. Why does the large intestine produce copious amounts of mucus and where is this mucus produced?

_____

_____

j. Indicate the physiological basis for the colour of the following stools:

i. Brown stools

_____

_____

ii. Black or dark brown stools

_____

_____

iii. White stools

_____

_____

iv. Green stools

_____

_____

v. Yellow stools

_____

_____

vi. Red stools

_____

_____

k. What is a mass movement?

_____

_____

l. Compare the structure and function of the internal and external anal sphincters.

_____

_____

m. Explain the processes occurring during the defecation reflex.

_____

_____

Apply the Concepts

1. Explain why a feeding tube may be inserted into the duodenum of an individual with oesophageal cancer rather than the stomach.

_____

_____

_____

2. How is intestinal gas or flatus produced in the large intestine?

_____

3. How does diarrhoea occur?

_____

_____

4. How does constipation occur?

_____

_____

5. Compare the actions of a bulk-forming laxative, a hyperosmotic laxative, and a stimulant laxative.

_____

_____

_____

6. What is irritable bowel syndrome (IBS) and how does it occur?

_____

_____

_____

7. Explain why faecal incontinence may occur in infants and adults.

_____

_____

_____

8. What are haemorrhoids and how do they occur?

_____

_____

_____

Additional Activities

For additional activities visit Activity 20D: A Model of Intestinal Absorption on Evolve˚.

For additional activities visit Activity 20E: Location and Auscultation of the Digestive Viscera on Evolve˚.

ACTIVITY 20.8: STRUCTURE AND FUNCTION OF THE ACCESSORY DIGESTIVE ORGANS

The accessory digestive organs – the salivary glands, liver, gall bladder and pancreas – are located externally to the gastrointestinal tract and produce secretions that aid the digestive process. These secretions are delivered to the gastrointestinal tract via a system of ducts (Fig. 20.7). The salivary glands produce and secrete saliva, which assists with the lubrication and mixing of food within the oral cavity. The **liver** is the heaviest internal organ of the body and produces **bile**, which is delivered to the gall bladder. From there, bile is secreted into the duodenum to assist with fat **emulsification**. As part of its exocrine function, the pancreas produces alkaline pancreatic juice that is rich in digestive enzymes and is also secreted into the duodenum.

This activity examines the structure and function of the accessory digestive organs.

1. Identify the structures of the salivary glands in Fig. 20.7A:

    a. Structure A: _____

    b. Structure B: _____

    c. Structure C: _____

    d. Structure D: _____

    e. Structure E: _____

    f. Structure F: _____

    g. Structure G: _____

    h. Structure H: _____

    i. Structure I: _____

2. Identify the structures associated with the liver, gall bladder and pancreas in Fig. 20.7B:

    a. Structure A: _____

    b. Structure B: _____

    c. Structure C: _____

    d. Structure D: _____

    e. Structure E: _____

    f. Structure F: _____

    g. Structure G: _____

    h. Structure H: _____

    i. Structure I: _____

    j. Structure J: _____

    k. Structure K: _____

    l. Structure L: _____

    m. Structure M: _____

    n. Structure N: _____

    o. Structure O: _____

    p. Structure P: _____

    q. Structure Q: _____

3. Consider the following questions:

    a. What is the role of saliva ? Explain its composition.

    _____

    _____

    _____

    _____

    b. Distinguish between intrinsic and extrinsic salivary glands.

    _____

    _____

    c. What causes salivation to occur?

    _____

    _____

    d. Identify the main functions of the liver.

    _____

    _____

    _____

    _____

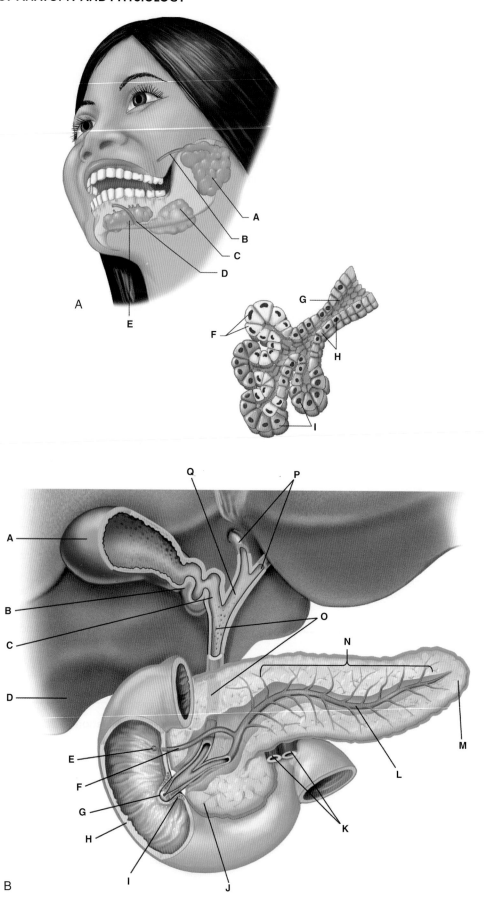

Figure 20.7 The accessory digestive organs. **A** Salivary glands. **B** Liver, gall bladder, pancreas and duodenum associations. *(Source: **A** Thibodeau, G. A., & T Patton, K. (2012). Anthony's textbook of anatomy and physiology. Mosby, Elsevier. **B** Lovaasen, K. R. (2019). ICD-10-CM/PCS coding: Theory and practice. Elsevier.)*

e. How does liver regeneration relate to the functions and overall homeostasis of the liver?

_____

_____

_____

f. Why is the liver dark red or brown?

_____

g. What are hepatocytes and how are they arranged within the liver?

_____

_____

h. Identify three structures found in liver portal triads.

_____

_____

i. Which ducts drain the liver?

_____

j. Trace the pathway of bile from the liver to the duodenum in Fig. 20.7B.

_____

k. What is the role of the gall bladder?

_____

l. Which duct drains the gall bladder?

_____

m. Which duct conveys bile into the duodenum and what is its origin?

_____

_____

_____

n. Is bile considered an enzyme? Explain.

_____

_____

o. What role does bile play in fat digestion?

_____

_____

p. Why is bile yellow to green in colour?

_____

_____

q. Identify the main functions of the pancreas.

_____

_____

r. Which population of pancreatic cells serves the digestive process?

_____

_____

s. Trace the pathway of pancreatic juice from the pancreas to the duodenum in Fig. 20.7B.

_____

t. At which structure does pancreatic juice enter the duodenum?

_____

u. What is the pH of bile and pancreatic juice? Relate this to their locations of secretion and action.

_____

_____

_____

Apply the Concepts

1. What is hepatitis and how might this affect digestive function?

_____

_____

_____

2. What is jaundice and how does it occur?

_____

_____

_____

3. Explain the effect on lipid metabolism if the gall bladder was removed (cholecystectomy).

_____

_____

_____

4. What are gallstones and how do they occur?

_____

_____

_____

Additional Activities

For additional activities visit Activity 20F: Microscopic Examination of the Accessory Digestive Organs on Evolve˙.

For additional activities visit Activity 20G: Digestive Function of Salivary Amylase on Evolve˙.

ACTIVITY 20.9: EMULSIFICATION OF FATS

The majority of ingested nutrients are water soluble; however, fats are water insoluble. This presents difficulties associated with chemical digestion within the gastrointestinal tract. In order for fats to mix with a watery solution, the addition of an emulsifier is required. Bile, produced by the liver, is the emulsifier of the gastrointestinal tract. It physically coats and separates fat droplets so that they can be dispersed within a watery solution, resulting in emulsification. Emulsification increases the overall surface area of the fat droplets, allowing for chemical digestion by lipase. Detergents also act as emulsifiers and can be utilised to simulate the action of bile.

This activity visually demonstrates the emulsification of fat.

 To conduct this activity, it is important to ensure the following safety precautions:

- _Scarlet R (Sudan IV) dye is a strong stain and can cause irritation._

- _Ensure disposable gloves are worn at all times during the activity._

1. This activity is best conducted individually.

2. Obtain two 1.5 mL microcentrifuge tubes with caps, pencil, paraffin oil, deionised water, colourless dishwashing liquid, scarlet R dye (Sudan IV), disposable pipettes, stopwatch, microscope slides, coverslips, compound microscope and disposable gloves.

3. Label the tubes 1 and 2 with the pencil.

4. To each tube, add 0.5 mL paraffin oil.

5. To each tube, add 0.5 mL deionised water.

6. To each tube, add 5 drops scarlet R dye.

7. Close the caps on the tubes and agitate the contents for 10 seconds.

   a. Which process in the gastrointestinal tract does agitation represent?

   _____

8. Allow the tubes to stand for 2 minutes and note any changes.

   a. What was observed in both tubes after 2 minutes?

   _____

   _____

   b. Which component of the mixture does the scarlet R dye stain red?

   _____

   _____

   c. How does the solubility of the scarlet R dye assist in identifying the chief components of the mixture?

   _____

   _____

9. To tube 2, add 5 drops of detergent.

10. Close the cap on tube 2 and agitate the contents of both tubes for 10 seconds.

11. Note any changes in both tubes.

12. Allow the tubes to stand for 5 minutes and note any changes.

   a. Which tube did not indicate emulsification and why?

   _____

   _____

   b. What was the purpose of tube 1?

   _____

   _____

   c. Which tube indicated emulsification and why?

   _____

   _____

   d. Describe the appearance of the emulsified product.

   _____

   _____

   e. What component of the mixture was responsible for emulsification?

   _____

   f. Which substance is responsible for the emulsification of fats within the human gastrointestinal tract?

   _____

13. Agitate the contents of tube 1 for 10 seconds.

14. Withdraw a sample from tube 1 and place two drops of the mixture on a microscope slide and add a coverslip.

15. Agitate the contents of tube 2 for 10 seconds.

16. Withdraw a sample from tube 2 and place two drops of the mixture on a microscope slide and add a coverslip.

17. View the sample from tube 1 under low power.

18. Draw a diagram of what you can see in the space below, labelling the oil, water and dye components.

Magnification of diagram: ✕ _____

   a. Which component of the mixture is the paraffin oil and which component is the water?

   _____

   _____

   b. Did the oil and water appear to mix cohesively? Explain.

   _____

   _____

c. What colour did the oil droplets appear and why?

_____

_____

d. Estimate the size of a single oil droplet:

_____

19. View the sample from tube 2 under low power, progressing to high power.

20. Draw a diagram of what you can see in the space below, labelling the oil, water and dye components.

Magnification of diagram: × _____

a. How does the appearance of the mixture differ from sample 1?

_____

_____

b. Did the oil and water appear to mix more cohesively than sample 1?

_____

_____

c. Estimate the size of a single oil droplet:

_____

21. Consider the following questions:

a. How does emulsification change the size of the oil droplets?

_____

b. What are the emulsified oil droplets called?

_____

c. Does emulsification have the effect of increasing or decreasing the surface area of the oil?

_____

_____

d. Does emulsification physically or chemically break down fats?

_____

_____

e. Explain how emulsifiers cause the emulsification of fats.

_____

_____

_____

_____

f. How are fats chemically broken down?

_____

_____

_____

_____

g. Are fats able to be absorbed in the gastrointestinal tract prior to emulsification? Explain.

_____

_____

_____

_____

Apply the Concepts

1. Would cholecystectomy affect fat digestion? Explain.

_____

_____

_____

Additional Resources

Atlas of Gastrointestinal Video Endoscopy
The Atlas of Gastrointestinal Video Endoscopy presents a high-resolution video atlas of gastrointestinal endoscopy based on research from the Republic of El Salvador.

www.gastrointestinalatlas.com/english/english.html

Continence Foundation of Australia: Bristol Stool Chart
The Bristol Stool Chart, or Bristol Stool Scale was developed as a clinical assessment tool. It is a medical aid designed to classify faeces into seven groups.

www.continence.org.au/bristol-stool-chart

Histology Guide Virtual Microscopy Laboratory: Gastrointestinal Tract, Liver and Gall Bladder
Histology Guide is an online resource providing a virtual microscopy laboratory experience by allowing users to view microscope slides from professional collections for the purpose of interpreting cellular and tissue structures, as seen through a microscope.

histologyguide.com/slidebox/14-gastrointestinal-tract.html

histologyguide.com/slidebox/15-liver-and-gallbladder.html

Independence Australia: Understanding the Colour of Your Poo
Independence Australia aims to improve the quality of lives by providing access to products, resources and encouragement that allow people to make choices to enhance their wellbeing and lifestyle. Stool colour can provide an indicator of underlying physiological processes.

www.independenceaustralia.com.au/health-articles/understanding-the-colour-of-your-poo/

Innerbody Research: Digestive System
Innerbody Research provides objective, science-based advice to help readers make more informed choices about home health products and services with the most up-to-date reviews, guides and research, including information about the digestive system.

www.innerbody.com/image/digeov.html

Osmosis – Gastrointestinal System
The Gastrointestinal System module of Osmosis provides videos, notes, quiz questions and links to further resources related to the gastrointestinal system.

www.osmosis.org/library/md/foundational-sciences/physiology#gastrointestinal_system

Pictorial Atlas of Gastroenterological Endoscopy
The Pictorial Atlas of Gastroenterological Endoscopy contains endoscopic pictures and videos with clinical findings for both learners and experienced researchers.

www.endoskopiebilder.de/en/endoskopie-atlas

The Histology Guide: Digestive System
The Histology Guide is a virtual experience of using a microscope with zoom features divided into topics and offering histological slides with labels and quizzes for each topic, including the digestive system. It is provided by the University of Leeds.

www.histology.leeds.ac.uk/digestive/index.php

Visible Body: The Digestive System
Visible Body provides interactive and highly accurate visualisations and apps for learning and teaching anatomy and physiology for students and healthcare professionals. These include body systems such as the digestive system.

www.visiblebody.com/learn/digestive

CHAPTER 21
The Urinary System and Electrolyte Balance

The volume and composition of the fluids that bathe the body's cells affect the functions of those cells. The kidneys are the organs chiefly involved in regulating body fluid volume, the constituents of extracellular fluids, acid–base balance, and osmotic relationships between body fluid compartments. (Refer to Chapter 3: Basic Chemistry, for further information on pH and electrolytes.)

The kidneys receive over 1700 litres of blood per day and extract about 180 litres of fluid from it for processing. This results in the removal of excess ions, toxins and metabolic wastes, while returning the substances needed by the body back into the blood. The role of the kidneys in homeostasis also includes producing substances for regulating red blood cell production and blood pressure, converting vitamin D to its active form, and synthesising glucose during prolonged fasting.

LEARNING OUTCOMES

On completion of these activities, the student should be able to:

1. distinguish between intracellular and extracellular fluids and their compositions
2. describe the anatomy of the urinary system and its component organs
3. describe the organisation of the kidney
4. identify the nephron as the unit of kidney function and describe its parts
5. describe the processes of filtration, reabsorption and secretion occurring at each part of the nephron
6. explain the ability of the kidney to form dilute and concentrated urine
7. understand hormonal influences on kidney function
8. define electrolyte balance and describe the mechanisms that regulate it
9. describe the renal and respiratory mechanisms that maintain acid–base balance
10. conduct a simple chemical analysis of urine.

KEY TERMS

Acid–base balance
Acidosis
Alkalosis
Afferent arteriole
Aldosterone
Antidiuretic hormone (ADH)
Atrial natriuretic peptide (ANP)
Bowman's capsule
Buffer
Collecting duct
Cortical nephron
Distal convoluted tubule
Efferent arteriole
Electrolyte
Extracellular fluid (ECF)
Filtrate

Glomerular filtration
Glomerulus
Hilum
Interstitial fluid (IF)
Intracellular fluid (ICF)
Juxtamedullary nephron
Kidney
Loop of Henle
Major calyx
Micturition
Minor calyx
Nephron
Non-electrolyte
Peritubular capillary
Plasma
Proximal convoluted tubule
Renal artery
Renal capsule

Renal columns
Renal cortex
Renal medulla
Renal pelvis
Renal pyramids
Renal vein
Renin-angiotensin-aldosterone system (RAAS)
Rugae
Trigone
Tubular reabsorption
Tubular secretion
Ureter
Urethra
Urethral sphincter
Urine
Urinalysis
Urinary bladder

ACTIVITY 21.1: BODY FLUIDS AND FLUID COMPARTMENTS

Body fluids and their compostion are essential to every aspect of physiological function. Body fluids are composed of water and solutes in the form of **electrolytes** and **non-electrolytes**, and are categorised into two main compartments. The **intracellular fluid (ICF)** is the largest fluid compartment, comprising nearly two-thirds of all body fluid, and is located within tissue cells. The **extracellular fluid (ECF)** is located outside the tissue cells and is comprised of the **interstitial fluid (IF)** between tissue cells, and blood **plasma**. The regulation of body fluid volume and concentration across compartments is largely achieved by the urinary system.

This activity explores the terms and concepts important in urinary system function.

1. Why are the contents of all body cells considered to be a single fluid compartment?

_____

_____

2. What are the two sub-compartments of the extracellular fluid (ECF)?

_____

3. Identify the specific type of ECF found in each of the following structures:

    a. Brain _____

    b. Eye _____

    c. Knee _____

    d. Stomach _____

4. Distinguish between an electrolyte and a non-electrolyte.

_____

_____

_____

    a. Provide an example of an electrolyte within the human body.

    _____

    b. Provide an example of a non-electrolyte within the human body.

    _____

FOUNDATIONS OF ANATOMY AND PHYSIOLOGY

5. The table below shows substances present in both ICF and ECF. Tick the box that correctly indicates the relative concentration of each in those fluid compartments.

Ion	Higher in ICF	Higher in ECF	Similar in both
Na^+			
K^+			
Ca^{2+}			
Mg^{2+}			
HCO_3^-			
Cl^-			
SO_4^{2-}			
Protein			

6. Complete the following sentences by filling in the blanks with the terms provided.

Decrease
Increase
Hydrostatic pressure
Osmosis
Lower
Higher

Permeable
Diffusion
Semipermeable
Osmotic pressure
Diffusible
Non-diffusible

a. When a membrane separating two fluid compartments is permeable to water but not to some of the dissolved solutes, it is called a _____ membrane.

b. Water will move by _____ across the membrane in both directions, but there will be a net movement towards the compartment with the _____ concentration of _____ solutes.

c. This phenomenon is called _____ and it causes the _____ within that compartment to rise.

d. This, in turn, causes the movement of water out of that compartment to _____, until there is no nett water movement across the membrane.

e. The amount of pressure required to achieve this is called the _____.

7. Explain why females tend to contain proportionately less body water than males.

_____
_____
_____

Apply the Concepts

1. Explain what happens to the volume of extracellular fluid after eating a bag of salted chips.

_____
_____

2. What is pitting oedema and what is a possible consequence?

_____
_____

3. What is dehydration and what is a possible consequence?

_____
_____

ACTIVITY 21.2: STRUCTURE AND FUNCTION OF THE URINARY SYSTEM

The urinary system is comprised of a number of structures responsible for the formation, storage and transport of **urine** (Fig. 21.1). Paired **kidneys** filter blood plasma, form **filtrate** and modify the filtrate into urine. Paired **ureters** convey the urine into the **urinary bladder** at the **trigone** for temporary storage (Fig. 21.2). The bladder is eventually drained by a single **urethra** in the process of **micturition**, which involves the actions of the **urethral sphincters**.

This activity provides an overview of the structures forming the urinary system, and their functions.

1. Obtain a model or chart of the human urinary tract and identify the following structures:

   ☐ Kidneys (with associated renal arteries and veins)

   ☐ Ureters (leading posteriorly from the kidneys)

   ☐ Urinary bladder (in the lower abdomen)

   ☐ Urethra (passing posteriorly from the bladder)

2. Examine Fig. 21.1, identify each labelled structure, and provide its function:

   a. Structure A: _____

      i. Function: _____

      _____

   b. Structure B: _____

      i. Function: _____

      _____

   c. Structure C: _____

      i. Function: _____

      _____

   d. Structure D: _____

      i. Function: _____

      _____

   e. Structure E: _____

      i. Function: _____

      _____

   f. Structure F: _____

      i. Function: _____

      _____

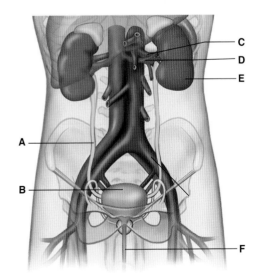

Figure 21.1 Organs of the urinary system.
(Source: El-Hussein, M. T., Power-Kean, K., Zettel, S. et al. (2023). Huether and McCance's understanding pathophysiology, second Canadian edition. Elsevier.)

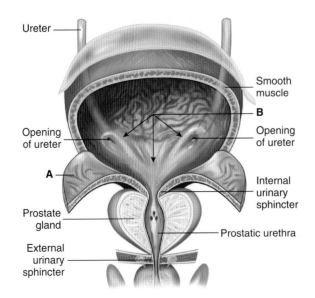

Figure 21.2 The urinary bladder of the male.
(Source: Cooper, K., & Gosnell, K. (2022). Adult health nursing. Elsevier.)

3. Refer back to the model or chart of the human urinary tract and Fig. 21.2.

4. Note the angle of entry of the ureters into the bladder.

   a. What is the function of this arrangement?

   _____

   _____

   b. Which muscle type is found in the walls of the ureters?

   _____

   c. What is the purpose of this muscle?

   _____

   _____

   d. What name is given to the smooth muscle in the wall of the bladder?

   _____

5. The folds on the interior aspect of the bladder wall (**A**) disappear as the bladder fills and becomes distended.

   a. What are these folds called?

   _____

   b. What name is given to the triangular region of the bladder (**B**) delineated by the openings of the two ureters and the urethra?

   _____

6. Complete the table below to highlight the differences between the internal and external urethral sphincters.

a. What is the function of these sphincters?

   _____

   _____

   _____

b. Which sphincter is responsible for voiding?

   _____

c. Is voiding achieved by relaxation or contraction of this sphincter?

   _____

d. What term is given to the process of voiding?

   _____

e. Explain how voiding of urine is achieved.

   _____

   _____

   _____

7. How does the length of the urethra differ between males and females?

   _____

   _____

8. The urethra forms part of which other organ system in males?

   _____

9. Which structure in Fig. 21.2 is not found in females?

   _____

Characteristic	Internal urethral sphincter	External urethral sphincter
Voluntary or involuntary control		
Type of muscle forming the sphincter		
Inferior or superior to the bladder		

Apply the Concepts

1. Explain why urinary tract infections are more common in women and mostly occur in sexually active women.

   _____

   _____

2. Urinary incontinence is normally prevented by which structure(s) in the urinary tract?

   _____

   _____

3. Why does coughing or sneezing sometimes result in leakage of urine in people who are not otherwise incontinent?

   _____

   _____

4. Why is incontinence a normal phenomenon in children under 2 years old?

   _____

   _____

5. What may lead to incontinence in the adult?

   _____

   _____

6. Is there a distinction between diuresis and enuresis? Explain.

   _____

   _____

   _____

7. Explain what is meant by the following terms:

   a. Oliguria: _____

   _____

   b. Anuria: _____

   _____

   c. Haematuria: _____

   _____

   d. Uraemia: _____

   _____

   e. Dysuria: _____

   _____

ACTIVITY 21.3: STRUCTURE OF THE KIDNEY

The kidneys are supported externally by three layers of tissue – the outermost renal fascia, the middle perirenal fat capsule, and the innermost **renal capsule** – and bear a noticeable cleft on their vertical surface referred to as the **hilum**. This serves as an entry point for blood vessels, the **renal artery** and the **renal vein**, and the ureters entering the internal kidney tissue. Internally, the kidneys consist of three distinct regions (Fig. 21.3): the outermost **renal cortex**; the middle **renal medulla**, which consists of the cone-shaped **renal pyramids** separated by the **renal columns**; and the innermost **renal pelvis**, which consists of branching **major calyces** and **minor calyces**, and is continuous with the ureters leaving the kidneys.

This activity examines the gross structure of the kidney.

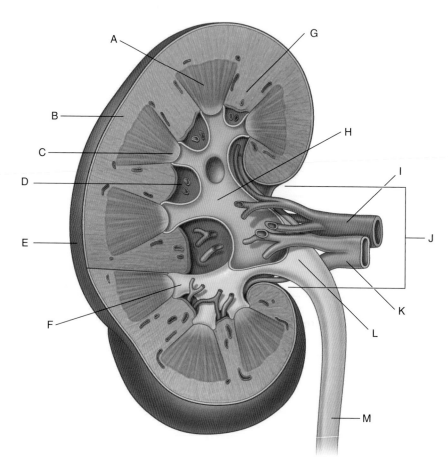

Figure 21.3 Internal anatomy of the kidney.
(*Source: Drake, R., Vogl, A. W., & Mitchell, A. W. (2020). Gray's anatomy for students. Elsevier.*)

1. Obtain a model or chart of a kidney.

   a. Describe the location of the kidneys within the human body.

   _____

   _____

   _____

2. Note the following external features:

   ☐ Hilum

   ☐ Perirenal fat capsule

   ☐ Renal artery

   ☐ Renal capsule

   ☐ Renal fascia

   ☐ Renal vein

   ☐ Ureter

3. The renal fascia is the outermost connective tissue layer, while the perirenal fat capsule lies just underneath the renal fascia and is heavily infiltrated with fat.

   a. What is the function of the renal fascia?

   _____

   _____

   _____

   b. What is the function of the perirenal fat capsule?

   _____

   _____

4. The renal capsule is a smooth membrane that adheres tightly to the surface of the kidney.

   a. What is the function of the renal capsule?

   _____

   _____

   _____

   b. Identify three ways in which the kidneys are protected from external damage.

   _____

   _____

   _____

5. The hilum is the indented surface of the kidney from which blood vessels and the ureter emerge.

6. The renal artery, renal vein, and ureter are all found within the hilum.

7. Open up the model of the kidney or examine a chart of a cross-section of the kidney.

8. Identify the three main regions within the kidney:

   ☐ Renal cortex

   ☐ Renal medulla

   ☐ Renal pelvis

9. The outermost region immediately inferior to the capsule is the light-coloured *renal cortex*.

   a. What is found within the renal cortex?

   _____

   _____

10. Beneath the cortex is the darker renal medulla, which contains cone-shaped masses of tissue called renal pyramids.

   a. What is found within the renal pyramids?

   _____

   _____

11. The inward-pointing tip of each pyramid is its *papilla*.

12. Between the pyramids are inward extensions of cortical tissue called *renal columns*, each of which abuts a fluid-filled space called a *renal sinus*.

   a. What is found within the renal columns?

   _____

   _____

13. The innermost region is the renal pelvis, a cavity which is continuous with the ureter.

   a. What is the function of the renal pelvis?

   _____

   _____

   b. The renal pelvis extends into which structure?

   _____

   c. Explain why the wall of the renal pelvis contains smooth muscle.

   _____

   _____

   _____

14. Large branches of the renal pelvis are the major calyces (singular: calyx) which divide into the smaller minor calyces.

    a. What is the function of the calyces?

    _____

    _____

15. Examine Fig. 21.3, and identify each of the structures labelled:

    a. Structure A: _____

    b. Structure B: _____

    c. Structure C: _____

    d. Structure D: _____

    e. Structure E: _____

    f. Structure F: _____

    g. Structure G: _____

    h. Structure H: _____

    i. Structure I: _____

    j. Structure J: _____

    k. Structure K: _____

    l. Structure L: _____

    m. Structure M: _____

Apply the Concepts

1. What are renal calculi and where do they occur?

   _____

   _____

2. Describe the composition of renal calculi.

   _____

   _____

3. What is most likely to cause the formation of renal calculi?

   _____

   _____

4. What property of the ureters would allow renal calculi to become lodged, blocking urine drainage and causing excruciating pain?

   _____

   _____

5. Explain why a patient with renal calculi is usually advised to increase their water consumption.

   _____

   _____

ACTIVITY 21.4: EXAMINATION OF KIDNEY STRUCTURE (KIDNEY DISSECTION)

A sheep kidney provides a convenient approximation of the human kidney, and its dissection allows a study of the major human anatomical features. Although the kidneys of other mammals are often specially adapted to the diet or environment in which the animal lives, their overall organisation is consistent with that of human kidneys.

This activity demonstrates the internal and external structures of the kidney through dissection.

⚠️ To conduct this activity it is important to ensure the following safety precautions:

- *Wear disposable gloves at all times during the activity as fresh biological tissues may harbour pathogenic microorganisms.*
- *Exercise care when handling dissection tools.*
- *Additional precautions, including safe disposal of dissected animal material, may be required by your demonstrator.*

1. This activity is best conducted in pairs and may be completed with a:

   - pre-dissected kidney for the purpose of observation.
   - preserved or fresh kidney, which will need to be dissected following the procedure below.

2. Obtain a sheep kidney, gloves, dissecting tray, dissecting lamp and dissecting instruments.

3. Place the sheep kidney in the dissecting tray under a dissecting lamp.

4. Identify the following external features:

   ☐ Renal artery

   ☐ Renal capsule

   ☐ Renal hilum

   ☐ Renal vein

   ☐ Ureter

5. The renal capsule adheres tightly to surface of the kidney.

   a. Describe the appearance of the renal capsule.

   _____

   _____

   b. Of which type of tissue is the renal capsule composed?

   _____

6. The *renal hilum* is located on the inner surface of the kidney and contains the remains of the *renal artery* and *renal vein*.

   a. The renal hilum leads into which structure?

   _____

7. The remains of the *ureter* exit the hilum at a point immediately inferior to the artery and vein.

   a. Of which types of tissue is the ureter composed?

   _____

   b. The ureter is a continuation of which structure?

   _____

8. Make an incision through the longitudinal axis of the kidney.

9. The incision should cut the kidney completely in half lengthways and should pass through the hilum.

10. Compare the internal features of the kidney with Fig. 21.3, and identify each of the following structures:

    ☐ Major calyces

    ☐ Minor calyces

    ☐ Papillae

    ☐ Renal columns

    ☐ Renal cortex

    ☐ Renal medulla

    ☐ Renal pelvis

    ☐ Renal pyramids

11. The *renal cortex* lies beneath the fibrous capsule and is light in colour.

    a. Describe the external appearance of the renal cortex.

    _____

    _____

    b. The renal corpuscles in this location obtain their blood supply from which arteries?

    _____

12. The renal medulla lies deeper in the kidney and is a darker red-brown colour.

    a. What are the medullary rays located in this region and what is their composition?

    _____

    _____

    b. What are the vasa recta located in this region and how do they appear?

    _____

    _____

13. The *renal pyramids* lie within the medulla and their *papillae* point to the interior of the kidney.

    a. Describe the appearance of the renal pyramids.

    _____

    _____

    b. What is contained within the renal pyramids?

    _____

    _____

    c. Which portion of the nephron extends into the papillae?

    _____

14. The *renal pelvis* is a flat cavity that is continuous with the ureter.

    a. Describe the appearance of the renal pelvis.

    _____

    _____

    b. Of which types of tissue is the renal pelvis composed?

    _____

15. The large extensions of the renal pelvis are the *major calyces* and the smaller branches are the *minor calyces*.

    a. Which structures merge and project into the calyces?

    _____

    b. The calyces converge and project into which structure?

    _____

16. In the space provided, draw a line diagram of the kidney section showing as many of the above features as you can see.

17. The diagram should not attempt to show details, but simply the outlines of the regions and structures listed above.

18. Label your diagram and show its magnification.

Magnification of diagram: ✕ _____

19. Once you have completed your examination, dispose of the kidney as indicated by your instructor.

Apply the Concepts

1. What is chronic kidney disease and how does it occur?

   _____

   _____

   _____

   a. How is chronic kidney disease usually treated?

   _____

   b. How does this treatment work?

   _____

   _____

   _____

   c. What changes would you expect to see in the chemical composition of the blood in chronic kidney disease?

   _____

   _____

2. During dialysis, identify the substances that would need to be:

   a. Removed from the blood: _____

   _____

   b. Added to the blood: _____

   _____

3. Kidney disease, unlike many other diseases, needs to be treated urgently. Explain why.

   _____

   _____

ACTIVITY 21.5: STRUCTURE AND FUNCTION OF THE NEPHRON

Nephrons are the functional units of the kidney, carrying out the filtration of blood plasma and the formation of urine (Fig. 21.4). About 2 million are found in the paired kidneys, as either **cortical nephrons** or **juxtamedullary nephrons**. Blood supply to each nephron occurs via an **afferent arteriole** serving the **glomerulus** and blood exits via an **efferent arteriole**. Filtrate collecting in the **Bowman's capsule**, or glomerular capsule, flows through and is modified by the **proximal convoluted tubule**, the **loop of Henle**, the **distal convoluted tubule**, and the **collecting duct**. These form urine through the processes of **tubular reabsorption** and **tubular secretion** between the tubule system and the **peritubular capillaries** (Fig. 21.5).

This activity examines the structure and function of the nephron.

Part 1: Nephron Structure

1. Identify each of the labelled structures shown in Fig. 21.4, by matching each structure with its correct term.

Ureter
Branch of renal vein
Distal tubule
Efferent arteriole
Peritubular capillaries
Urinary bladder

Vasa recta
Branch of renal artery
Afferent arteriole
Proximal tubule
Minor calyx
Bowman's capsule

Glomerulus
Loop of Henle
Urethra
Major calyx
Renal pelvis
Collecting duct

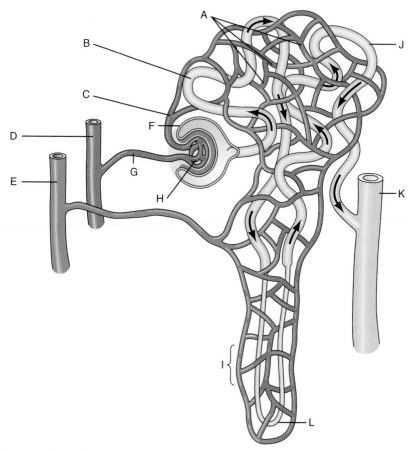

Figure 21.4 Schematic diagram of a nephron.
(Source: Copstead-Kirkhorn, L. E. C., & Banasik, J. L. (2019). Pathophysiology. Elsevier.)

a. Structure A: _____

b. Structure B: _____

c. Structure C: _____

d. Structure D: _____

e. Structure E: _____

f. Structure F: _____

g. Structure G: _____

h. Structure H: _____

i. Structure I: _____

j. Structure J: _____

k. Structure K: _____

l. Structure L: _____

2. Using the terms provided above, and starting with the structure where blood is filtered, list the structures through which the filtrate moves in their correct sequence.

   a. Structure 1: _____

   b. Structure 2: _____

   c. Structure 3: _____

   d. Structure 4: _____

   e. Structure 5: _____

   f. Structure 6: _____

   g. Structure 7: _____

   h. Structure 8: _____

   i. Structure 9: _____

   j. Structure 10: _____

   k. Structure 11: _____

3. Identify the two major types of nephron found in the kidneys and how they differ in terms of their location and structure:

   a. Nephron type 1:

      i. Location: _____

      _____

      ii. Structure: _____

      _____

   b. Nephron type 2:

      i. Location: _____

      _____

      ii. Structure: _____

      _____

4. Identify the collective term given to the glomerulus and Bowman's capsule.

   _____

Part 2: Nephron Function

Nephrons function to filter blood plasma by forming filtrate through the process of glomerular filtration. The formed filtrate is then modified as substances are reabsorbed into the blood through the process of tubular reabsorption, and as substances are actively secreted into the filtrate through the process of tubular secretion, regulated through the **renin-angiotensin-aldosterone system (RAAS)**. Exchange of substances between the filtrate in the nephron tubules and the blood involves the peritubular capillaries.

1. Which three processes are involved in the formation of urine?

   _____

   _____

   _____

   a. Identify three items that are reabsorbed during tubular reabsorption.

   _____

   _____

   _____

   b. Identify three items that are secreted during tubular secretion.

   _____

   _____

   _____

   c. How does the composition of blood plasma differ from that of glomerular filtrate?

   _____

   _____

   _____

d. What is meant by glomerular filtration rate (GFR)?

_____

_____

_____

e. Explain how glomerular filtration rate (GFR) relates to renal clearance.

_____

_____

_____

2. Complete the following sentences by filling in the blanks:

a. Filtration of the blood occurs within the

_____ capsule, where fluid from the

blood is forced by _____ pressure to

leave the _____ capillaries and enter

the lumen of the capsule.

b. This fluid, which is now called _____, is

similar in composition to blood, but does not normally

contain any _____ and only very small

amounts of _____.

c. The filtrate then passes into the _____

tubule, where reabsorption of water and inorganic

ions, such as _____, _____ and

_____ occurs.

d. Many organic solutes are also reabsorbed here, such

as _____, _____,

_____ and _____.

e. These substances move into the _____

capillaries.

3. Describe the structure of the filtration membrane.

_____

_____

_____

a. What type of capillaries form the glomerulus?

_____

b. What is the function of the podocytes and pedicels?

_____

_____

c. What is the function of the filtration slits?

_____

_____

4. Examine Fig. 21.5, which shows osmotic concentrations of the filtrate and surrounding interstitial fluid in milliosmoles per litre.

5. In Fig. 21.5A, what is the name of the process that produces highly concentrated urine (1200 mOsm/L)?

_____

a. Describe how this osmotic gradient is established and maintained in the medulla of the kidney.

_____

_____

_____

b. What energy-consuming process in the ascending limb of the loop of Henle is essential to the establishment of the gradient?

_____

c. By what mechanism does the vasa recta help to maintain the gradient?

_____

d. Differentiate between osmotic gradient and osmotic pressure.

_____

_____

_____

_____

e. Why does the filtrate become hypotonic as it flows through the ascending limb of the loop of Henle?

_____

_____

_____

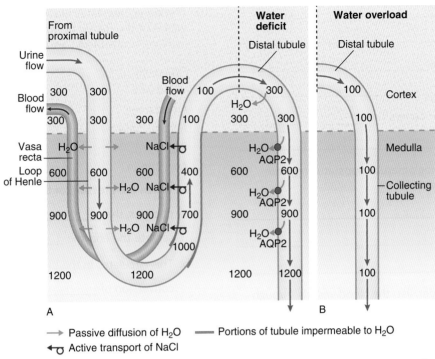

Figure 21.5 Mechanisms for producing concentrated and dilute urine. **A** The production of concentrated urine. **B** The production of dilute urine.
(Source: Miller-Hodges, E., Sullivan, D. R., Mather, A. (2023). Davidson's principles and practice of medicine. Elsevier.)

f. What is occurring in the collecting duct to cause the urine to be concentrated?

_____

_____

_____

g. Which pituitary hormone controls this process?

_____

h. Explain what the unit mOsm/L refers to.

_____

_____

i. What is the difference between osmolarity and osmolality?

_____

_____

_____

_____

6. With reference to Fig. 21.5B:

a. Why does the osmolality of the fluid in the collecting duct not increase as it moves through the region of high osmolality?

_____

_____

_____

b. What is the role of the distal convoluted tubule in urine formation?

_____

_____

_____

7. Define the following terms:

a. Glycosuria: _____

_____

b. Proteinuria:_____

_____

c. Renal clearance:_____

_____

d. Juxtaglomerular apparatus:_____

_____

8. How does the juxtaglomerular apparatus regulate systemic blood pressure?

_____

_____

_____

9. In their correct order, list the blood vessels through which an erythrocyte moves from the time it enters a renal artery to the time it leaves the kidney.

a. Renal artery

b. _____

c. _____

d. _____

e. _____

f. _____

g. _____

h. _____

10. The kidney regulates blood pressure indirectly by means of the RAAS. Complete the following sentences by filling in the blanks with the terms provided.

Potassium	Sodium
Vasodilator	Vasoconstrictor
Aldosterone	Juxtaglomerular
Juxtamedullary	Angiotensin II
Renin	Angiotensin
Angiotensin I	Increase

a. When the pressure of blood in the renal artery declines, the _____ cells of the kidney secrete the enzyme _____.

b. This circulates in the blood and catalyses the conversion of _____ to _____, which is then converted to _____.

c. This substance is a powerful _____, and also stimulates the adrenal cortex to secrete the hormone _____, which increases the renal reabsorption of _____, causing water to follow and blood volume to _____, restoring blood pressure to normal.

11. What three nitrogenous wastes are excreted by the kidneys?

_____

Apply the Concepts

1. Is there a distinction between nephritis and pyelonephritis? Explain.

_____

_____

2. What is a diuretic?

_____

a. How and where does a diuretic exert its effect?

_____

_____

3. Is there are distinction between a countercurrent exchanger and a countercurrent multiplier? Explain.

_____

_____

_____

ACTIVITY 21.6: MICROSCOPIC EXAMINATION OF THE URINARY STRUCTURES

The paired, bean-shaped kidneys are composed of three functional regions – the renal cortex, the renal medulla and the renal pelvis (Fig. 21.6). Each kidney consists of an extensive tubule network, which converts filtrate into urine through the processes of tubular reabsorption and tubular secretion (Fig. 21.7). The production of filtrate and the urine-forming process commences at the glomerulus, a high-pressure capillary bed which leads into Bowman's capsule (Fig. 21.8). Paired ureters drain urine from the renal pelvis of the kidneys (Fig. 21.9), entering the urinary bladder at the trigone through the posterior bladder wall. The urinary bladder is a highly muscular organ that is capable of withstanding stretch and tearing by means of internal folds or **rugae**, which allow for internal expansion associated with bladder filling.

This activity examines the microscopic structure of the components of the urinary system.

Kidney (LS)

1. Obtain a slide of a kidney LS (H&E) and hold it up to the light.

2. Identify the renal cortex, renal medulla and hilum, if present.

3. Examine the slide under the low power of a compound microscope and locate the renal cortex.

4. Compare the structures visible on the slide with Fig. 21.6.

    a. Which structures are visible in the renal cortex?

    _____

    b. What type of nephrons dominate this region?

    _____

    c. Which structures are visible in the renal medulla?

    _____

    d. Which structures are visible at the hilum?

    _____

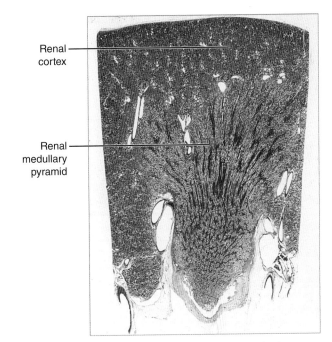

Figure 21.6 The renal cortex and renal medulla under low power.
(Source: Lowe, J. S., et. al. (2020). Stevens and Lowe's human histology. Elsevier.)

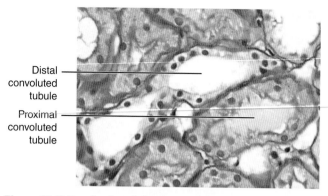

Distal convoluted tubule

Proximal convoluted tubule

Figure 21.7 Proximal and distal convoluted tubules under high power.

(Source: Young, B., Woodford, P., & O'Dowd, G. (2014). Wheater's functional histology: A text and colour atlas. Elsevier.)

5. Identify the *glomeruli* and *renal tubules*, which will be sectioned at different angles.

6. Examine a renal tubule under high power.

7. Compare the structures visible on the slide with Fig. 21.7.

   a. What type of epithelium lines the renal tubules?

   _____

   b. How many layers of epithelial cells can be seen?

   _____

   c. Relate the number of layers seen to the function of the tubules.

   _____

   _____

   d. What structural features of some tubule epithelial cells enhance their function?

   _____

   _____

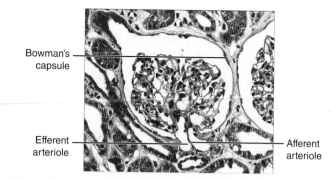

Bowman's capsule

Efferent arteriole

Afferent arteriole

Figure 21.8 The glomerulus.
(Source: Lowe, J. S., et. al. (2020). Stevens and Lowe's human histology. Elsevier.)

Glomerulus

1. Examine a glomerulus (H&E) under high power.

2. Compare the structures visible on the slide with Fig. 21.8.

3. Identify the thin-walled glomerular capillaries, the lumen of the Bowman's capsule and the capsule wall.

   a. What type of epithelium forms the walls of the capillaries?

   _____

   b. How is this type of epithelium suited to the function of the capillaries?

   _____

   _____

   c. Explain why the glomerulus is a high-pressure capillary bed.

   _____

   _____

   d. How does the high pressure of the glomerulus aid its function?

   _____

   _____

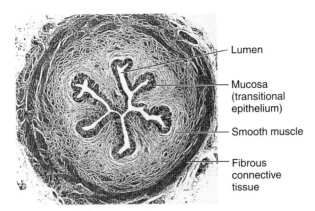

Figure 21.9 Transverse section of the ureter.
(Source: Patton, K. T., Thibodeau, G. (2012). Structure and function of the body. Elsevier.)

Ureter (TS)

1. Obtain a prepared slide of a ureter TS (H&E).

2. Examine it under the low power of a compound microscope.

3. Compare the structures visible on the slide with Fig. 21.9.

4. Identify the *lumen* (central space) of the ureter, the layers of *transitional epithelial cells*, the layers of *smooth muscle* and the *adventitia*, a fibrous connective tissue.

   a. Why is transitional epithelium well suited to the function of the ureter?

   _____

   _____

   _____

   b. Explain why the wall of the ureter contains layers of both circular and longitudinal smooth muscle.

   _____

   _____

   _____

   c. Explain the presence of mucosal folds in the walls of an empty ureter.

   _____

   _____

   _____

5. Draw a diagram of what you can see in the space below, labelling all identified structures.

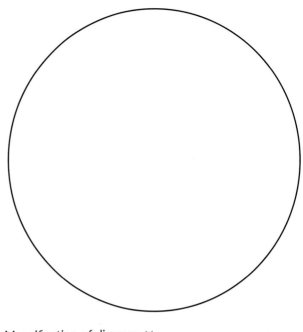

Magnification of diagram: × _____

Urinary Bladder (TS)

1. Obtain a slide of a urinary bladder wall TS (H&E).

2. Examine it under the low power of a compound microscope.

3. Observe and identify the three tissue layers present:

   ☐ Mucosa

   ☐ Muscularis

   ☐ Adventitia

   a. What type of epithelium lines the mucosal layer?

   _____

   b. What is the term given to the folds present in the mucosal layer?

   _____

c. What is the function of these folds?

_____

_____

_____

4. Study the arrangement of smooth muscle tissue.

   a. How many layers can be seen?

   _____

5. Examine the slide under high power.

   a. How many layers of epithelial cells can be seen?

   _____

   b. Describe the arrangement of the layers of smooth muscle tissue.

   _____

   _____

   c. Describe the expansion of the bladder as urine accumulates.

   _____

   _____

   _____

6. Draw a diagram of what you can see in the space below, labelling all identified structures.

Magnification of diagram: × _____

7. Compare your sketch of the bladder wall to your sketch of the ureter.

   a. What differences can be seen?

   _____

   _____

   _____

ACTIVITY 21.7: ELECTROLYTE BALANCE

A major role of the kidneys is to help maintain blood plasma concentrations of electrolytes within normal ranges. This usually refers to salt balance but also includes **acid–base balance**, in which the kidneys are aided by a number of other organs. Sodium comprises nearly 95% of all solutes in the extracellular fluid (ECF), having a major role in controlling the distribution of water in the body, and thus a central role in fluid and electrolyte balance. Potassium is the major cation in the intracellular fluid (ICF) and the ICF–ECF potassium balance is of great importance to both nerve and muscle function. Calcium in the ECF plays an important role in blood clotting and cell membrane permeability in addition to nerve and muscle function, with about 99% of the body's calcium stored as calcium salts in the bones. The maintenance of water and solute concentrations within normal ranges is regulated through the actions of **aldosterone, antidiuretic hormone (ADH)**, and **atrial natriuretic peptide (ANP)**.

This activity examines the mechanisms associated with regulation of the body's electrolyte balance.

Part 1: Ionic Balance

1. Explain how ADH and aldosterone differ in their regulation of water output.

_____

_____

_____

_____

2. Explain why the retention of sodium in a body fluid compartment, such as extracellular fluid, causes that compartment to increase in volume.

_____

_____

_____

3. A number of hormones are involved in the regulation of sodium balance. In the table below, state the source of each hormone and its effect on the function of the kidney nephron.

Hormone	Aldosterone	Atrial natriuretic peptide (ANP)	Oestrogen
Source			
Effect on the nephron			

4. Which anion is most closely associated with sodium in the ECF?

_____

5. Like sodium, potassium is reabsorbed from the glomerular filtrate in the proximal tubule, but unlike sodium, potassium can be secreted into the filtrate.

   a. In what part of the nephron does this happen?

   _____

   b. Under what conditions is the kidney stimulated to increase the excretion of potassium?

   _____

   _____

   c. What is the effect of aldosterone on potassium excretion?

   _____

6. Which hormone regulates ECF calcium levels?

_____

   a. Identify the effect of this hormone on the following organs:

      i. Bones: _____

      _____

      ii. Kidneys: _____

      _____

      iii. Small intestine: _____

      _____

   b. Which anion is most closely associated with calcium balance?

   _____

7. Anions such as sulphates and nitrates are reabsorbed in the proximal convoluted tubule by transport maximum-limited processes.

   a. Explain what this means.

   _____

   _____

   b. What happens to these ions if their concentration in the filtrate exceeds the transport maximum?

   _____

   _____

Part 2: Acid–Base Balance

Nearly all chemical processes in the body are affected by the pH of the surrounding medium, which needs to be maintained within narrow limits. The maintenance of acid–base balance is achieved through the actions of chemical **buffer** systems. Renal and respiratory buffering form the basis of physiological buffering within the body and play a vital role in long-term acid–base balance, and the responses to **acidosis** and **alkalosis**.

1. Define the following terms:

   a. Respiratory acidosis: _____

   _____

   b. Respiratory alkalosis: _____

   _____

2. What causes the fall in blood pH during respiratory acidosis?

_____

_____

3. What is the effect of hyperventilation on blood pH?

_____

   a. Explain this effect.

   _____

   _____

   _____

4. A person experiences acidosis due to the accumulation of lactic acid in their body.

   a. What effect do you think this would have on their respiratory rate? Explain.

   _____

   _____

   _____

5. The pH of the urine varies widely as a result of renal acid–base regulation.

   a. Which two ions are secreted or reabsorbed to adjust blood pH levels?

   _____

   b. Which part(s) of the nephron are involved in these adjustments?

   _____

6. Identify four factors that can cause:

   a. Metabolic acidosis: _____

   _____

   _____

   b. Metabolic alkalosis: _____

   _____

   _____

Apply the Concepts

1. What is Addison's disease and how does it occur?

_____

_____

   a. Which hormones are deficient in this disease?

   _____

   b. Why does this deficiency cause a craving for salty foods?

   _____

   _____

   c. Explain why this deficiency may also cause low blood pressure.

   _____

   _____

2. What is syndrome of inappropriate ADH secretion (SIADH), and what are its effects on urine output?

_____

_____

3. What is diabetes insipidus and how does it occur?

_____

_____

ACTIVITY 21.8: URINALYSIS

Urine is the end-product of the processes of glomerular filtration, tubular reabsorption and tubular secretion in the nephrons of the kidneys, and varies enormously in its chemical composition. The testing of the physical and chemical characteristics of urine is called **urinalysis** and is a useful diagnostic tool.

This activity demonstrates some common clinical tests on samples of urine.

 To conduct this activity it is important to ensure the following safety precautions:

- _Body fluids and sharps will be used in this activity. Exercise caution at all times._

- _Wear disposable gloves, disposable apron, and safety glasses at all times during this activity, as urine may harbour biological hazards._

- _When you have finished, disinfect all working surfaces and place all disposable urine containers, pipettes, tissues, test strips and paper towels into the biohazard container provided._

- _Place used glassware in the special container provided._

- _Treat all urine samples, whether real or artificial, as biohazards._

- _Additional precautions, including safe disposal of biological materials, may be required by your demonstrator._

1. This activity is best conducted in pairs.

2. Collect two 'normal' but different samples of urine (A and B) and two unknown pathologic samples (C and D).

3. Conduct the tests below and record your results in the table provided.

Colour and Transparency

4. Hold each sample up to the light and determine its colour and transparency.

pH

5. Pour 10 mL of each sample into small, labelled containers and use strips of pH paper to determine the pH of each.

6. Dip the paper into the urine two or three times and compare its colour to the colours shown on the dispenser.

Specific Gravity

7. Label four wide test tubes A, B, C and D and half-fill each with the corresponding urine sample.

8. Obtain a hydrometer and determine how to read its markings. Carefully lower the hydrometer into tube A and let it float freely.

9. Read and record the specific gravity of the urine, then remove the hydrometer, rinse it with distilled water and dry it with tissues.

10. Repeat for the other three samples.

Sulphates

11. Dispense 5 mL of each urine separately into labelled test tubes and to each add a few drops of 1.0 M hydrochloric acid and 2 mL of 10% barium chloride solution.

12. Gently shake the mixture.

13. The appearance of a white precipitate of barium sulphate indicates the presence of sulphates in the urine.

Chlorides

14. Dispense 5 mL of each urine into labelled test tubes and to each add a few drops of silver nitrate.

15. The appearance of a white precipitate of silver chloride indicates the presence of chlorides in the urine.

Nitrites, Glucose, Albumin, Ketones and Blood

16. Dispense 10 mL of each urine into labelled test tubes and use a combination urinalysis dipstick to test for the presence of nitrites, glucose, albumin, ketones and blood.

17. Familiarise yourself with the colours that indicate the presence of these substances by comparing the resulting colours to those shown on the dispenser.

Observation or test	Normal range	Normal sample A	Normal sample B	Pathologic sample C	Pathologic sample D
Colour	Medium yellow				
Transparency	Transparent				
pH	4.5–8.0				
Specific gravity	1.001–1.030				
Sulphates	Present				
Chlorides	Present				
Nitrites	Absent				
Glucose	Absent				
Albumin	Absent				
Ketones	Absent				
Blood	Absent				

18. Compare your results with those of other students and note any differences.

    a. Suggest a possible reason for any differences noted.

    _____

    _____

    _____

19. What is specific gravity and on what standard is it based?

    _____

    _____

    _____

a. What factors may cause differences in urine colour and specific gravity between samples?

_____

_____

b. Explain the relationship between urine colour and specific gravity.

_____

_____

c. The yellow colour of urine is due to which pigment?

_____

d. What is the source of this pigment?

_____

_____

20. What factors may cause differences in pH between urine samples?

_____

_____

21. Based on glucose transport mechanisms in the nephron:

a. Explain why glucose is not normally present in urine.

_____

_____

b. What technical name is given to the presence of glucose in the urine?

_____

c. What does the presence of glucose in the urine indicate?

_____

_____

22. Based on protein transport mechanisms in the nephron:

a. Why are proteins not normally present beyond trace amounts in urine?

_____

_____

b. What could cause significant amounts of protein to be found in the urine?

_____

_____

23. Based on ketone transport mechanisms in the nephron:

a. Why are ketones not normally present in urine?

_____

_____

b. What might cause the presence of ketones in the urine?

_____

_____

24. What can you infer from your results for samples C and D?

_____

_____

Apply the Concepts

1. Why is urinalysis a routine part of any good physical examination?

_____

_____

2. Explain why urine may appear cloudy or develop an ammonia odour.

_____

_____

a. Should urine with these characteristics be tested? Explain.

_____

_____

3. Indicate possible causes of the following items appearing in the urine:

   a. Haemoglobin: _____

   _____

   b. Bile pigments: _____

   _____

   c. Erythrocytes: _____

   _____

   d. Leukocytes: _____

   _____

Additional Resources

Course Hero: Overview of the Urinary System
Course Hero is an online learning platform for course-specific study resources where students can access step-by-step explanations for a variety of anatomy and physiology subjects, such as the urinary system, urine characteristics, elimination, and fluid-electrolyte balance.

www.coursehero.com/study-guides/boundless-ap/overview-of-the-urinary-system/
www.coursehero.com/study-guides/boundless-ap/water-balance/

GetBodySmart: Urinary System
GetBodySmart presents fully animated, illustrated, and interactive eBooks about human anatomy and physiology body systems.

www.getbodysmart.com/urinary-system

Histology Guide Virtual Microscopy Laboratory: Urinary System
Histology Guide is an online resource providing a virtual microscopy laboratory experience, by allowing users to view microscope slides from professional collections for the purpose of interpreting cellular and tissue structures as seen through a microscope.

histologyguide.com/slidebox/16-urinary-system.html

Innerbody Research: Urinary System
Innerbody Research provides objective, science-based advice to help readers make more informed choices about home health products and services with the most up-to-date reviews, guides and research, including information about the urinary system.

www.innerbody.com/image/urinov.html

NursesLabs: Urinary System Anatomy and Physiology
NursesLabs is an educational resources for student nurses covering care plans, exams, test banks, and study notes on a variety of health-related topics.

nurseslabs.com/urinary-system/

Osmosis – Renal System
The Renal System module of Osmosis provides videos, notes, quiz questions, and links to further resources related to the renal system.

www.osmosis.org/library/md/foundational-sciences/physiology#renal_system

Stem Learning: Kidney Dissection
Stem Learning provides a range of resources and courses across various scientific disciplines for teachers, students, and professionals seeking to supplement their learning.

www.stem.org.uk/resources/elibrary/resource/31240/let%E2%80%99s-dissect-%E2%80%93-kidney

The Histology Guide: Urinary System
The Histology Guide is a virtual experience of using a microscope with zoom features divided into topics and offering histological slides with labels and quizzes for each topic, such as the urinary system. It is provided by the University of Leeds.

www.histology.leeds.ac.uk/urinary/index.php

Urology Care Foundation: Urine Colour
The Urology Care Foundation provides information related to urinary health and resources to facilitate patient education.

www.urologyhealth.org/documents/Product-Store/English/Urine-Color-Fact-Sheet.pdf

Visible Body: Urinary System
Visible Body provides interactive and highly accurate visualisations and apps for learning and teaching anatomy and physiology for students and healthcare professionals, including body systems such as the urinary system.

www.visiblebody.com/learn/urinary

CHAPTER 22

The Reproductive System and Heredity

Like most vertebrate animals, humans show sexual dimorphism; that is, differences in form between males and females. The purpose of both male and female reproductive systems is to produce offspring that are genetically different from each other and from their parents through physiological and genetic mechanisms. (Refer to Chapter 4: Biological Chemistry, for further information on genes and their function.)

Unlike other organ systems, the reproductive system is not functional throughout the life of the individual. Although they grow in size as other organs grow, reproductive organs remain largely dormant until puberty, at which time the gonads, the primary sex organs, start producing sex cells (gametes) and a range of steroid sex hormones. The other reproductive organs, called accessory reproductive organs, are concerned with uniting male and female gametes (fertilisation) and the development of the resulting embryo until birth. Although male and female reproductive systems are quite different, they have the common purpose of producing viable and genetically diverse offspring.

LEARNING OUTCOMES

On completion of these activities, the student should be able to:

1. identify the primary and accessory male reproductive organs and describe their functions

2. examine the microscopic structures of selected male reproductive organs and relate these to their roles

3. relate the structure of spermatozoa to their role in reproduction

4. identify the primary and accessory female reproductive organs and describe their functions

5. describe the microscopic structure of the ovary and relate changes in structure to the ovarian cycle

6. examine the structure of the uterine wall and explain changes seen during the menstrual cycle

7. outline the roles of hormones in the female reproductive cycle

8. describe the structure and function of mammary glands

LEARNING OUTCOMES—cont'd

9. trace the early stages of development of the embryo and foetus
10. understand and use the language of genetics
11. distinguish between mitosis and meiosis in terms of their processes and genetic consequences
12. understand interactions between alleles and predict the outcomes of simple genetic crosses
13. distinguish between autosomal and sex-linked inheritance
14. derive genotypes for some single-gene traits.

KEY TERMS

Allele
Anaphase
Autosome
Bulbourethral glands
Centromere
Cervix
Chromatid
Chromatin
Chromosome
Co-dominant
Corpus luteum
Cytokinesis
Diploid
Dominant
Embryo
Endometrium
Epididymis
Fallopian tube
Fertilisation
Foetus
Gamete
Gene
Genotype

Gestation
Gonad
Haploid
Heterozygous
Homologous
Homozygous
Interphase
Locus
Mammary gland
Meiosis
Metaphase
Mitosis
Myometrium
Oestrogen
Oocyte
Oogenesis
Ovary
Ovulation
Ovum
Parturition
Penis
Perimetrium
Phenotype

Placenta
Progesterone
Prophase
Prostate gland
Recessive
Recombination
Semen
Seminal vesicle
Seminiferous tubule
Sex chromosome
Sex-linked
Sperm
Spermatogenesis
Spermatozoa
Spermiogenesis
Telophase
Testis
Testosterone
Uterus
Vagina
Vas deferens
Zygote

ACTIVITY 22.1: STRUCTURE OF THE MALE REPRODUCTIVE SYSTEM

In the male reproductive system (Fig. 22.1), the primary reproductive organs or **gonads** are the **testes** (Fig. 22.2), which produce **spermatozoa** (sperm cells) via the **seminiferous tubules** under the influence of the hormone **testosterone**. All other organs are accessories, such as the **penis** which helps to deliver **sperm** to the female reproductive tract, and the **prostate gland**, **bulbourethral glands** and **seminal vesicle** which produce secretions that form semen.

This activity examines the structure and components of the male reproductive tract.

1. Obtain a model or chart of the male reproductive tract and identify the structures labelled in Fig. 22.1.

   a. Structure A: _____

   b. Structure B: _____

   c. Structure C: _____

   d. Structure D: _____

   e. Structure E: _____

   f. Structure F: _____

   g. Structure G: _____

   h. Structure H: _____

   i. Structure I: _____

   j. Structure J: _____

   k. Structure K: _____

   l. Structure L: _____

   m. Structure M: _____

   n. Structure N: _____

   o. Structure O: _____

   p. Structure P: _____

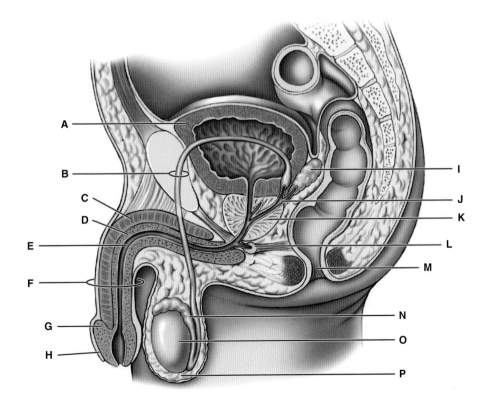

Figure 22.1 Male reproductive structures and perineum.
(Source: Wilson, S. F., & Giddens, J. F. (2022). Health assessment for nursing practice. Elsevier.)

2. Identify the function of the following male reproductive system structures:

a. Prostate gland _____

_____

b. Epididymis _____

_____

c. Vas deferens _____

_____

d. Seminal vesicle _____

_____

e. Corpus cavernosum _____

_____

3. Examine Fig. 22.2 and use the terms provided to identify each of the labelled structures.

Epididymis   Septum of testis
Lobule   Spermatic cord
Rete testis   Tunica albuginea
Scrotum   Tunica vaginalis
Seminiferous tubules Vas deferens
Septum of scrotum

a. Structure A: _____

b. Structure B: _____

c. Structure C: _____

b. Structure D: _____

e. Structure E: _____

f. Structure F: _____

g. Structure G: _____

h. Structure H: _____

i. Structure I: _____

j. Structure J: _____

k. Structure K: _____

4. Match the following structures with their correct description.

Cremaster muscles   Rete testis
Efferent ductules   Seminiferous tubules
Leydig cells   Spermatic cord

a. The site of spermatogenesis

_____

b. Contains blood vessels and nerves supplying the testis

_____

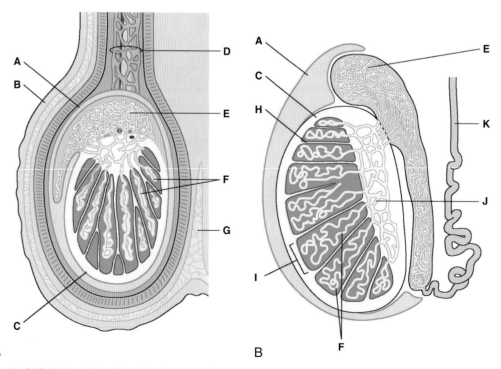

Figure 22.2 The testis (LS). **A** Frontal section showing coverings. **B** Lateral section.
(Source: Waugh, A., & Grant, A. (2014). Ross & Wilson anatomy and physiology in health and illness. Elsevier.)

c. Cause the testis to rise toward the abdomen

_____

d. Produce testosterone

_____

e. Tubular network between seminiferous tubules and epididymis

_____

f. Carry sperm to the epididymis

_____

5. What occurs during spermatogenesis?

_____

_____

_____

a. Where does spermatogenesis occur?

_____

6. What occurs during spermiogenesis?

_____

_____

_____

a. Where does spermiogenesis occur?

_____

7. Semen is an alkaline mixture of sperm cells, testicular fluid and the secretions of accessory glands.

a. Which glands contribute fluid to semen?

_____

b. Describe the contribution of each of these glands to semen.

_____

_____

_____

c. Why does semen need to be alkaline?

_____

d. Listed below are some of the chemicals found in semen. Briefly state the function of each:

i. ATP _____

_____

ii. Antibiotics _____

_____

iii. Clotting factors _____

_____

iv. Prostaglandins _____

_____

Apply the Concepts

1. What are male secondary sex characteristics? Identify three.

_____

_____

2. What is erectile dysfunction (ED) and how does it occur?

_____

_____

3. Explain the following common symptoms of prostatitis with reference to the male reproductive and urinary systems.

a. A burning sensation or pain when urinating.

_____

_____

b. Difficulty in passing urine.

_____

_____

c. The need to urinate frequently.

_____

_____

d. Painful ejaculation.

_____

_____

ACTIVITY 22.2: MICROSCOPIC EXAMINATION OF MALE REPRODUCTIVE STRUCTURES

The seminiferous tubules within the testes are the site where spermatozoa are formed via the processes of **spermatogenesis** and **spermiogenesis** (Fig. 22.3). Mature spermatozoa are then delivered to the **epididymis** and **vas deferens**, where they are transferred to the penis for expulsion (Fig. 22.4).

This activity examines the microscopic structure of the testis, epididymis, penis and spermatozoa.

Testis (TS)

1. Obtain a prepared slide of a testis TS (H&E) and examine it under the low power of a microscope. Refer to Fig. 22.3 to assist with identification of the structures examined.

2. Note the dense connective tissue *capsule*, which forms the boundary of the testis, the *tunica albuginea*. Within this can be seen many *seminiferous tubules* cut in cross-section.

3. Examine a single *seminiferous tubule* under high power and identify its basement membrane, wall and lumen. Within the *lumen* can be seen numerous immature *spermatozoa*.

4. Identify the *interstitial cells* between the seminiferous tubules. Note the large, pale cells in the tubule walls, the *Sertoli cells*.

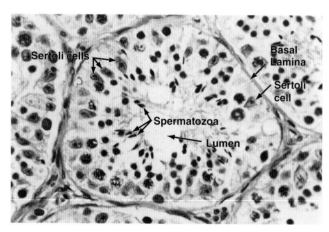

Figure 22.3 A seminiferous tubule of the testis.
(Source: Koeppen, B. M., & Stanton, B. A. (2018). Berne and Levy physiology. Elsevier.)

5. Draw an outline sketch showing as many of these features as you can see in the space below and label your diagram.

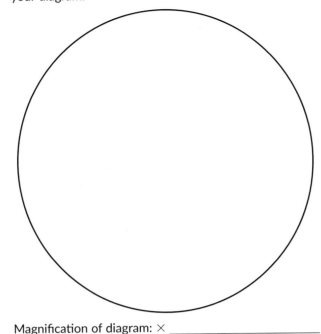

Magnification of diagram: × _____

a. What is the function of the Sertoli cells?

_____

_____

b. The majority of cells in the tubule walls are germ cells. In what activity are they engaged?

_____

Epididymis (TS)

1. Obtain a prepared slide of epididymis TS (H&E) and examine it under low power.

2. Note the many seminiferous tubules cut in cross-section.

a. What differences can be distinguished between the tubules of the epididymis and those of the testis?

_____

_____

3. Examine a single *seminiferous tubule* under high power. Note the *microvilli* extending into the lumen of the tubule.

a. What is the function of these microvilli?

_____

_____

4. Note the layer of smooth muscle in the wall of each seminiferous tubule.

a. What is the function of this smooth muscle?

_____

_____

5. Draw an outline sketch showing as many of these features as you can see in the space below and label your diagram.

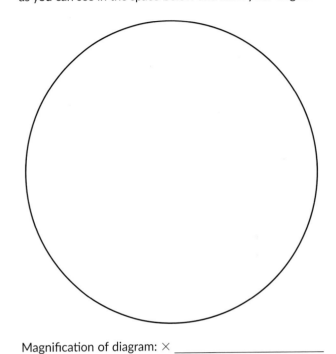

Magnification of diagram: × _____

Penis (TS)

1. Obtain a prepared slide of a penis TS (H&E) and scan it under low or extra low power. Refer to Fig. 22.4 to assist with identification of the structures.

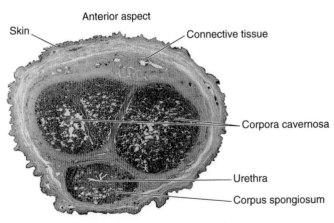

Figure 22.4 Transverse section of the penis.
(Source: Peate, I. (ed.). (2019). Learning to care: The nurse associate. Elsevier.)

2. Identify the *corpora cavernosae*, the *corpus spongiosum* and the *urethra*. Note that the corpus spongiosum surrounds the urethra.

    a. What is the function of the corpus spongiosum?

    _____

    _____

3. Examine the wall of the urethra under high power.

    a. What type of epithelium lines most of the urethra?

    _____

4. Draw an outline sketch showing as many of these features as you can see in the space below and label your diagram.

Magnification of diagram: × _____

Spermatozoa (Smear)

1. Obtain a prepared sperm smear and observe it under high power.

2. Note that each sperm cell has a head, a midpiece and a tail.

3. Identify the intracellular structures found within the:

    a. Head _____

    b. Midpiece _____

    c. Tail _____

4. What is the acrosome and what is its function?

    _____

    _____

    _____

5. Draw an outline sketch showing as many of these features as you can see in the space below and label your diagram.

Magnification of diagram: × _____

6. About one-third of sperm cells in a normal specimen may be deformed and may show multiple or misshapen heads or tail kinks.

    a. Explain why this might occur.

    _____

    _____

    _____

    b. Identify any obvious deformities in your specimen and describe their appearance.

    _____

    _____

    _____

    c. Would this proportion of deformities be likely to result in reduced fertility?

    _____

    d. Explain why or why not.

    _____

    _____

Apply the Concepts

1. Explain why the testes are suspended superficially within the scrotum.

   _____

   _____

2. Explain why the epithelium of the epididymis is lined with stereocilia.

   _____

   _____

3. Explain why an absence of dynein in semen can render an individual infertile.

   _____

   _____

4. What is cryptorchidism and why does it lead to sterility?

   _____

   _____

5. What is benign prostatic hyperplasia (BPH) and how does it occur?

   _____

   _____

6. What is orchiectomy and why might it be performed?

   _____

   _____

ACTIVITY 22.3: STRUCTURE OF THE FEMALE REPRODUCTIVE SYSTEM

In the female, the primary reproductive organs or gonads are the **ovaries**, which produce **ova** via **oogenesis** and the hormones **oestrogen** and **progesterone** (Fig. 22.5). Additional structures associated with copulation are the external genitalia, such as the **vagina** (Fig. 22.6). While the male reproductive organs are concerned only with the production and delivery of **gametes**, the reproductive role of the female is much more complex. In addition to the production of gametes, her role includes housing and nurturing a developing **foetus** for about nine months, as well as feeding the child after birth.

This activity examines the organisation and structures of the female reproductive system.

1. Obtain a model or chart of the female reproductive system and locate the structures labelled in Fig. 22.5.

2. Identify the structures labelled in Fig. 22.5:

   a. Structure A: _____

   b. Structure B: _____

   c. Structure C: _____

   d. Structure D: _____

   e. Structure E: _____

   f. Structure F: _____

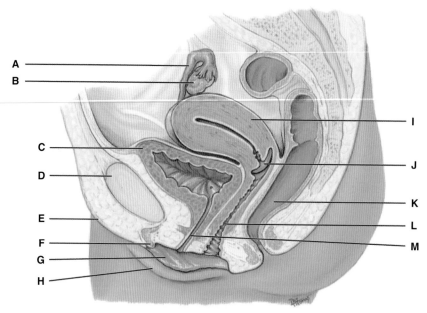

Figure 22.5 Female reproductive system.
(Source: Applegate, E. M. (2010). The Anatomy and physiology learning system. Elsevier.)

g. Structure G: _____

h. Structure H: _____

i. Structure I: _____

j. Structure J: _____

k. Structure K: _____

l. Structure L: _____

m. Structure M: _____

3. Which structures hold the ovaries in place within the pelvic cavity?

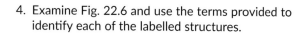

4. Examine Fig. 22.6 and use the terms provided to identify each of the labelled structures.

Mons pubis	Urethral orifice
Prepuce	Vaginal orifice
Clitoris	Hymen
Vestibule	Opening of greater vestibular gland
Anus	Perineal body
Labia majora	Fourchette
Labia minora	

a. Structure A: _____

b. Structure B: _____

c. Structure C: _____

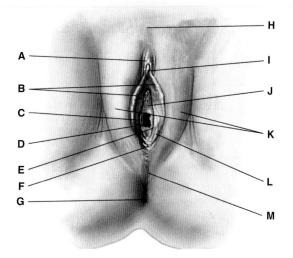

Figure 22.6 Female external genitalia.
(Source: Ball, J. W., Dains, J. E., Flynn, J. A., et al. (2021). Seidel's guide to physical examination: An interprofessional approach. Elsevier.)

d. Structure D: _____

e. Structure E: _____

f. Structure F: _____

g. Structure G: _____

h. Structure H: _____

i. Structure I: _____

j. Structure J: _____

k. Structure K: _____

l. Structure L: _____

m. Structure M: _____

5. Assign each of the following structures the letter of its correct description from the list provided.

   A. Cervix   F. Uterus

   B. Fallopian tube   G. Vagina

   C. Fimbriae   H. Vestibule

   D. Mons pubis   I. Vulva

   E. Ovary

   a. The site of oogenesis _____

   b. The usual site of fertilisation _____

c. The birth canal _____

d. Central part of the chamber into which the vagina and urethra open

   _____

e. The collective term for the external genitalia _____

f. A fatty mound over the pubic symphysis _____

g. Hollow, thick-walled organ in which foetal development occurs

   _____

h. Found at the junction of the uterus and vagina _____

i. Finger-like projections of the fallopian tubes _____

Apply the Concepts

1. What is the hypothalamic-pituitary-gonadal (HPG) axis and when does it first become activated?

   _____

   _____

   _____

2. What are female secondary sex characteristics? Identify three.

   _____

   _____

   _____

3. A woman has both her right ovary and left fallopian tube removed surgically because of tumours found in them. Two years later she gives birth to a healthy child.
   Explain how this is possible.

   _____

   _____

   _____

4. A 28-year-old mother of three decides on tubal ligation to prevent further pregnancies but is concerned that the procedure will result in menopause.

   a. What is tubal ligation?

      _____

      _____

b. Are her concerns justified? Explain.

_____

_____

5. What is an oophorectomy and when might it be required?

_____

_____

ACTIVITY 22.4: THE OVARY

Reproduction begins with the production of **ova** from **oocytes** within the **ovaries**, paired ovoid organs at the termini of the female reproductive tract (Fig. 22.7). Mature ova are released from follicles in the ovaries under the influence of oestrogen in the process of **ovulation**. The remaining follicle then forms the **corpus luteum** which secretes progesterone.

This activity examines the structure and function of the ovaries.

1. Obtain a model or chart of an ovary and compare it to Fig. 22.7A.

2. Note that the ovary is surrounded by a fibrous tunic, the *tunica albuginea*, and that the interior of the ovary has two regions, a dark-staining outer *cortex* and a lighter staining inner *medulla*.

   a. Which structures in the ovary are concerned with the production of oocytes?

   _____

   b. In which region of the ovary are they found?

   _____

   c. What important structures are found within the ovarian medulla?

   _____

3. Obtain a prepared slide of an ovary in sagittal section (H&E) and examine it under the low power of a microscope. Refer to Fig. 22.7 to assist with identification of the structures examined.

4. In the space below, make an outline sketch of your specimen and label as many of the following structures as you can identify:

   ☐ Blood vessels

   ☐ Cortex

☐ Follicles

☐ Hilum

☐ Medulla

☐ Tunica albuginea

Magnification of diagram: ✕ _____

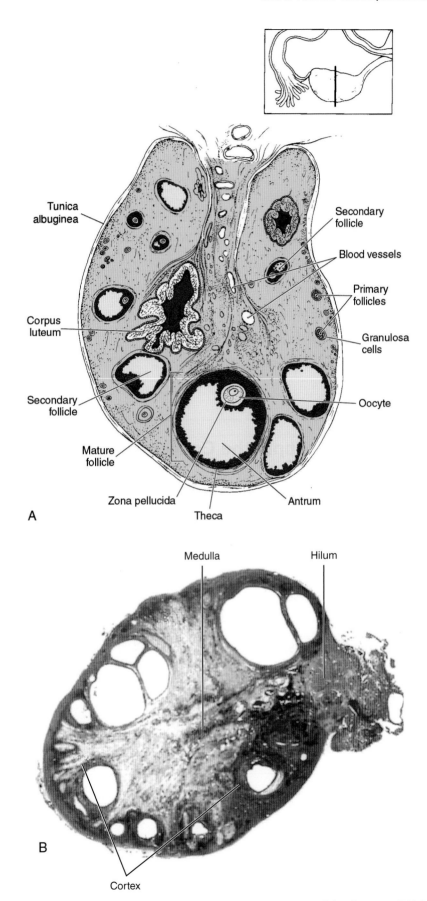

Figure 22.7 Sagittal section of an ovary. **A** Diagram showing follicles in different stages of development. **B** Light micrograph of an ovary. (*Source: Patton, K. T., Bell, F. B., Matusiak, D. J. et al. (2019). Anatomy and physiology laboratory manual. Elsevier.*)

5. Complete the following sentences by filling in the blanks with the terms provided.

Anterior pituitary   Luteinising hormone
Corpus luteum   Oestrogen
Follicular   Ovulation
FSH   Posterior pituitary
Luteal   Progesterone

a. The development of an ovarian follicle is stimulated by oestrogen produced by the _____ cells in the ovary and by the hormone _____ secreted by the _____ gland.

b. The release of an egg from a mature follicle, called _____, is triggered by the hormone _____ secreted by the anterior pituitary.

c. The empty follicle then develops into an endocrine organ called the _____, which produces the hormone _____.

d. The 28-day ovarian cycle comprises two phases. The first lasts about 14 days and is called the _____ phase, and the second is the _____ phase. The event which separates these two phases is _____.

6. What is the function of luteinising hormone (LH)?

_____

_____

7. What is the function of follicle stimulating hormone (FSH)?

_____

_____

Apply the Concepts

1. Explain the processes involved in the development of a vesicular (antral) follicle from a primordial follicle.

_____

_____

_____

2. During ovulation, where is the ovum released?

_____

3. What is polycystic ovarian syndrome (PCOS) and how does it occur?

_____

_____

_____

4. Differentiate between menarche and menopause.

_____

_____

5. What is amenorrhoea and how does it differ from menopause?

_____

_____

_____

6. When is menopause considered complete?

_____

7. What are the possible consequences of menopause?

_____

_____

8. Why is the use of hormone replacement therapy (HRT) in post-menopausal women controversial?

_____

_____

ACTIVITY 22.5: THE UTERUS

The **uterus** is a thick-walled muscular chamber that terminates at the **cervix**. It receives a **fertilised** egg or **zygote** and nurtures the resulting **embryo** to full term (Fig. 22.8). It is composed of three layers – the **perimetrium**, the **myometrium** and the **endometrium**.

This activity examines the structure and function of the uterus.

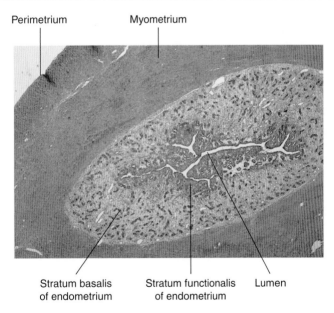

Figure 22.8 Uterine wall (TS).
(Source: Raskin, R. E., Meyer, D., & Boes, K. M. (2021). Canine and feline cytopathology: A color atlas and interpretation guide. Elsevier.)

1. Obtain a prepared slide of uterine wall TS (H&E) and examine it under the low power of a microscope. Refer to Fig. 22.8 to assist with identification of the structures.

2. Identify the three tissue layers of the uterine wall:

   ☐ Perimetrium (outer serosal layer)

   ☐ Myometrium (middle layer composed of bundles of smooth muscle)

   ☐ Endometrium (inner layer which forms the mucosal lining of the uterine cavity)

3. Draw an outline sketch showing as many of these features as you can see in the space below and label the tissue layers and the lumen of the uterus.

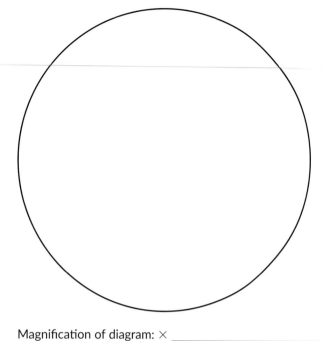

Magnification of diagram: × _____

4. Switch to high power and focus on the myometrium.

   a. How are the muscle fibres arranged?

   _____

   _____

b. What is the function of these muscles and how does their arrangement relate to their function?

_____

_____

_____

5. Return to low power and focus on the endometrium. Notice that it is composed of two layers – a thick superficial layer, the *stratum functionalis*, or *functional layer*, and a deeper layer, the *stratum basalis*, or *basal layer*.

   a. Which of these layers is shed during menstruation?

   _____

   b. What is the function of the other layer?

   _____

   c. What is the function of the numerous uterine glands that can be seen?

   _____

   _____

Apply the Concepts

1. What is endometriosis and what are its consequences?

   _____

   _____

   _____

2. What is a hysterectomy and why is it performed?

   _____

   _____

   _____

3. What is a prolapsed uterus and how does it occur?

   _____

   _____

   _____

4. What is pelvic inflammatory disease (PID) and how does it occur?

_____

_____

_____

ACTIVITY 22.6: MAMMARY GLANDS

Mammary glands are found within the breasts of both sexes, but are normally functional only in females and only when reproduction and birth have been successful (Fig. 22.9).

This activity explores the structure and function of the mammary glands.

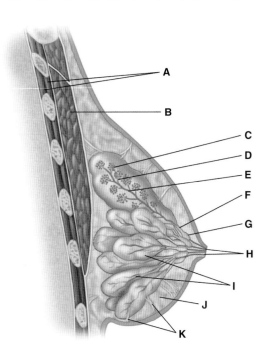

Figure 22.9 The female breast.
(*Source: Cooper, K., & Gosnell, K. (2022). Adult health nursing. Elsevier.*)

1. Examine Fig. 22.9 and use the terms provided to identify each of the labelled structures.

Adipose tissue	Lactiferous sinus
Alveolus	Lobes
Duct	Nipple pores
Ductule	Pectoralis major muscle
Intercostal muscle	Suspensory ligaments
Lactiferous duct	

a. Structure A: _____

b. Structure B: _____

c. Structure C: _____

d. Structure D: _____

e. Structure E: _____

f. Structure F: _____

g. Structure G: _____

h. Structure H: _____

i. Structure I: _____

j. Structure J: _____

k. Structure K: _____

2. Consider the following questions:

a. What is the function of the areola?

_____

_____

_____

b. Which structures produce milk during lactation?

_____

_____

c. What is the function of the lactiferous ducts?

_____

_____

d. How is the breast attached to underlying tissue?

_____

e. List in order the structures through which milk passes from its formation to the suckling child's mouth.

_____

_____

b. Milk production after giving birth

_____

c. The milk let-down reflex

_____

3. Identify the hormone that stimulates:

a. Development of mammary glands in puberty

_____

Apply the Concepts

1. Mammary glands are modifications of which type of glands?
_____

2. What is gynaecomastia and how does it occur?
_____

_____

_____

3. What is galactorrhoea and how does it occur?
_____

_____

_____

4. What is prolactinoma and how does it occur?
_____

_____

_____

ACTIVITY 22.7: HUMAN DEVELOPMENT

The fertilisation of an ovum by a sperm cell occurs within the **fallopian tubes** and triggers a series of events which create a zygote, embryo and foetus during the period of **gestation**. This culminates in **parturition**, or birth of a baby, about 9 months later. During pregnancy and development, the **placenta** is a temporary organ produced by both embryonic and maternal tissue (Fig. 22.10). The early embryology of sea urchins can be used as a model for early human development.

This activity explores the stages of development from a fertilised egg into a fully formed human.

The Zygote

1. Obtain a compound microscope and a set of slides showing the early development of the sea urchin.

   a. In humans, where does fertilisation occur?

   _____

   b. Explain how the zygote is transferred to the uterus.

   _____
   _____
   _____

   c. Describe what occurs during implantation.

   _____
   _____
   _____

2. Examine a slide of a sea urchin's fertilised egg, or zygote, surrounded by a jelly-like region, the zona pellucida.

   a. What is the zona pellucida and what is its function?

   _____
   _____

   b. What is the role of the zona pellucida in preventing polyspermy?

   _____
   _____

3. In the space below, make an outline sketch of a zygote and label as many of the structures as you can identify:

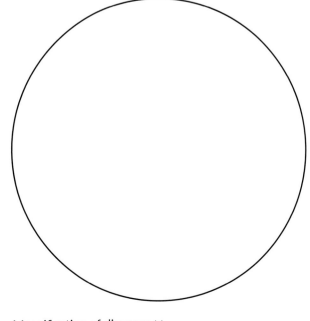

Magnification of diagram: × _____

4. Examine slides of the 2-cell, 4-cell, 8-cell and 16-cell stages resulting from *cleavage* of the *zygote*.

5. In the space below, make an outline sketch of each stage and label as many of the structures as you can identify:

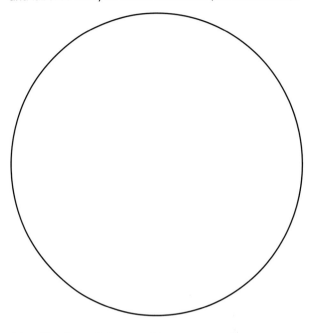

Magnification of diagram: × _____

   a. What name is given to the small cells resulting from cleavage?

   _____

   b. How does cleavage differ from the mitotic cell divisions that occur later in life?

   _____
   _____

   c. What name is given to the ball of cells at the 32-cell stage?

   _____

6. The final product of cleavage is the *blastula* (called a *blastocyst* in mammals).

   a. What is different between the blastocyst and the 32-cell stage?

   _____
   _____

7. In the space below, draw an outline sketch of a gastrula and label the tissue layers that can be identified.

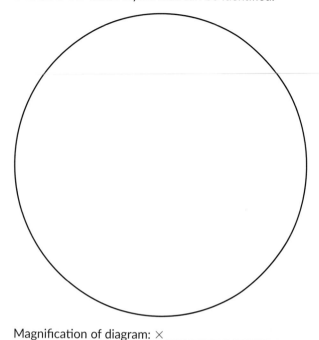

Magnification of diagram: × _____

a. What are the three primary germ layers that result from gastrulation?

_____

b. Which germ layer is sandwiched between the other two?

_____

c. Which germ layer gives rise to each of the following body structures?

   i. Liver _____

   ii. Skeletal muscle _____

   iii. Stomach _____

   iv. Brain _____

   v. Epidermis _____

   vi. Pulmonary alveoli _____

   vii. Lens of the eye _____

   viii. Blood vessels _____

   ix. Nasal cavity _____

   x. Thyroid gland _____

The Placenta

1. List the four extra-embryonic membranes that form during early development of the embryo.

_____

_____

a. Which membrane helps to form the placenta?

_____

b. Which membrane helps to form the umbilical cord?

_____

c. Which membrane helps to protect the embryo?

_____

d. What is the function of the yolk sac in humans?

_____

2. Obtain a prepared slide of a placenta (H&E) and examine it under the low and high power of a compound microscope. Refer to Fig. 22.10 to assist with identification of the structures.

3. Identify the *chorionic villi* and note their rich blood supply. Note the *intervillous spaces* which are normally filled with maternal blood.

a. What tissue forms the maternal portion of the placenta?

_____

b. What structures form the foetal portion of the placenta?

_____

4. In the space below, draw an outline sketch of a representative part of the placenta and label any structures that you can identify.

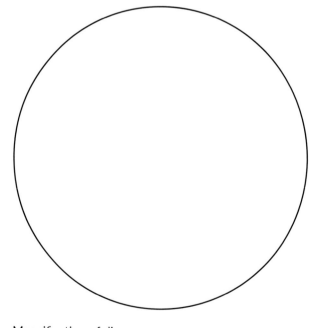

Magnification of diagram: × _____

a. What is the function of the placenta?

_____

_____

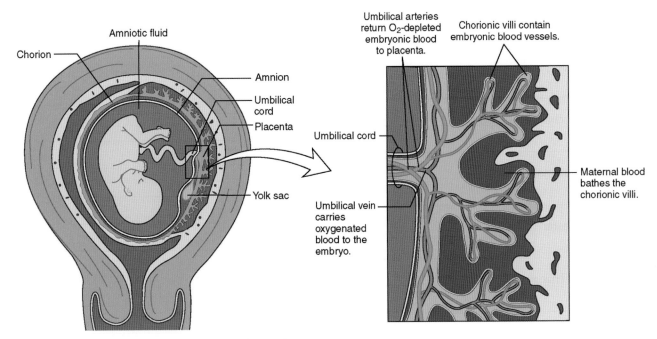

Figure 22.10 Diagrammatic representation of placental structure.
(Source: Carroll, R. G. (2007). Elsevier's integrated physiology. Elsevier.)

b. Which embryonic membranes have very different functions in birds and reptiles, which do not have a placenta?

_____

_____

5. Match each of the following structures and events with its correct description below. (Note: Terms may be used once, more than once, or not at all.)

Allantois	Embryo	Mesoderm
Amnion	Endoderm	Morula
Blastocyst	Fertilisation	Parturition
Chorion	Foetus	Yolk sac
Cleavage	Gastrulation	Zygote
Ectoderm	Gestation	

a. The formation of a three-layered embryo

_____

b. A solid ball of blastomeres

_____

c. Developmental stage from week 9 to birth

_____

d. Structure that implants in the uterine wall

_____

e. Occurs at the end of pregnancy

_____

f. Event which forms the zygote

_____

g. Event which forms the embryo

_____

h. A hollow ball of cells

_____

i. Encloses the fluid bathing the embryo

_____

j. Cell division resulting in blastocyst formation

_____

6. List the stages of human development from zygote to embryo.

_____

_____

7. For each trimester of pregnancy, identify the duration, maternal changes, and the developmental changes occurring in the embryo:

  a. First trimester

    i. Duration: _____

    ii. Maternal changes: _____

    _____

    iii. Developmental changes: _____

    _____

  b. Second trimester

    i. Duration: _____

    ii. Maternal changes: _____

    _____

    iii. Developmental changes: _____

    _____

  c. Third trimester

    i. Duration: _____

    ii. Maternal changes: _____

    _____

    iii. Developmental changes: _____

    _____

8. Why is the multicellular blastocyst only slightly larger than the single-celled zygote?

  _____

  _____

  _____

9. Identify the three stages of labour and the processes that occur in each stage:

  a. First stage: _____

    i. Processes: _____

    _____

    _____

  b. Second stage: _____

    i. Processes: _____

    _____

    _____

  c. Third stage: _____

    i. Processes: _____

    _____

    _____

10. What is the function of oxytocin?

  _____

  _____

  _____

Apply the Concepts

1. What is an ectopic pregnancy and what are its consequences?

  _____

  _____

  _____

2. Distinguish between the origins of identical and fraternal twins.

_____

_____

_____

3. Distinguish between abruptio placenta and placenta previa.

_____

_____

_____

4. Explain why oxytocin may be administered intravenously during labour.

_____

_____

5. What is human chorionic gonadotropin (hCG) and what is its role?

_____

_____

_____

ACTIVITY 22.8: INTRODUCTION TO GENETICS

Human cells possess 46 chromosomes, of which 23 are inherited from each parent. Of these 46 chromosomes, 44 are paired autosomes and the remaining two are **sex chromosomes**. Heredity refers to the inheritance of body traits and its mechanisms fall within the field of genetics, which is the study of specific **genes** and **alleles** found within an individual's DNA.

This activity introduces the basic concepts of genetics.

1. Define the following terms:

   a. Gene _____

   _____

   b. Allele _____

   _____

   c. Chromosome _____

   _____

   d. Autosome _____

   _____

   e. Genome _____

   _____

2. Complete the following sentences by filling in the blanks with the terms provided.

Alleles	Homologous
Co-dominant	Homozygous
Diploid	Phenotype
Dominant	Recessive
Genotype	Sex
Haploid	Somatic
Heterozygous	

   a. All the body's _____ cells contain 46 chromosomes, called the _____ number of chromosomes.

   b. The _____ cells contain half this number, called the _____ number.

c. Paired chromosomes, which carry genes that code for the same traits, are called _____ chromosomes.

d. Genes therefore come in pairs, which are referred to as _____ of each other.

e. When both genes in a pair are identical, the individual is said to be _____ for that trait.

f. When the paired genes are different, the individual is _____ for that trait.

g. When an individual is heterozygous and only one allele is expressed, that allele is said to be _____ and the other is _____.

h. If both alleles in a heterozygous individual are expressed, the alleles are said to be _____.

i. An individual's genetic makeup for a characteristic is called their _____, while the actual expression of that characteristic is their _____.

ACTIVITY 22.9: MITOSIS

Human **chromosomes** are composed of **chromatin**, a complex of DNA, histone proteins and RNA strands. Chromosomes contain genes, which are expressed as alleles and give rise to the physical characteristics of an individual. **Mitosis** is the process of somatic cell division, and results in the production of two genetically identical daughter cells from a parent cell (Fig. 22.12). It is the process by which all parts of the body grow and replace their component cells. The process of mitosis includes the stages of **interphase**, **prophase**, **metaphase**, **anaphase**, and **telophase**, followed by **cytokinesis**.

This activity examines the events of mitosis.

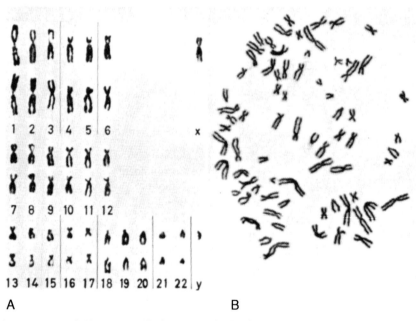

Figure 22.11 Human chromosomes. **A** Karyotype of a human male. **B** Chromosomes in prophase of mitosis.
(Source: Puck, TT, (1960). In vitro studies on the radiation biology of mammalian cells. Progress in Biophysics and Molecular Biology, 10, 237–258.)

1. Obtain a prepared slide of human chromosomes (Giemsa stain) and examine it under the low and high power of a compound microscope. Refer to Fig. 22.11 to assist with identification of the structures.

2. Explain what is meant by the following terms:

   a. Chromatin _____

   _____

   b. Chromatid _____

   _____

   c. Centromere _____

   _____

3. Consider the following questions:

   a. What is the diploid (2*n*) number of chromosomes in humans?

   _____

   b. How many of these are autosomes? _____

   c. How many of these are sex chromosomes? _____

4. Explain why images of chromosomes are normally only possible when cells are dividing.

   _____

   _____

5. Obtain a prepared slide of onion root tips and examine it under low power to identify the mitotic cells. Once a mitotic cell has been found, change to high power. Refer to Fig. 22.12 to assist with identification of the stages.

   a. What stages of mitosis are visible on the slide?

   _____

   _____

6. In the space below, make an outline sketch of each stage of mitosis that you can identify:

Magnification of diagram: × _____

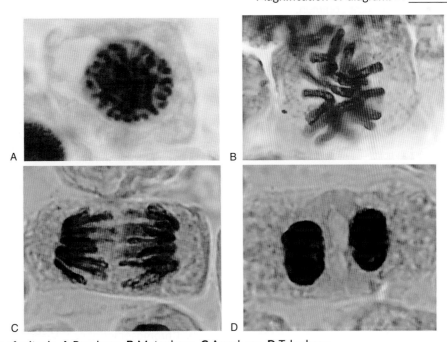

Figure 22.12 Stages of mitosis. **A** Prophase. **B** Metaphase. **C** Anaphase. **D** Telophase.
(Source: Mercado, S. A. S., & Caleño, J. D. Q. (2020). Cytotoxic evaluation of glyphosate, using Allium cepa L. as bioindicator. Science of the Total Environment, 700, 134452.)

7. In the low power field of view, count the number of cells in each of the mitotic stages identified, recording your results in the table provided.

Mitotic stage	Number of cells	Percentage of cells (%)[1]	Time taken (min)[2]
Interphase			
Prophase			
Metaphase			
Anaphase			
Telophase			
Total			N/A

Notes:
1. Percentage of cells (%) = (Number of cells ÷ Total number of cells) × 100
2. Time taken (min) = (Percentage of cells ÷ 100) × 80

8. Calculate the percentage of cells in each mitotic stage using the information provided and record your results in the table provided.

9. Considering that mitosis in an onion cell takes approximately 80 minutes, calculate the time taken (minutes) for each mitotic stage using the information you have gathered and record your results in the table.

   a. Which phase of mitosis was most common?

   _____

   b. Which phase of mitosis was least common?

   _____

   c. Based on the results, which mitotic phase took the greatest time?

   _____

   i. Suggest a reason for this observation.

   _____

   _____

   _____

   d. Based on the results, which mitotic phase took the least time?

   _____

   i. Suggest a reason for this observation.

   _____

   _____

   _____

e. Can the results be considered reliable? Explain.

_____

_____

_____

10. Complete the sentences below by assigning terms to the letters shown.

   a. Replication and division of the cell's nuclear material is called ___ a ___, while division of the cytoplasm is called ___ b ___.

   b. The four stages of mitosis in chronological order are ___ c ___, ___ d ___, ___ e ___ and ___ f ___.

   c. The period during which the cell is not dividing is called ___ g ___.

   d. Two types of cells in the body that do not usually divide are ___ h ___ and ___ i ___ cells.

   a. _____

   b. _____

   c. _____

   d. _____

   e. _____

   f. _____

   g. _____

   h. _____

   i. _____

11. Assign each of the following structures the letter that corresponds to its correct description from the list provided below.

   A. Telophase   D. Early prophase
   B. Anaphase   E. Late prophase
   C. Interphase   F. Metaphase

   a. The mitotic spindle forms _____

   b. The nuclear membrane disappears _____

   c. Chromatids separate and move towards the poles _____

   d. Chromosomes line up at the cell's equator _____

   e. DNA replication occurs _____

   f. The cleavage furrow forms _____

   g. Chromatin condenses to form chromosomes _____

   h. Chromosomes appear V-shaped _____

   i. Cytokinesis begins _____

   j. Nuclear membranes re-form _____

Apply the Concepts

1. What is a karyotype?

   _____

   _____

2. When a might a karyotype be beneficial medically?

   _____

   _____

   _____

ACTIVITY 22.10: MEIOSIS

Meiosis is the process by which the sex cells, or gametes, are produced (Fig. 22.13). The resulting sperm and ova have only half the normal number of chromosomes (represented by *n*), and are **haploid**, compared to somatic cells with the normal number of chromosomes (represented by *2n*), which are **diploid**. Most importantly, gametes are genetically different from each other, due to the processes of **recombination** and independent assortment.

This activity compares the events of mitosis and meiosis.

1. Consider the following questions with reference to Fig. 22.13:

   a. Identify the number of daughter cells produced from one parent cell in:

      i. Mitosis _____

      ii. Meiosis _____

   b. Why are two cell divisions required in meiosis?

      _____

      _____

      _____

2. With reference to meiosis explain the terms:

   a. Equating division _____

      _____

   b. Reducing division _____

      _____

3. What important event occurs during prophase I of meiosis, but is absent in the prophase of mitosis?

   _____

   a. What is the genetic significance of this event?

      _____

      _____

b. In which organs does meiosis take place?

   _____

4. Complete the following sentences by filling in the blanks with the terms provided. (Note: Terms may be used once, more than once, or not at all.)

Centromere	Haploid
Chiasma	Homologous
Chromatids	Homologues
Crossing over	Reducing
Diploid	Synapsis
Equating	Tetrad

   a. During prophase I of meiosis, duplicated

      _____ chromosomes line up next each

      other in a process called _____.

   b. Genetic rearrangement between non-sister

      _____ then occurs in a process known as

      _____.

   c. In late prophase I, the four structures of a

      homologous pair become visible in a microscope as a

      structure called a _____.

   d. Each of these normally contains at least one X –

      shaped region called a _____.

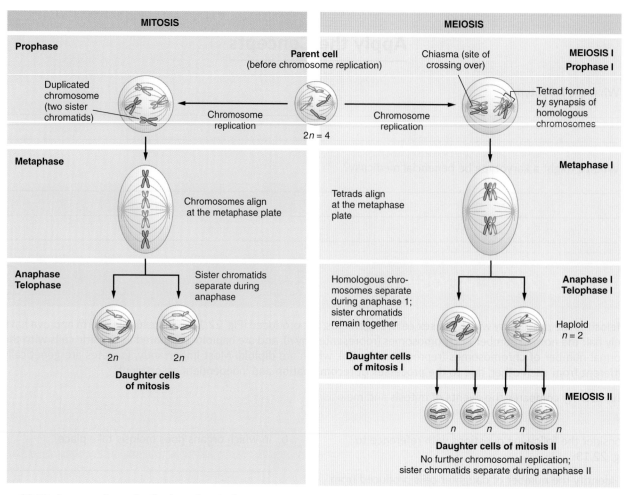

Figure 22.13 A comparison of mitosis and meiosis.
(Source: Craft, J., Gordon, C., Huether, S. E. et al. (2014). Understanding pathophysiology – ANZ adaptation. Elsevier.)

e. By the end of meiosis I, each daughter cell has two copies of one member of each _____ pair of chromosomes and has the _____ number of chromosomes.

f. In meiosis II the _____ of each pair of sister _____ splits and the chromosomes are distributed equally to each daughter cell, which now has the _____ number of chromosomes.

g. Meiosis I is an example of a(n) _____ division and meiosis II is an example of a(n) _____ division.

5. Consider the following questions:

a. In males, what cell type results from meiosis?

_____

b. When does meiosis I occur in females?

_____

_____

c. When does meiosis II occur in females?

_____

_____

d. Explain what is meant by independent assortment with reference to gamete production.

_____

_____

_____

ACTIVITY 22.11: DOMINANCE, RECESSIVENESS AND SEX-LINKED INHERITANCE

Genes that code for the same trait on **homologous** chromosomes are called alleles of each other. As chromosomes come in pairs, so do alleles.

This activity examines the effect of interactions between alleles on their expression.

Part 1: The Language of Genetics

1. Define the following terms:

a. Gene _____

_____

_____

b. Allele _____

_____

_____

c. Homozygous _____

_____

_____

d. Heterozygous _____

_____

_____

e. Dominant _____

_____

_____

f. Recessive _____

_____

_____

g. Genotype _____

_____

_____

h. Phenotype _____

_____

_____

2. Two alleles determine flower colour in a snapdragon plant. The dominant allele (R) produces red flowers and the recessive allele (r) produces white flowers.

a. Using the terms defined above, describe each of the genotypes provided and give its phenotype:

Genotype	Description	Phenotype
RR		
Rr		
rr		

Part 2: Dominant-Recessive Inheritance

The results of genetic crosses can be predicted by the use of a device called a Punnett square, which relies on the fact that each parent contributes one allele of its pair to each offspring. A Punnett square is a grid showing the alleles of one parent across the top and those of the other parent down the side.

1. If a homozygous red-flowered plant is crossed with a white-flowered plant, the following Punnett square would be drawn:

RR x rr

Parents	R	R
r		
r		

Combining the gametes from each parent, all offspring would be heterozygous and would have red flowers:

Parents	R	R
r	Rr	Rr
r	Rr	Rr

Now two of the heterozygous offspring can be crossed (a monohybrid cross):

Rr x Rr

Parents	R	r
R	RR	Rr
r	Rr	rr

a. What genotypes are present in the offspring of this cross, and what is the percentage of each genotype?

_____

b. What phenotypes are present and what is the percentage of each?

_____

2. For each of the following crosses, draw a Punnett square in the space provided and determine the percentages of genotypes and phenotypes that result.

a. RR x Rr

i. Punnett square:

ii. Genotypes: _____

iii. Phenotypes: _____

b. rr x Rr

i. Punnett square:

ii. Genotypes: _____

iii. Phenotypes: _____

Part 3: Co-dominance

When two different alleles are present and the **dominant** allele is expressed, the individual is **heterozygous** dominant; however, when two different alleles are both expressed, they are said to be incompletely dominant or **co-dominant**. In humans, group A blood is produced by the allele A and group B blood by the allele B. When both alleles are present, group AB blood results. A third allele (i) is found in the human ABO blood group system. i is **recessive** to both A and B. Individuals who are **homozygous** for this allele (ii) have group O blood.

1. Draw a Punnett square in the space provided to show the predicted blood groups of the offspring of two AB parents.

a. Punnett square:

b. Identify the percentage of children that will have:

i. Group A blood _____

ii. Group B blood _____

iii. Group AB blood _____

2. Draw Punnett squares in the spaces provided for the following crosses and predict the percentages of genotypes and phenotypes in the offspring.

a. Ai x Bi

i. Punnett square:

ii. Genotypes: _____

iii. Phenotypes: _____

b. AB x ii

i. Punnett square:

ii. Genotypes: _____

iii. Phenotypes: _____

c. AA x Bi

i. Punnett square:

ii. Genotypes: _____

iii. Phenotypes: _____

3. In many Western countries, O is the most common blood type. Explain how this is possible if the allele i is recessive to both A and B.

_____

_____

_____

Part 4: Sex-linked Inheritance

Autosomal inheritance involves interactions between pairs of alleles on homologous chromosomes, but sex-linked inheritance can be different. **Sex-linked** characteristics are determined by genes on the X chromosome.

1. A human male carries which combination of sex chromosomes?

_____

2. A human female carries which combination of sex chromosomes?

_____

3. In females the inheritance of sex-linked traits is identical to that of autosomal traits, but this is not true of males. Explain why.

_____

_____

_____

a. From which parent does a male child inherit his X chromosome?

_____

4. A gene for normal blood clotting (H) is found on the human X chromosome. The recessive allele (h), when expressed, causes haemophilia. Since these alleles are sex linked, they are usually represented as X^H and X^h. Females, having two X chromosomes, may be homozygous or heterozygous for this characteristic. Males, having only one X chromosome, will express whichever allele they have.

a. Draw a Punnett square in the space provided for the following cross between a heterozygous female and a phenotypically normal male.

$X^H X^h$ x $X^H Y$

i. Punnett square:

b. Identify the percentage of the offspring that will be:

i. Homozygous normal females _____

ii. Heterozygous females _____

iii. Normal males _____

iv. Haemophiliac males _____

c. Females who are heterozygous for sex-linked conditions are phenotypically normal but are said to be carriers of the condition. Explain why.

_____

_____

_____

d. Why are males much more likely than females to display a sex-linked condition such as haemophilia or red-green colour blindness?

_____

_____

_____

Apply the Concepts

1. What is Klinefelter's syndrome and what are the outcomes?

_____

_____

_____

2. What is Turner's syndrome and what are the outcomes?

_____

_____

_____

3. A colour-blind man and a woman with normal colour vision decide to have children. The woman's father was also colour-blind. The gene for colour vision is carried on the X chromosome. The pair seek the advice of a genetic counsellor. Consider the following questions:

a. What is the chance that their first child will be a colour-blind son?

_____

b. What is the chance that any daughter they have will be colour-blind?

_____

c. What is the chance that any son they have will be colour-blind?

_____

d. Is it possible that they could produce a daughter who does not have the allele for colour-blindness?

_____

4. Huntington's disease is a neurodegenerative disorder caused by an autosomal dominant allele. It usually only becomes apparent after the age of 40. Mary's father, who is 43, has Huntington's disease, but her mother, who is 36, shows no symptoms. Mary has no knowledge of the family history of either of her parents.

a. What is the highest probability that Mary will develop Huntington's disease herself?

_____

b. What is the lowest probability of this?

_____

ACTIVITY 22.12: INVESTIGATING HUMAN GENOTYPES AND PHENOTYPES

Most human traits, such as skin and hair colour, are determined by more than one pair of alleles and have a complex inheritance pattern, but some can be traced to a single **locus** on a chromosome. An individual's **phenotype** represents the physical expression of a trait and is determined by the **genotype** of the individual's alleles.

This activity investigates some traits whose inheritance involves a single pair of alleles.

Part 1: Sense of Taste

1. Obtain a sodium benzoate taste strip and chew it. The ability to taste something sweet, salty or bitter is dominant.

2. Obtain a PTC (phenylthiocarbamide) taste strip and chew it. The ability to taste something bitter is dominant.

3. Obtain a Thiourea test strip and chew it. The ability to taste something bitter is dominant.

4. Record your observations in the table provided, showing all possible genotypes you may have for that trait.

Part 2: Cheeks

1. The presence of a dimple in one or both cheeks is dominant.

2. Record your observations in the table provided, showing all possible genotypes you may have for that trait.

Part 3: Features of the Hand

1. The ability to noticeably bend the distal joint of the thumb backwards (hitchhiker's thumb), is a recessive trait.

2. The presence of any hair on the middle joint of the third or fourth fingers is dominant.

3. Record your observations in the table provided, showing all possible genotypes you may have for that trait.

Part 4: Earlobes

1. Attachment of the earlobes along their length to the skin of the neck is recessive.

2. Record your observations in the table provided, showing all possible genotypes you may have for that trait.

Part 5: Tongue

1. The ability to roll the tongue as it is extended from the mouth is dominant.

2. Record your observations in the table provided, showing all possible genotypes you may have for that trait.

Part 6: Hairline

1. A downward V-shaped hairline in the middle of the forehead (widow's peak) is dominant.

2. Record your observations in the table provided, showing all possible genotypes you may have for that trait.

Part 7: Freckles

1. The presence of facial freckles is due to a dominant allele.

2. Record your observations in the table provided, showing all possible genotypes you may have for that trait.

Part 8: Blood Types

1. Consider your ABO blood type.

2. Consider your rhesus (Rh+ or Rh−) factor. The presence of the Rh antigen is dominant.

3. If you know your ABO and rhesus blood types, record them in the table provided below, showing all possible genotypes you may have for that trait.

Trait	Dominant allele	Recessive allele	Your phenotype	Possible genotypes
Sodium benzoate	S	s		
PTC	P	p		
Thiourea	T	t		
Cheeks	D	d		
Hitchhiker's thumb	H	h		
Joint hair	J	j		
Earlobes	A	a		
Tongue	R	r		
Hairline	W	w		
Freckles	F	f		
ABO blood group	A, B	i		
Rh blood group	R	r		

3. Consider the following questions:

   a. Compare your results with those of other students. Are you all genetically different?

   _____

   _____

   b. Are these results likely to be typical of the frequency of these traits within the human population? Explain.

   _____

   _____

   _____

   c. Does the recessiveness of a trait reflect how rare it is within the population? Explain.

   _____

   _____

   _____

Apply the Concepts

1. Identical twins are genetically identical because they have developed from a single zygote.

   a. Is it possible for an individual who is not an identical twin to be genetically identical to anyone else? Is this likely? Explain.

   _____

   _____

   _____

2. What is a pedigree and how can it assist with the identification of genetic conditions?

   _____

   _____

   _____

3. Explain what is meant by polygene inheritance and provide an example of such a trait.

   _____

   _____

   _____

Additional Resources

Embryology

Embryology is an educational research website providing information, scientific explanations, and imaging related to reproductive cycles, fertilisation, embryonic and systems development, diagnosis and abnormalities, and neonatal issues.

embryology.med.unsw.edu.au/embryology/index.php/Main_Page

Histology Guide Virtual Microscopy Laboratory: Reproductive Systems

Histology Guide is an online resource providing a virtual microscopy laboratory experience by allowing users to view microscope slides from professional collections for the purpose of interpreting cellular and tissue structures as seen through a microscope.

histologyguide.com/slidebox/18-female-reproductive-system.html
https://histologyguide.com/slidebox/19-male-reproductive-system.html

Innerbody Research: Female and Male Reproductive Systems

Innerbody Research provides objective, science-based advice to help readers make more informed choices about home health products and services with most up-to-date reviews, guides and research, including information about the reproductive systems.

www.innerbody.com/image/repfov.html
www.innerbody.com/image/repmov.html

NursesLabs: Female and Male Reproductive Systems

NursesLabs is an educational resource for student nurses, covering care plans, exams, test banks, and study notes on a variety of health-related topics.

nurseslabs.com/female-reproductive-system/
nurseslabs.com/male-reproductive-system/

Osmosis – Reproductive System

The Reproductive System module of Osmosis provides videos, notes, quiz questions and links to further resources related to the reproductive system.

www.osmosis.org/library/md/foundational-sciences/physiology#reproductive_system

The Histology Guide: Reproductive System

The Histology Guide is a virtual experience of using a microscope with zoom features divided into topics and offering histological slides with labels and quizzes for each topic such as the reproductive system. It is provided by the University of Leeds.

www.histology.leeds.ac.uk/female/index.php
www.histology.leeds.ac.uk/male/index.php

The Virtual Human Embryo

The Virtual Human Embryo is a project that aims to increase understanding of human embryology and human embryonic development by providing students and researchers with reliable resources for human embryo morphology.

virtualhumanembryo.lsuhsc.edu/

Visible Body: Reproductive System

Visible Body provides interactive and highly accurate visualisations and apps for learning and teaching anatomy and physiology for students and healthcare professionals, including body systems such as the reproductive system.

www.visiblebody.com/learn/reproductive

Your Genome: Mitoses Versus Meiosis and Inheritance

Your Genome is a website provided by the Wellcome Trust UK, that provides information about genetics and genomics allowing users to explore topics, facts, and stories relating to mitosis, meiosis and inheritance.

www.yourgenome.org/facts/mitosis-versus-meiosis
www.yourgenome.org/facts/what-is-inheritance

INDEX

C

FOUNDATIONS OF
ANATOMY and PHYSIOLOGY
A workshop manual with laboratory applications

An all-inclusive resource for health science and nursing students within anatomy and physiology courses

This new practice manual is designed to provide students with the conceptual foundations of anatomy and physiology, as well as the basic critical thinking skills they will need to apply theory to practice in real-life settings.

Written by lecturers Dr Ellie Kirov and Dr Alan Needham, who have more than 60 years teaching experience between them, the manual caters to nursing, health science and allied health students at varying levels of understanding and ability. Learning activities are scaffolded to enable students to progress to more complex concepts once they have mastered the basics.

A key advantage of this manual is that it can be used by instructors and students in conjunction with any anatomy and/or physiology core textbook, or as a standalone resource. It can be adapted for learning in all environments, including where wet labs are not available.

KEY FEATURES

- Can be used with any other textbook or on its own – flexible for teachers and students alike
- Scaffolded content – suitable for students' varying learning requirements and available facilities
- Concept-based practical activities – can be selected and adapted to align with different units across courses
- Provides a range of activities to support understanding and build knowledge, including theory, application and experimentation
- Activities can be aligned to learning requirements and needs – may be selected to assist pre-class, in-class, post-class, or for self-paced learning
- Easy to navigate – icons identify content type contained in each activity, as well as safety precautions
- An eBook included in all print purchases

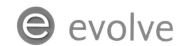 **evolve**

Additional resources on Evolve:
- eBook on VitalSource

Instructor resources:
- Answers to all Activity questions
- List of suggested materials and set up requirements for each Activity

Instructor and Student resources:
- Additional activities
- Image collection

About the authors

Ellie Kirov, *BSc (BiolSc) Hons, PhD*
Unit Coordinator & Lecturer
(Health Sciences)
School of Science
Edith Cowan University
Perth, Australia

Alan Needham, *BSc (Hons), PhD*
Former Senior Lecturer and
Course Co-ordinator
Edith Cowan University
Perth, Australia

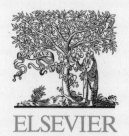

ELSEVIER

ISBN 978-0-7295-4401-6

9 780729 544016